Advanced Micropipette
Techniques for Cell Physiology

IBRO HANDBOOK SERIES:
METHODS IN THE NEUROSCIENCES

General Editor: **A. D. Smith**
Department of Pharmacology
University of Oxford

Advanced Micropipette Techniques for Cell Physiology

Kenneth T. Brown and Dale G. Flaming
Department of Physiology
University of California
San Francisco, CA 94143
USA

A Wiley–Interscience Publication

JOHN WILEY & SONS
Chichester · New York · Brisbane · Toronto · Singapore

Copyright © 1986 by The International Brain Research Organization

Reprinted January 1992

British Library Cataloguing in Publication Data:

Brown, Kenneth T.

  Advanced micropipette techniques for cell
  physiology.—(IBRO handbook series. Methods in
  the neurosciences; v. 9)
  1. Cell Physiology   2. Pipettes
  I. Flaming, Dale G.   II. Series
  574.87'6   QH631

ISBN 0 471 90952 1 (cloth)

Library of Congress Cataloging in Publication Data:

Brown, Kenneth T. (Kenneth Taylor), 1922–

  Advanced micropipette techniques for cell physiology.

  (IBRO handbook series. Methods in the
neurosciences; v. 9)
  Bibliography: p.
  Includes index.
  1. Micropipettes.   2. Cell physiology—Technique.
I. Flaming, Dale G.   II. Title.   III. Series.
QH585.5.M52B76   1986   574.87'028   85-29481
ISBN 0 471 90952 1 (cloth)

Printed and bound in Great Britain by
Biddles Ltd, Guildford and King's Lynn

Contents

Preface for IBRO Handbook Series

During the last 50 years there have been two changes in the way in which scientists have studied the nervous system. First of all, the traditional and largely independent major scientific disciplines of physics, chemistry, physiology, pharmacology, and pathology gave rise to the more specialized subdisciplines of neurophysiology, neurochemistry, neuropharmacology, etc., and the science of experimental psychology was born. Then, after about another generation, it became clear that a deeper understanding of the brain could not be achieved by separate and unrelated studies in each of these subdisciplines. Rather, a unified approach was needed in which the specialized methods were applied in a coordinated way to solve a particular problem. Indeed, combinations of methods could often yield results not obtainable by the application of any individual technique. Thus, scientists studying the nervous system began to call themselves neurobiologists or neuroscientists because they did not wish to be identified with any particular experimental discipline. Very soon meetings took place (e.g. in 1955 the First International Meeting of Neurobiologists) and organizations (Neuroscience Research Program, MIT) were founded to give formal recognition of this new approach to the study of the brain. In 1958 the decision was taken in Moscow to establish the International Brain Research Organization (IBRO), which became incorporated as an independent organization through a Bill in the Parliament of Canada at Ottawa in 1961.

IBRO now has 2000 members, most of whom hold senior positions in research or teaching, in 52 countries of all political complexions. Through its National Corporate members, many of which are academies of sciences or national societies for neuroscience, the body of neuroscientists reflected in IBRO must be of the order of 15,000. One of the programmes of IBRO, all of which aim to serve the international community of neuroscientists, is the publication programme. IBRO publications include *IBRO News, Neuroscience* and the *IBRO Symposia Series*. With the present *Handbook Series*, IBRO aims to fill a major gap in the world literature. The neuroscientist needs to be able to turn to whichever specialized method that is most suited for the problem he is currently studying.

The series on *Methods in the Neurosciences* will help to provide expert advice on exactly how to carry out the experiments, on what difficulties can occur and on the limitations of the method. It is planned as a continuing series, so that new volumes can be published as and when new methods are developed, tested, and found useful. It is my hope that books in this series will have a significant impact on neuroscience throughout the world, by helping to provide the tools with which the scientist can tackle his problems.

A. David Smith,
Director of Publications, IBRO,
University Department of Pharmacology,
South Parks Road,
Oxford OX1 3QT, UK.

Preface

Because fine glass micropipettes can provide channels into cells, they have become instruments of primary importance in cell physiology and have had particularly intensive applications in neurophysiology. Their importance stems partly from their versatile capabilities, which permit many kinds of intracellular and extracellular research, and partly from the fundamental nature of many of the questions to which they can provide answers.

Following the initial application of micropipettes as intracellular microelectrodes (Graham and Gerard, 1946), research in relatively large cells proceeded rapidly. Some useful improvements of technique were also introduced, but efficient and high quality work remained limited to relatively large cells, and the making of micropipettes adapted to various types of intracellular work in varied preparations remained largely a trial-and-error process. In 1973, when we began intracellular work in vertebrate photoreceptors, it quickly became evident that limitations of micropipette technique were still major barriers to research in relatively small cells. And these limitations seemed crucially significant, because almost all cells in the central nervous system of higher vertebrates are small from the standpoint of intracellular work. We thus undertook a systematic attempt to improve the capabilities and efficiency of intracellular work, an effort that has continued to the present time.

This book aims to make available the most advanced current knowledge on the fabrication and use of micropipettes for intracellular research. This account will draw heavily upon our own work, which has touched upon all of the main aspects of micropipette techniques that are covered. Some of this work has been published previously in various journals. Since 1979, however, most of our findings have been so closely interrelated that they have been retained for publication in book form, and those findings are presented here for the first time. This procedure permits evolving findings to be presented in as near final a form as is possible and with adequate opportunity to clarify relations between the various aspects of micropipette techniques. Wherever feasible, we have evaluated micropipette techniques by examining and measuring micropipettes with high-resolution scanning electron microscopy, or by testing the performance of micropipettes and other aspects of technique during intracellular recording in vertebrate photoreceptors. In some cases these tests have amounted to experiments in themselves, and they will be presented as such, so that the evidence underlying our conclusions can be understood and critically evaluated by the reader. An attempt will also be made to present and evaluate all other work that in our judgement has contributed significantly to the aspects of micropipette technique covered in this book.

Our general approach will be to describe a theory of how glass micropipettes are formed and to present both observations and quantitative evidence supporting that theory. New strategies of micropipette design have already been developed from this theory, the applications of which will be discussed. Emphasis will also be placed upon practical techniques, especially the design and use of instruments for intracellular work with micropipettes. Practical aspects of extracellular work with relatively large micropipettes will likewise be treated, including patch clamping. Attention will be given to the capabilities and limitations of any given instrument, any given mode of operating an instrument such as a micropipette puller, or any given procedure. This combination of theoretical and practical information should prove helpful to anyone performing research with micropipettes, from the graduate student conducting a first project to the most experienced investigator. In particular, this information should assist in meeting the requirements of different types of research in highly varied preparations, thus permitting the conduct of research with minimal technical limitations and with optimal efficiency in the use of experimental animals, research funds, and the investigator's own time.

CHAPTER 1

A Brief History of Micropipette Techniques and Their Applications

PART I THE INTRODUCTION OF MICROPUNCTURE TECHNIQUES FOR INTRACELLULAR WORK IN EXCITABLE CELLS

The demonstration that glass micropipettes could be used as intracellular microelectrodes was profoundly important to the neural sciences and also to the more general field of cell physiology. The critical initial steps were taken by Graham and Gerard (1946) and Ling and Gerard (1949) in measuring resting membrane potentials of muscle cells. By the time of their work, resting membrane potentials had been measured by other methods, most notably by filling a glass pipette of 0.1 mm tip diameter with sea water and inserting it 8–9 mm into a squid giant axon by threading it in from the cut end (Hodgkin and Huxley, 1945). That technique yielded accurate results and provided the basis for important work, but it was obviously limited to exceptionally large cells. Graham and Gerard (1946) used glass micropipettes with external tip diameters of 2–5 μm, which were inserted directly through the membrane into single cells at the surface of the frog sartorius muscle; this was done under visual control with the aid of a dissecting microscope. Their micropipettes had previously been filled with a conducting salt solution (isotonic KCl), so the tip of the micropipette became a microelectrode. When the electrical signal between this intracellular microelectrode and an extracellular reference electrode was amplified, the membrane potential was recorded from whatever cell had been penetrated. Graham and Gerard showed that even tips of 2–5 μm diameter, especially the smaller ones, could occasionally penetrate through the membrane of a muscle cell and

1

into the intracellular compartment without seriously damaging the cell. They thus demonstrated the feasibility of this micropuncture method of intracellular recording. Their relatively large tips gave considerable variability of results, the measured resting membrane potentials averaging 62 mV and varying from 41–80 mV. It was recognized, of course, that in these measurements the higher values should best represent the normal ones. Ling and Gerard (1949) refined this technique by using finer micropipette tips only a 'few tenths' μm in outer diameter. When applied to the same preparation, measurements on 1350 fibers in the muscles of 148 frogs gave an average resting membrane potential of 78.4 mV, very close to the highest values obtained by Graham and Gerard. This resulted mainly from the finer tips eliminating most of the low values, and the consistency of results was sufficiently improved that the variation between resting membrane potentials from different fibers of the same muscle 'was rarely over 2–3 mV.'

Though the successful use of micropipette electrodes for measuring membrane potentials is usually dated from Ling and Gerard (1949), it seems abundantly clear from the above account that such work began with Graham and Gerard (1946). Indeed, the demonstration that a technique is feasible is a particularly critical step, and the necessary refinements usually follow quickly unless they are excessively difficult. In addition, the introduction of this technique appears even in retrospect to have been a bold step. Though Graham and Gerard are both deceased and cannot be questioned about their thoughts at the time, they must have been quite skeptical of the approach, since it required the penetration of a delicate and living cell membrane by a foreign body, with many possibilities for damage to the integrity and normal functions of that membrane. Whatever their level of skepticism, they did not allow it to deter them from making the attempt, and in so doing they became scientific pioneers. It thus seems appropriate to credit Graham and Gerard with the introduction of this technique, while also recognizing the contribution of Ling and Gerard in more fully demonstrating its power. This point of view was taken by Ling and Gerard themselves, who credited Graham and Gerard with having introduced the basic technique, and whose only claimed technical contribution was the use of smaller tips to obtain more consistent results. It is not clear why Ling and Gerard have generally been credited with the technique itself, but it is likely that an early incorrect attribution simply became habitual. In fact, we have also perpetuated this incorrect view on some occasions, and regrettably it has become well established.

As is so often the case with major innovations, the original idea of introducing glass micropipettes into cells of living tissues began much earlier than Graham and Gerard. According to Bretag (1983) this concept was being explored by Barber as early as 1902, and various applications were attempted between then and 1946. In summary of Bretag's account, it seems that the main successes of this earlier work were in large plant cells, and there was no prior claim of definitive success in measuring the resting or active electrical properties of cell membranes.

Following the pioneering work in Gerard's laboratory, some of the enormous possibilities of cellular micropuncture were quickly recognized by many investigators. This led to a growth in intracellular work that was relatively slow at first, but which has accelerated along a roughly exponential course up to the present time. In fact, this technical innovation laid the primary basis for the modern flowering of neural science, which has already become one of the most rapid and fundamental advances of knowledge in the history of the biological sciences.

Like many great achievements, this one had a simplicity that was both practical and aesthetically appealing. After penetrating a cell, of course the micropipette becomes a channel into that cell, and this is its primary function. Since glass is an excellent electrical insulator, the glass not only confines the solution filling the micropipette, but electrical signals as well. The solution contained by the micropipette thus becomes a versatile medium for communicating with the interior of the cell. Indeed, there is a stark simplicity in the fact that so many secrets, which were locked within cell interiors until rather recently, have now been revealed by these extremely fine and tenuous liquid channels of information flow. Various methods of using these information channels have now been devised and new ones continue to be developed.

PART II   MICROPIPETTES AS INTRACELLULAR MICROELECTRODES

In early work with intracellular micropipettes, they were used exclusively as microelectrodes. In this application they can provide a continuous record of the electrical potential across the membrane of the cell penetrated, and their initial use to study resting membrane potentials was quickly expanded to include the transmembrane signals evoked during normal cellular activity (Nastuk and Hodgkin, 1950). Through extensive intracellular studies of nerve impulses and postsynaptic slow potentials, some of which have been revealed for the first time, great advances have now been made in understanding how nerve cells generate and transmit the signals by which they carry out their functions of rapid information flow within the body.

PART III   THE EJECTION OF SUBSTANCES FROM MICROPIPETTES

The next major technical step was to fill micropipettes with charged substances that could be ejected iontophoretically from the tip. This technique was introduced by Nastuk (1951, 1953) in studying synaptic transmission at the neuromuscular junction. When a micropipette was filled with acetylcholine, and its tip was located in the extracellular space close to the neuromuscular junction, an electrical current could be applied to the micropipette to drive acetylcholine out of the tip and deliver it close to the neuromuscular junction. The acetylcholine could be delivered either continuously (Nastuk, 1951) or by brief pulses of current (Nastuk, 1953). The more natural brief pulses proved superior because the cell becomes depolarized during continuous delivery of acetylcholine; also, the amount of acetylcholine delivered could be controlled rather accurately by the strength and duration of a brief current pulse.

By using a second micropipette to record intracellularly from the muscle cell, the effects of the acetylcholine pulses could be recorded accurately. This type of work, as elaborated by Del Castillo and Katz (1955), showed that externally applied pulses of acetylcholine evoked end-plate potentials quite similar to those evoked by stimulation of the motor nerve innervating a muscle cell. It was also shown that when acetylcholine was delivered after inserting the ejecting micropipette into the muscle cell, it no longer evoked a response. This work became an important part of the evidence identifying acetylcholine as the transmitter at vertebrate skeletal neuromuscular junctions and demonstrating that the molecular receptor sites for the acetylcholine are located only on the external surface of the postsynaptic membrane of the muscle cell.

From the standpoint of micropipette techniques, this introduced a second realm of possibilities. Not only could micropipettes be used to listen in on the private electrical language of single cells, but henceforth they could also be used to ask cells a variety of questions such as 'What about this putative synaptic transmitter? Is it the one customarily received, or at least so similar chemically that the cell cannot tell the difference?' With this development the investigator could both ask questions and receive answers through the use of micropipettes, thus ushering in the use of these instruments for two-way conversations between the investigator and the cell.

PART IV   METHODS OF IDENTIFYING CELLS STUDIED

Another great advantage of micropipettes is their ability to penetrate not only cells that may be visualized, but cells deeply buried in masses of tissue such as the spinal cord and brain. Since deep cells can be penetrated only by blind probing, however, it became necessary to develop methods for identifying the exact type of cell that had been penetrated. This problem was first solved by Brock *et al.* (1952) in intracellular work on spinal motoneurons of the cat. These cells were identified as motoneurons by their antidromic activation from electrical stimulation of proximal ends of cut ventral roots, while the muscle normally innervated was determined by orthodromic activation of the impaled motoneuron from stimulation of a sensory nerve in the monosynaptic reflex pathway of a specific muscle. This method of identifying impaled cells can be quite accurate, and adaptations of this method have proved useful in a variety of preparations, but there are two specific requirements. In blind probing there is always a 'target cell', defined as the cell that the experimenter wishes to impale; the neuroanatomy of this target cell, and of the cells that synaptically influence it, must be well established. In addition, there must be at least one accessible site at which electrical stimulation will activate the target cell, but only that type of cell, among all the cells that might be impaled in the nervous tissue being probed. Of course this requires further anatomical information concerning the other types of cells that might be impaled and the pathways by which they are innervated. These requirements are seldom met rigorously for cells of the central nervous system, so a more general method was required for identifying impaled cells. Such a method was supplied by filling the micropipette with an intracellular marker dye, of which Procion yellow became one of the most successful following its introduction by Stretton and Kravitz (1968). After obtaining an intracellular recording, the marker dye is iontophoretically injected into the cell, which is thus made visible for later identification during a histological examination of the tissue. In this case the same micropipette may be used both for marking the cell and for recording its electrical activity. Using techniques of this type, great advances have been made in studying details of cell connectivity in cell systems serving specific functions, such as the visual system. Progress has also been made in learning how signals are processed as they pass through a series of cells. Of course much work of that type can be done by extracellular metal electrodes recording the impulse discharges of identifiable single cells. But in the retina, for example, the early stages of signal processing involve cells that generate only slow potentials. In the absence of impulses, signal processing can be studied only by intracellular methods. And even if a cell does fire impulses, its postsynaptic potentials that reveal so much about its functions can be revealed only by intracellular work.

PART V   SUMMARY OF MICROPIPETTE APPLICATIONS IN NEURAL SCIENCES

Though micropipettes have now been used in many specific ways, all these applications fall into two broad categories. Either the micropipette is used to record an electrical signal, or it is used to eject a specific substance from the tip. The requirements of these two broad applications are quite different, as will be dealt with in some detail in this book. Within each of these broad categories are many variations, and each of these also has its own requirements. For example, dual-channel micropipettes have been used for voltage- and current-clamping studies, while multi-channel micropipettes have been used for studying synaptic transmission, one channel being used to record the electrical responses of the cell while it is challenged with a variety of putative synaptic transmitters ejected from the other barrels. By using an appropriate ligand, a micropipette can also be converted into an ion-specific electrode that gives a voltage signal proportional to the concentration of a specific ion such as Na^+, Cl^-, K^+ or Ca^{2+}. This provides a method for measuring highly local ionic concentrations and the alterations of those concentrations during cellular activity. Most recently, relatively large micropipettes have been applied to the new and powerful technique of patch clamping, which permits the study of single ionic channels in cell membranes. Moreover, micropipettes have become critical tools in the field of genetic engineering, which carries such great promise for both increased knowledge and practical applications in human medicine. In this case micropipettes are used, for example, to insert man-made forms of genetic material into cells, which then multiply and produce specific substances that can be harvested for medical applications. With new uses of micropipettes still evolving, it seems likely that this process will continue into the indefinite future, as new findings produce further needs for these channels into cells.

Though any given application of micropipettes is conceptually simple, the actual use of micropipettes in meeting the requirements of a given application is rarely simple. Most applications require careful consideration of many aspects of how micropipettes are best fabricated and used. Hence the major aspects of this subject will now be discussed in turn.

CHAPTER 2

Early Methods of Fabricating Micropipettes

PART I   MICROPIPETTE TERMINOLOGY

The discussion of micropipettes requires a consistent terminology, and the terms suggested by Frank and Becker (1964) have been followed by many but not all authors. For this book we have adopted a modification of the Frank and Becker terminology that conforms as closely as possible to established usage. The *shaft* of a micropipette is defined as the straight portion of capillary tubing, while the *shoulder* is the rapidly tapering segment that is formed initially during pulling. Frank and Becker introduced the term *shank* for the tapered segment extending from the outermost tip to the point on the shoulder where the diameter of the capillary tubing has been reduced by half. Though arbitrary and little used, this term is also occasionally helpful. The term *tip* often refers to a micropipette's outer terminal. But there is frequent need to refer to the entire tapered portion of a micropipette, which is also customarily called the *tip*, and we shall follow this usage. The exact meaning of 'tip' is usually clear from the context, and where needed the meaning will be assisted by appropriate modifiers. For example, the *entire tip* will refer to the complete tapered segment of the micropipette, and *tip length* will refer to the length of the entire tip. *Tip size* will refer to the diameter of the micropipette terminal, and it will always mean the outer diameter unless otherwise specified. A special category of tip size is *ultrafine tips*, which we define as tips with outer diameters of 0.1 μm or less. This definition has proved convenient and useful because ultrafine tips provide the requisite range of tip size for high quality intracellular work in small cells such as vertebrate photoreceptors (see Chapter 13). Tip sizes ranging from 0.1–0.5 μm will be referred to as *fine tips*. This category covers the remaining tip sizes that are below the resolving power of a light microscope, and tips larger than 0.5 μm are used for intracellular work only in exceptionally large cells.

PART II   HAND MADE MICROPIPETTES

The earliest intracellular micropipettes were formed by hand, as described by Nastuk and Hodgkin (1950).

> Pyrex tubing (7 mm O.D.) was heated in an oxy-gas flame and drawn out into uniform lengths of 1 mm O.D. A short length of the 1 mm tube was heated in a very small oxy-gas flame and drawn out to about 0.3 mm O.D. The narrow section was again heated and the tube drawn apart very rapidly. Under favorable conditions the last operation produced a microelectrode of suitable dimensions. Throughout the whole process the heating was kept at a minimum in order to ensure that the electrode had reasonably thin walls. The electrodes were examined with a microscope and about 5% selected for further use. These were filled by boiling in KCl solutions and examined carefully with a water immersion objective at an overall magnification of $\times 800$.

Based upon observations with the light microscope, they estimated that this procedure yielded tips of outer diameters varying from 0.2–1.0 μm, with the commonest value being about 0.5 μm. But they also emphasized large errors in these measurements. In fact, the limit of resolution with the light microscope is about 0.5 μm, and this has always been a major problem in measuring tips of micropipettes. Electron microscopy offered better resolution and was applied by Nastuk and Hodgkin (1950), who published the first electron photomicrograph of a micropipette tip that was suitable for intracellular work. This photograph, reproduced as Figure 1, shows a hand-pulled tip of outer diameter about 0.4 μm.

Though hand-made micropipettes served certain purposes, it was very difficult to make the tips sufficiently small, short, and straight to be useful. Success depended upon both native skill and considerable practice. Even among those few who could make usable intracellular micropipettes by hand, the results were highly variable; Nastuk and Hodgkin (1950) note that they only attempted intracellular work with about 5% of their hand-made micropipettes, and undoubtedly some of those were not satisfactory. In addition, even the best hand-made tips fell quite short of ideal and thus placed severe restrictions upon the types of research that could be performed. It was obvious that better and more consistent

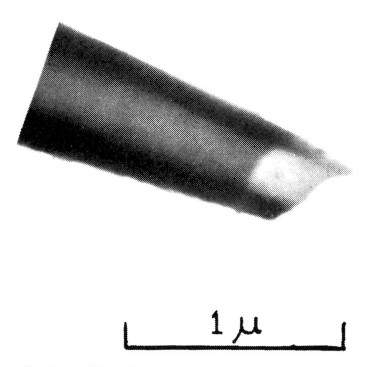

Figure 1. The first published electron photomicrograph of the tip of a micropipette suitable for intracellular electrical recording. Tip formed by hand pulling, as described in text. (From Nastuk and Hodgkin (1950), reproduced by permission of Alan R. Liss, Inc., New York, N.Y.)

micropipettes should be obtainable by forming them with instruments designed specifically for the purpose. Efforts were quickly directed toward that end, and it was only in a few laboratories that hand methods persisted into the mid- or late 1950's.

Based upon our experience with machine-pulled micropipettes, it appears that the greatest problem with hand-pulling was the control of glass temperature when a rapid pull was applied to form the tip. If the glass was too hot, the tip formed was too long and flimsy to be useful. But if the glass was too cool at the beginning of the pull, it broke too soon during pulling and the tip was too large. Since the glass was heated in a flame, the temperature of the glass was a complex function of several variables concerning how the flame was formed and the position of the pipette in relation to the flame. Timing was also particularly crucial, whether it concerned the length of time the pipette was in the flame or how long it was removed from the flame before pulling the tip. Glass changes temperature rapidly when a flame is applied or removed, and the glass temperature at the beginning of pulling is very critical for tip formation. Hence it was not possible to achieve the requisite accuracy of timing with hand-pulled tips, aside from those rare cases that enjoyed the complicity of great good luck.

PART III   INSTRUMENTS FOR PULLING MICROPIPETTES

III.1   The Du Bois Micropipette Puller

In designing devices for the machine-pulling of fine micropipettes, attention was turned to earlier instruments that had been developed to form pipettes for different purposes. The earliest instrument of this type was described by Du Bois (1931). It fulfilled the basic requirements and thus became the prototype that influenced all later designs. The original illustration of this device was not very clear, so it has been enlarged and redrawn as Figure 2.

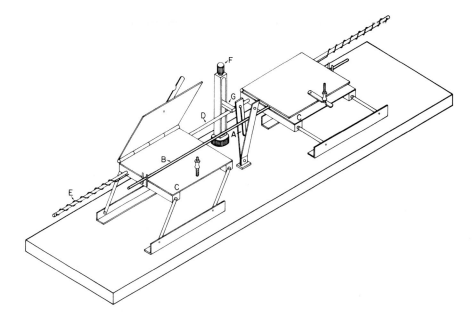

Figure 2. Redrawn and enlarged diagram of the Du Bois micropipette puller. Labeling is as follows: (A) platinum wire filament; (B) glass capillary tubing; (C) pipette clamps; (D) alignment rod; (E) coil spring; (F) knurled knob; (G) locking bar. For further description, see text. (From Du Bois (1931), Copyright 1931 by the AAAS, which granted permission for this reproduction)

The Du Bois micropipette puller was developed by studying the hand movements of an expert in hand-pulling micropipettes. It was noted that the main requirements were an appropriate glass temperature at the moment of pulling the tip and a rapid pull to form the tip. As shown in Figure 2, these requirements were met by using a platinum wire filament (A) to heat a narrow segment of a glass tubing (B), which was clamped at both ends by special holders (C). The two symmetrical pipette holders were mounted to the base of the instrument by hinges, which were so attached as to assure that the bottom plates of the pipette clamps remained parallel with the baseplate of the instrument as the pipettes were pulled. Furthermore, an alignment rod (D) through the lower plates of the pipette clamps assured that both clamps were always at the same height above the instrument's baseplate as the pipettes were formed. At each end of this alignment rod, a spring (E) was attached to the adjacent pipette clamp to provide power for pulling the pipettes. In using this instrument the two pipette clamps were manually drawn together, thus stretching the springs and lowering the alignment rod, which could be locked down by rotating a knob (F) to position a locking bar (G) over the alignment rod. A piece of glass tubing long enough to make two micropipettes was then lowered into the pipette clamps, which included pins for aligning the glass tubing with the horizontal axis of the instrument. The upper hinged plate of each pipette clamp was next locked over the capillary tubing, which was held between leather and rubber facings on the surfaces of the pipette clamps, and the locking bar was removed from above the alignment rod. The spring tension tending to pull the pipette clamps apart was then prevented from doing so only by the glass tubing that was firmly held by the clamps, and this glass tubing was correctly located to be heated by the platinum wire filament. When current was applied to this filament, it heated and softened a short segment of the glass tubing, and when the glass became sufficiently soft that the pipette clamps could be pulled apart by the applied spring tension, pulling began; this started slowly at first and then accelerated. The acceleration was partly because of the geometry of the hinges attaching the pipette clamps to the instrument base. In addition, the connection between the pipette clamps was rapidly weakened as the glass tips became smaller. As the micropipette tips were pulled they were also lifted out of the heating filament. The heating current was then turned off to complete the cycle.

This early design exhibited a number of features that have been incorporated in some form in all later instruments for pulling micropipettes. (1) A source of tension was provided for pulling the micropipettes, and this tension could be set accurately. (2) An electrical heating filament was used to heat a short segment of the glass tubing. The heat output could be regulated by the current through the filament, and the distance of the glass from the filament was kept relatively constant. (3) Pulling began immediately and automatically when the glass was warmed to a temperature at which it could be pulled apart by the preset tension. This assured that temperature of the glass at the onset of pulling was well controlled, depending mainly upon the preset tension and being relatively independent of many other factors that were difficult to control when micropipettes were pulled by hand. In consequence, it became possible to begin pulling at a reliable glass temperature. (4) Pulling began relatively slowly and then accelerated. While a slow initial pull causes a rapid reduction of capillary diameter that keeps the tips from being too long, a rapid pull is then necessary to form fine tips. In the Du Bois design this was obtained by a smooth and continuous acceleration of the pull, while some later designs provided separate stages of slow and rapid pulling. (5) As pulling occurred the glass tubing was lifted out of the heating filament, so that the tips themselves were formed outside of the heating filament. Unless the tip is removed from the heating filament before the ultimate tip is formed, or unless the tip is cooled in some other manner, the glass temperature during tip formation remains too high and the tips are much too long to be usable. So the upward motion of the glass capillary in the Du Bois puller was an important intrinsic aspect of the design, rather than an incidental aspect of the pulling motion. (6) The alignment rod through the pipette carriers kept the glass tubing straight as the tips were formed, thus facilitating the formation of straight tips, a goal that was very difficult to attain with hand-pulled micropipettes.

It is not clear what type of research was originally conducted with the Du Bois pipette puller, but it was used by a Dr. Chambers at New York University (Du Bois, 1931). We were surprised to learn recently that this puller design has long been available from Leitz; we are not aware of any applications to intracellular recording, but it appears to be used to form microneedles for fine dissections. In any event, this pipette puller solved the main problems that pertained to hand-pulled micropipettes, and it thus became the direct ancestor of other designs that have been widely used. So this instrument was quite important, based more upon the published design than upon the extent to which it has been applied.

III.2　The Livingston Micropipette Puller

The next step was a modification of the Du Bois design by Livingston and Duggar (1934), who used their instrument to form tip 'openings' estimated at 0.5–1.0 μm in diameter. These micropipettes were used to obtain samples of fluid from cells of tobacco plants infected with the tobacco mosaic virus. The potency of these fluid samples for infecting other plants was then assessed in an attempt to locate the site where the infection was most concentrated. Livingston and Duggar (1934) mentioned briefly the use of a micropipette puller modified from the Du Bois design, and they promised a later description of the device by Livingston. It thus appears that the modified design was by Livingston, and it has become known as the Livingston puller. In fact, no published description of the instrument ever appeared. The following description is based upon the version of this micropipette puller that became available to other laboratories in the early 1950's.

As shown in Figure 3, the Livingston puller employs a single spring to rotate a pair of wheels holding the pipette clamps. The rate at which the wheels rotate is determined by the tension of the spring, which may be adjusted by altering its initial length. The two wheels are geared together to rotate in opposite directions at the same speed. The two pipette clamps are thus pulled apart over identical time courses, forming two tips of similar length and configuration. The pulling motion of the Livingston instrument is much like that of the Du Bois, a smooth acceleration being provided in both cases, but the wheels accomplish this with a simpler method that probably reduces the cost of construction. The feature of an alignment rod was retained in the Livingston design, and rubber shock absorbers were added to cushion the shock at the end of the pulling motion. These are helpful in avoiding breakage of fine micropipette tips. In the Livingston instrument the platinum heating filament is mounted in an insulated block, which in turn is clamped into a metal block that can be adjusted vertically. The heating filament is usually a platinum wire or band formed into a deep trough, so vertical adjustment of the heating block controls how close the glass capillary is to the bottom of the trough of the heating filament. This adjustment is useful because it influences the rate at which the filament delivers heat to the glass capillary. Interchangeable blocks can be used for different heating filaments, thus providing for rapid and convenient changing of heating filaments.

In operating the Livingston puller, a glass capillary is first aligned in the pipette clamps, only one of which is initially tightened. The two wheels are then manually rotated to bring the pipette clamps together and lower the glass capillary into the heating filament. This motion also stretches the spring, and the endpoint of this motion is a stop on the back of one of the wheels. While holding the wheels against that stop with one hand, the other hand is used to

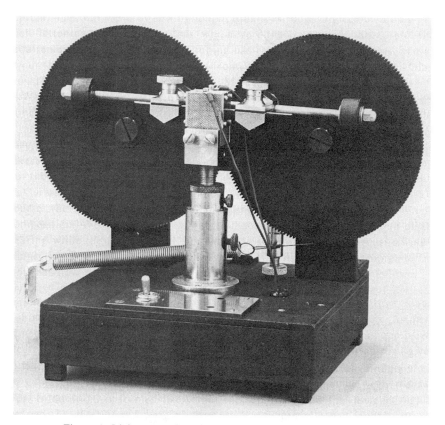

Figure 3. Livingston micropipette puller made by Otto K. Hebel.

tighten the second pipette clamp, and upon releasing the wheels they are held only by the glass capillary. The heating filament is then turned on, and pulling proceeds when the glass becomes sufficiently softened, the pipettes being lifted up and out of the heating filament as they are formed.

Figure 4 shows a typical pair of micropipette tips just after they have been pulled. The two tips are quite similar in length and in the profile of their tapers. As originally used, this puller did not produce especially fine tips. Investigators later modified the instrument by using a band of platinum–iridium (90%–10%) several mm wide as the heating filament and by greatly strengthening the spring to increase the pulling velocity. When thus modified the Livingston puller can form ultrafine tips, as we have determined by scanning electron microscopy. Two difficulties have persisted, however, both of which are shown in Figure 4. The tips formed are longer than desired for many purposes because of their great flexibility. For example, it is very difficult to form ultrafine tips shorter than about 25 mm, when measured from the beginning of the taper to the ultimate tip. There is also a distinct tendency for the tips to be bent. The amount of bending illustrated in Figure 4 is near the minimum and it is often more severe. Though the direction of bending is not consistent, it is frequently upward, as shown. This probably results from the tip being lifted upward as it is formed, so that when the pulling motion suddenly ceases the tip tends to be thrown slightly upward until it fully hardens. Bending is typically greatest at the base of the long tip, where the glass is considerably thicker than at the tip itself and where the glass will thus require longer to cool and fully harden.

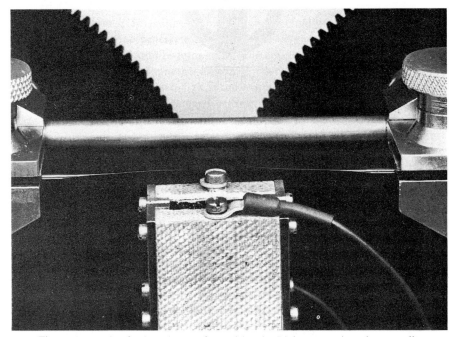

Figure 4. A pair of micropipettes formed by the Livingston micropipette puller.

Shortly after the original application of micropipettes as intracellular electrodes, there was renewed interest in this Livingston design. Livingston himself was then in the Biology Department at Swarthmore College, and Otto K. Hebel, an instrument maker in the department, began making this pipette puller in his spare time. It is not clear when this instrument was first used in neurophysiology, but a Livingston micropipette puller was already being used in the laboratory of Stephen W. Kuffler when one of us (KTB) began working there in 1955. So this instrument was adopted very early for making intracellular micropipette electrodes. Beginning in 1963, Hebel was assisted by F. S. Hockman, another instrument maker at Swarthmore College. In 1970 Mr. Hebel retired from making this device, which was then taken over by Hockman, who still makes it at 638 Flagler Blvd., Lake Park, FL 33403, USA. The design of the puller, as supplied by Hebel and Hockman, was never altered significantly. Slightly different versions of this device have also become available from other instrument companies, and a number of minor modifications have been made by various users for special purposes.

In summary, the history of the Livingston puller contrasts strongly with that of the Du Bois instrument, upon which it was based. Though the Du Bois was published but little used, the Livingston was never published but was adopted quite early for fabricating intracellular micropipette electrodes. Since then it has been used by many investigators and has made significant contributions to research with intracellular micropipettes.

III.3   The Alexander–Nastuk Micropipette Puller

Another micropipette puller, which became available commercially at about the same time as the Livingston, was developed and described by Alexander and Nastuk (1953). Though based in part upon the Du Bois and Livingston designs, it also introduced significant new features. Development of this micropipette puller was assisted by Mr. John della Pietra, who then made it available through Industrial Science Associates, Inc. (current address 25–44 163rd St., Flushing, NY 11358, USA). He informed us that the first three were sold in about 1954 to David Nachmansohn, C. Ladd Prosser, and Stephen W. Kuffler. Though Mr. della Pietra is now deceased, this instrument is still available from the same company without any major modification from the original design.

An overall view of the Alexander–Nastuk instrument is shown in Figure 5. Instead of a spring, the force for pulling micropipettes is supplied by an electromagnetic solenoid. This feature has proved so advantageous that it has been used in all subsequent pullers, aside from the recent design of Bertrand *et al.* (1983) which went back to coil springs. A solenoid permits the strength of pull to be controlled accurately and conveniently by altering the current through it. In the Alexander–Nastuk design it is also used to provide an initial weak pull followed by a much stronger one. Hence this was the first case in which pulling was divided into distinct slow and rapid phases to provide relatively fine tips that are not excessively long. As shown in Figure 5, the one end of a glass capillary (A) is clamped in a spring-loaded hinge (B) that is fixed in position, while the other end is gripped by a spring-loaded clamp (C) in the pulling rod (D) that is moved axially by the solenoid (E). Hence the pull is not symmetrical but one-sided. The desired current through the heating element is first set by a control (F) on the front panel of the instrument. When the starting switch is depressed, current begins to flow through the heating element, which is a band of platinum formed into a loop, as shown in Figure 6. Simultaneously, a current of 0.19 A is initiated through the pulling solenoid, which provides a weak pulling force of 100 grams. When the glass is sufficiently softened to be attenuated by this force, the slow pull begins. During the slow pull the arm of a microswitch (G), rides upon a cam (H) that is slipped concentrically over the pulling rod. As the pulling rod moves to the left, the leaf of the microswitch drops off the cam. This initiates an immediate rise of the solenoid current to 1.2 A, which increases the pulling force to 1700 grams. The cam may be adjusted axially along the pulling rod, which determines the length of the slow pull. A slow pull of predetermined length and strength is thus followed by a much more rapid pull, at the end of which the heating and solenoid currents are terminated.

Figure 6(A) shows a glass capillary mounted in the Alexander–Nastuk puller, while Figure 6(B) shows a pair of micropipettes just after being formed. Since the pull is one-sided, the tips are drawn to the left and formed outside the heating filament. This is another way to carry the forming tips out of the heating filament, thus preventing them from becoming too long and slender to be useful. This principle is utilized in all micropipette pullers in which only one pipette carrier moves. As shown in Figure 6(B), the strictly axial orientation

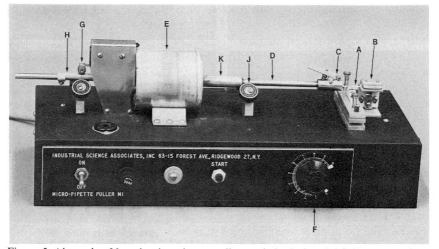

Figure 5. Alexander–Nastuk micropipette puller made by Industrial Science Associates. Labeling is as follows: (A) glass capillary; (B) spring-loaded hinge; (C) spring-loaded clamp; (D) pulling rod; (E) solenoid; (F) heating current control; (G) arm of microswitch; (H) cam on pulling rod. For further description, see text.

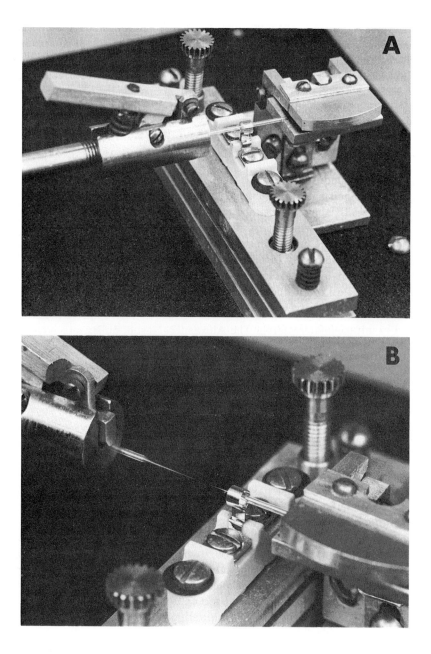

Figure 6. Details of the Alexander–Nastuk micropipette puller. (A) Glass capillary mounted in puller before applying heat. (B) Pair of micropipettes just after being formed.

of the pull results in tips that are reasonably straight. But the two tips are asymmetrical, with the one in the moving carrier being appreciably longer than the tip formed in the stationary clamp. This is not a critical consideration in most cases because the longer or shorter tips may be selected, depending upon the research in which they are applied. Figure 6(B) also shows that both tips are sufficiently short for many applications, even the longer one typically measuring about 12 mm from the beginning of taper to the ultimate tip. The tips are also small enough for many purposes, but ultrafine tips could not be obtained with the original design. Alexander and Nastuk (1953) illustrated a tip by electron microscopy that had an outer tip diameter of about 0.19 μm. We have modified an Alexander–Nastuk puller to provide a 25 sec delay between onset of the heating current and beginning of the slow pull; this raises the glass temperature at the beginning of pulling and provides somewhat smaller tips. Even with this modification, however, ultrafine tips were obtained only quite rarely (Brown and Flaming, 1974). As documented in Chapter 13, ultrafine tips become critically important for work in small cells.

III.4   Uses and Limitations of Livingston and Alexander–Nastuk Pullers

The Livingston and Alexander–Nastuk instruments, with minor modifications, served for many years as the basic designs of micropipette pullers employed in intracellular research. The Alexander–Nastuk puller was extensively employed for work in relatively large cells. For small cells (such as vertebrate photoreceptors, for example), the Livingston puller was required and proved useful, but the long and somewhat bent tips had distinct disadvantages.

Paradoxically, the different limitations of the two instruments probably result largely from the same cause. Ultrafine tips require attainment of a high velocity during the final pulling phase. This is because the tip is cooling as it attenuates, and the rate of cooling accelerates as the pipette wall becomes thinned toward the tip. Unless the final attenuation is very rapid, the pipette wall will cool to a temperature at which the two tips will form by separation before the ultrafine range of tip size is reached. Of course a high velocity requires overcoming both the inertia of the moving element and any friction that occurs during the movement. As shown in Figure 5, the pulling rod (D) of the Alexander–Nastuk instrument rides on ball bearings (J), which reduce friction to a negligible level. But the long pulling rod is stainless steel, with a soft steel collar (K) that extends into the solenoid so that the solenoid's electromagnetic action will be exerted upon the pulling rod. So the moving element is rather heavy, especially in view of the relatively weak force of 1700 gm (3.74 lb) that is applied during the rapid pull. Thus the Alexander–Nastuk design probably fails, largely because of inertia, to provide the requisite pulling velocity to form ultrafine tips.

Similarly, the rotating wheels of the Livingston design involve little friction, but the wheels have considerable inertia. Though ultrafine tips can be achieved by using a relatively wide filament and a suitably strong spring, their undesirably great length probably results from the relatively long time required to overcome the inertia of the wheels in reaching the requisite velocity to form ultrafine tips. In brief, the different limitations of these two early micropipette pullers for intracellular work probably resulted largely from the common factor of high inertia in the moving elements.

An additional difficulty with both instruments was their low reliability over the period of weeks or months required to complete most research projects. Though they were usually reliable for a few days at a time, investigators were plagued by sudden and inexplicable changes in the micropipettes formed, even when the conditions of operation were held as constant as possible. These inexplicable changes led to frustrating periods of readjusting the instrument, largely by trial-and-error, to obtain satisfactory micropipettes again. These unproductive periods seriously impaired the conduct of research, since they entailed losses of laboratory animals, while considerably increasing the time, effort and funds required to complete any given project.

III.5 The Winsbury Vertical Micropipette Puller

Micropipette pullers following the Alexander–Nastuk design were made available by a number of instrument companies. Most of the design modifications among these instruments were relatively minor and yielded little variation in performance, but a noteworthy variation was the mounting of this type of puller in a vertical orientation. It was noted that tips formed on an Alexander–Nastuk puller in the horizontal orientation exhibited some sagging of the tip, owing to the action of gravity as the micropipette was pulled, and a vertical orientation of the pulling axis was the earliest method used to eliminate that problem. The first vertical puller was described by Winsbury (1956), as shown in Figure 7(A). This design also provided the necessary modifications to handle heavy borosilicate (Pyrex ®) tubing with an outer diameter of 2.5–4.5 mm. Consequently, it proved especially useful in forming multi-barrel micropipettes to study the effects of putative synaptic transmitters upon the activity of a single cell. Figure 7(B) shows a 7-barrel assembly that has been made by a glass worker, pulled by hand in a preliminary way, and mounted in the Winsbury puller prior to forming the fine tips. Typically, the central micropipette is then used to record the activity of a single cell during the iontophoretic application of various putative transmitters through the other six channels. The Winsbury instrument supplies the necessary heat for pulling these relatively large glass assemblies. This is done by using heavy platinum wire (0.048 in. diameter) to form a heating coil of many turns, as shown in Figure 7(B); of course this heating coil draws a relatively high current, which is also provided.

III.6 Design Considerations in Vertical Micropipette Pullers

Following the Winsbury puller, other vertical pullers became available. For example, Figure 8 shows that the Alexander–Nastuk puller was offered in a vertical orientation by the simple expedient of a mounting bracket to turn it

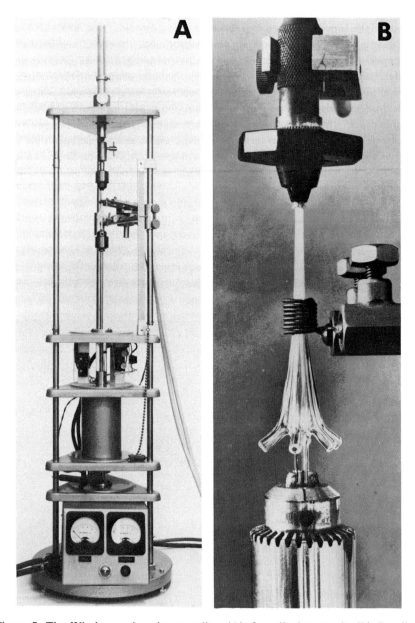

Figure 7. The Winsbury micropipette puller. (A) Overall photograph. (B) Detail of a 7-barrel assembly of pipettes that has been fabricated by a glass worker, pulled by hand in a preliminary way, and then mounted in the puller preparatory to forming the fine tips. (Photographs supplied by Prof. D. R. Curtis of the Australian National University, Canberra City, Australia, and published with his permission)

on end. As described by Frank and Becker (1964), the Instrument Section of the National Institutes of Health designed a puller specifically intended for vertical orientation, which appears to have influenced especially the early puller produced by David Kopf Instruments (7324 Elmo St., Tujunga, CA 91042, USA).

As shown in Figures 7 and 8, vertical pullers feature a fixed pipette clamp above the heating element and a moving element below. The initial slow pull is typically provided by the weight of the moving element, which is then supplemented by the solenoid to provide the fast pull. Gravity thus becomes a factor in both the slow and fast phases of pulling. This introduces a limitation that the slow pull cannot be conducted with less force than that resulting from the weight of the moving element. On the other hand, the effect of gravity would increase the pulling velocity during the fast phase, and this may have significantly

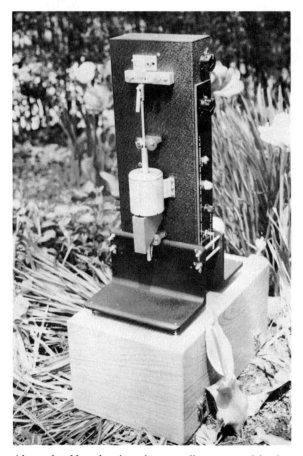

Figure 8. An Alexander–Nastuk micropipette puller mounted in the vertical orientation. This is the Model M-1 puller produced by Industrial Science Associates, Inc., 25–44 163rd St., Flushing, NY, 11358, USA. (Photograph supplied by Industrial Science Associates and published with their permission)

reduced tip size in the early vertical pullers, especially since they used solenoids of relatively low strength.

We have now shown that the problem of gravity-bent tips can be prevented in a horizontal puller, with tip lengths up to at least 27 mm, by using such a high pulling velocity that there is insufficient time for the tip to sag (Flaming and Brown, 1982). Hence it is no longer necessary to orient a puller vertically to solve this problem, provided that the strong pull is sufficiently rapid. It should be noted, however, that a horizontal puller usually requires some adjustment to attain straight tips, while this is not so critical with a vertical puller.

CHAPTER 3

The Brown–Flaming Micropipette Puller:
Its Background, Design, and Underlying Principles

PART I   BACKGROUND

I.1   Needs for an Improved Micropipette Puller

In 1973 we began intracellular research in vertebrate photoreceptors with the aim of further clarifying how electrical signals are initiated in these highly specialized cells. This work was first conducted in a turtle eyecup preparation, which was obtained by enucleating the eye, removing the front half of the eye, and then approaching the retina from the vitreous humor. In this preparation a microelectrode must traverse the layer of retinal ganglion cells and then the inner nuclear layer before reaching the photoreceptors. Nevertheless, Baylor and Fuortes (1970) had shown this preparation to be feasible for intracellular work in the inner segments of turtle photoreceptors, and this had been confirmed in both our own and other laboratories. The inner segments of turtle cones and rods are 8–12 μm in diameter (Copenhagen and Owen, 1976), which places them among the largest vertebrate photoreceptors that have been found, but even these are small from the standpoint of intracellular work.

Our intracellular techniques were initially those that other investigators had found most fruitful in this preparation. Micropipettes were formed on the Livingston puller to obtain fine enough tips to penetrate these small cells without severe damage. These micropipettes were then advanced through the retina by a Kopf stepping microdrive (see Part II of Chapter 11). When the tip of the micropipette was deep enough to be approaching the photoreceptors, further advances were made by 1.0 μm steps, which occasionally resulted in penetration of a photoreceptor. As first reported by Baylor *et al.* (1971), cell penetration may be facilitated by increasing the negative capacitance of a preamplifier until it goes into oscillation, thus imposing a high frequency oscillating current across the micropipette. The mechanism of this effect is not known, but the oscillating current presumably sets up very fine vibrations of the micropipette tip, which may be generated by reversing the mechanoelectric transducer properties of micropipettes that are discussed in Section IX.1a of Chapter 12. While traversing the photoreceptor layer, we thus applied frequent brief bursts of 60 Hz current across the microelectrode at a peak-to-peak amplitude of about 60 mV. The 60 Hz current was used to produce oscillations of controlled frequency and amplitude, and this procedure likewise proved an effective aid in cell penetration.

In common with other investigators, we found that these techniques could yield useful results. But intracellular recordings were difficult to obtain. More important, those that were obtained usually exhibited a steady decline of both the resting membrane potential and light-evoked responses. Intracellular recordings that were sufficiently stable to yield reliable data were very rare, so the acquisition of useful information was costly in both time and effort. Moreover, the stable recordings that were obtained seldom lasted more than 10–15 min, and this brief recording time limited both the quality of results and the types of experiments that could be performed. In short, although these intracellular methods had been adequate for many earlier studies in vertebrate photoreceptors, they were quite marginal for the kind of quantitative work required to produce a detailed understanding of the electrophysiology of these cells.

As an illustration of the changing requirements in this type of research, one of the earliest and most important observations was the hyperpolarization of these cells in response to light (Bortoff, 1964; Tomita, 1965). This was surprising, because all other types of receptors previously studied had exhibited depolarizing receptor potentials. The early findings were convincing, however, because they only required brief intracellular recordings from a small sample of photoreceptors. Response amplitude usually declined rapidly, but it was readily shown that the unexpected response polarity was not due to membrane damage. This was because hyperpolarizing light responses were found immediately after cell penetration, and the amplitude of these hyperpolarizing responses was sometimes maintained for a few minutes. So this type of finding did not require intracellular recording from very many photoreceptors, nor did it require accurate quantitative measurements or time-consuming control observations that demand intracellular recordings of high quality and stability.

By contrast, studies of how light-evoked responses are elicited and controlled require manipulation of cytoplasmic constituents, such as free Ca^{2+}. An early approach to this problem was to alter extracellular free Ca^{2+} (assumed to alter the intracellular concentration as well) while recording the extracellular 'dark current' that is reduced by light (Yoshikami and Hagins, 1971). A more ideal experiment to determine effects of Ca^{2+} upon photoreceptor sensitivity would be to first obtain intracellular responses to a range of light intensities under control conditions, with extracellular Ca^{2+} normal and with an adequate separation of responses to avoid significant light adaptation by the stimuli. Extracellular Ca^{2+} would then be altered and the entire procedure repeated, followed by a final series of responses under control conditions to see whether the cell had been damaged by the altered Ca^{2+}. Since this type of experiment requires stable recording conditions for a long period of time, it demands much better intracellular recording conditions than those that had sufficed for early intracellular work in photoreceptors. Though gradual improvements in technique had been made, our experience with turtle photoreceptors showed that intracellular techniques were still quite inadequate for this type of experiment, which is typical of many experiments that had become desirable in these cells.

When intracellular techniques were considered on a larger scale, it was also evident that their limitations had been a dominant factor influencing the entire broad field of intracellular research. Thus, research in the vertebrate nervous system had concentrated upon the relatively few cells sufficiently large to be readily accessible to available intracellular techniques. Since the vast majority of cells in the central nervous systems of vertebrates had proven too small for high quality intracellular work, equally vast problem areas in neurophysiology had been explored either little or not at all. In many small cells the limitations were similar to those in vertebrate photoreceptors, while many others (such as auditory hair cells) had not yielded at all to intracellular techniques. Taken together, these facts indicated a compelling need to overcome the technical barriers to high quality intracellular work in small cells.

On the one hand, we were somewhat daunted by the fact that techniques for recording in small cells had shown little improvement over a long period of time. On the other hand, it had become clear that the technical problems were sufficiently complex to require a determined program of work in which the improvement of intracellular techniques was regarded as a field of research in itself. Such an approach had not been tried, previous efforts having been either incidental to physiological studies or quite limited technique problems that were undertaken only as short term projects. We thus undertook a long term commitment to improving micropipette techniques, especially those required for intracellular work in small cells.

In our first project, techniques were developed for the rapid and precise beveling of micropipette tips with diameters as small as 0.1 μm (Brown and Flaming, 1974, 1975). Since beveling offers a variety of advantages, it will be treated in detail in Chapter 9. During that project it became evident that beveling could not be applied optimally to fine tips unless the tips were sufficiently short and stiff to contact the abrasive surface with significant pressure. Micropipette pullers available at that time could not form fine tips as short as desired for beveling, so this provided a further reason to develop an improved micropipette puller. Although this became our second main project, it will be treated first in this book because the formation of micropipettes is the most fundamental step in preparing them for research work. In addition, the development and refinement of this micropipette puller has taught us much about how micropipettes are formed, and this puller has been used in most of our additional work on other aspects of micropipette techniques.

I.2   The Chowdhury Micropipette Puller

It was first shown by Lux (1960) that the tip of a micropipette can be shortened by using a stream of air to accelerate its cooling while it is being formed. Chowdhury (1969) incorporated this principle into the design of a micropipette puller, which is illustrated schematically in Figure 9. The Chowdhury puller used a coil type of heating filament that consisted of four complete turns of platinum–iridium wire. Two nozzles directed air toward this heating filament from symmetrical positions in front of, and behind, the filament. Both pipette carriers moved on low-friction bearings, and from the back end of each pipette carrier a light steel cable passed around a pulley and thence to the plunger of a solenoid. The initial weak pull was provided by an adjustable spring, which was mounted in parallel with the solenoid plunger, while the solenoid itself provided the strong pull, with the symmetrical motions of the pipette carriers yielding two essentially identical micropipettes. Upon mounting a glass capillary in this puller and turning on the heating filament, the pulling motion began when the glass was sufficiently softened to be pulled apart by the weak pull. When the pipette carrier had moved about 2.0 mm, a microswitch was activated that triggered the strong pull, and after a delay of about 4.0 msec an electromechanical valve opened to release compressed air through the two nozzles. As a result, air was blown over the softened portion of the tips during the latter part of the strong pull.

The Chowdhury puller was reported capable of producing tips with diameters as small as about 0.05 μm. Though tip lengths were not stated, the tips were described as considerably shorter than those provided by other pullers available at that time, and the shorter tips were reported to offer a variety of advantages.

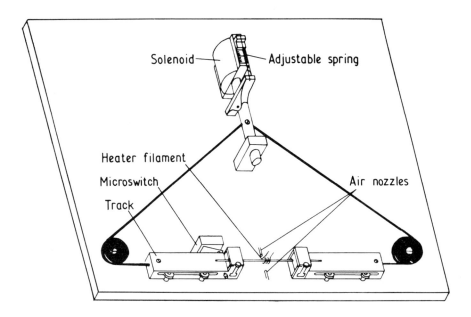

Figure 9. Diagram of the Chowdhury micropipette puller utilizing the airjet principle. (From Chowdhury (1969), reproduced by permission of The Institute of Physics, Bristol, England)

The cone angle of the tip, defined as the angle formed by the cone of the tip itself, was reported to be about $11°$, while the cone angle of micropipettes formed by conventional pullers was stated to be only about $1°$. It was computed that the increased cone angle should decrease the electrical resistance of electrodes by at least an order of magnitude, and measurements of electrode resistance were in reasonable agreement with that calculation (Chowdhury, 1969).

I.3 Testing of the Chowdhury Design

Since one of our major goals was ultrafine but short tips, we first built a micropipette puller following the Chowdhury design as closely as possible. Though the airjet principle seemed promising, it was puzzling why this design had not achieved any significant popularity among neurophysiologists. We quickly confirmed that the airjet principle was sound. Tip length could be shortened progressively by increasing the amount of air emitted from the nozzles, and the cooling air did not significantly increase the tip diameter. Ultrafine short tips could thus be obtained. But the tips provided by this puller were highly inconsistent in tip size and form. We learned that a few other neurophysiologists had experienced similar difficulties, and this probably explains the lack of popularity of the original Chowdhury design. Since this puller used a sound principle, we next undertook the refinements required to utilize its advantages. Among those that were identified, two were particularly critical. First, the wire coil filament made it difficult to prevent the puffs of air from deforming the micropipette tip. Second, the original solenoid operated on 60 Hz current, and the strong pull was initiated at random times, so the strength of this pull depended upon when it began within the 16.7 msec occupied by a single cycle of current. We later found that the entire period occupied by the strong pull, in the case of short tips formed by our own puller, was only 5–8 msec. Thus the strength of the strong pull varied markedly among the micropipettes formed by a 60 Hz solenoid.

PART II   THE BROWN–FLAMING MICROPIPETTE PULLER

II.1   Methods of Developing and Testing Design

In developing our own puller using the airjet principle (Brown and Flaming, 1977a), many specific design features were tested in one or both of two ways. High resolution scanning electron microscopy (SEM) was used to determine the effects of a given design feature upon tip size and configuration. In addition, tip performance was often tested by determining how well rod photoreceptors could be penetrated without damage in an isolated and inverted toad retina. Though onerous and time consuming, these methods of evaluating micropipettes were essential. In addition to revealing which design features are most important, they showed how design features could be manipulated to best advantage in both constructing and operating the micropipette puller.

II.2   The Design

As supplied by the Sutter Instrument Co. (P.O. Box 3592, San Rafael, CA 94912, USA), our original airjet puller was designated the Model P-77. After altering the airjet system it became the P-77A, and when the heating filament was also modified it became the P-77B. Figure 10 provides an overall view of Model P-77B, and Figure 11 is a schematic diagram of its mechanical aspects. Figure 12(A) shows further details of the heating filament and airjet, while Figure 12(B) shows that this puller forms a virtually identical pair of micropipettes, the tips of which are quite straight and short.

Figures 10 and 11 show that our instrument is basically a two-stage horizontal micropipette puller. Two forward-extending grips permit the pipette carriers to be held together by one hand, while the other hand inserts the glass tubing and clamps it into position (see Figure 10). Figure 12(A) shows that the glass tubing is then aligned by V-grooves in the pipette carriers and held by rubber-faced clamps. Figure 12(A) also shows that since the heating filament is a rectangular trough, the glass tubing may be dropped directly down into the clamps. Cutouts in the upper edges of the pipette clamps permit this to be done easily with either hand. Smooth and consistent pulling motions are facilitated by each pipette carrier being supported by three V-grooved wheels that rotate on ball bearings. From the back end of each pipette carrier, Figure 11 shows that a stranded stainless steel cable passes around an outboard pulley, then inward

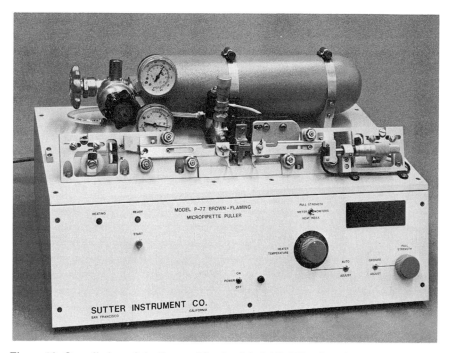

Figure 10. Overall view of the Brown–Flaming Model P-77B micropipette puller as it is supplied by the Sutter Instrument Co. For details, see text.

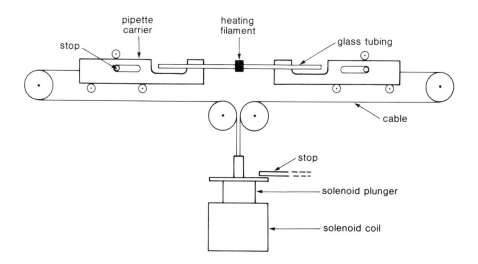

Figure 11. Schematic diagram of mechanical aspects of the Brown–Flaming Model P-77 micropipette puller (not to scale). For details, see text.

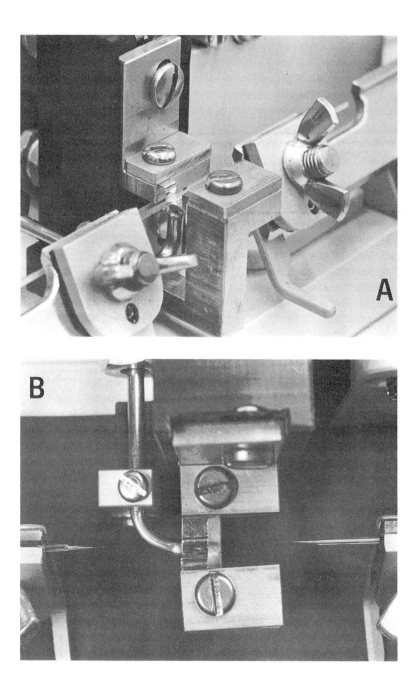

Figure 12. Detail photographs of the Brown–Flaming Model P-77B puller. (A) The heating filament and airjet, with a glass capillary mounted in the pipette clamps. (B) A pair of micropipettes that has just been formed.

to a second pulley, then downward to attach to the plunger of a solenoid. The weight of this plunger (80 gm) provides the slow pull, and this fixed strength of the slow pull has proved adequate for all of our purposes to date. For the fast pull, a DC solenoid is employed to eliminate the cyclical variations of pull strength inherent in AC solenoids. Our solenoid develops a pull of 50 lb when it is operated at 50 V, which we have adopted as a standard value because it has proved sufficient for most of our purposes to date. Such a strong pull is important to form ultrafine short tips, and this fast pull is considerably stronger than that used in other micropipette pullers. For example, it is about 13 times greater than the pull strength of the Alexander–Nastuk instrument and 2.5 times that of the Chowdhury design.

Figure 11 shows that each pipette carrier contains a slot that moves over a stationary pin, and this pin acts as a stop limiting the forward motion of the pipette carrier. When inserting a piece of glass tubing, the pipette carriers are held together against these stops. Both of the outboard pulleys may be adjusted laterally, and these adjustments are made when the instrument is assembled. While holding each pipette carrier forward against its stop, its associated outboard pulley is positioned so that the solenoid plunger does not quite touch the stop limiting its upward motion (see Figure 11). These aspects of the design are quite important, as will now be explained.

A stainless steel cable is used for its strength and resistance to corrosion, and it must be stranded for adequate flexibility. But a stranded cable is also elastic and may be stretched to a significant extent. If stops did not limit the forward motion of the pipette carriers, the carriers could be held together with their motion limited only by the stop on the solenoid plunger. In that event both cables would have identical tensions at the beginning of the slow pull, as desired to form two identical micropipettes. But the cables would be stretched, which would contribute to the initial strength of the weak pull, and the extent of this contribution would depend upon how firmly the pipette carriers were held together while clamping the glass tubing. As a result, the initial strength of the weak pull would vary greatly from one pull to the next. It is not clear from Chowdhury's description whether this problem was avoided in his instrument (Chowdhury, 1969); if not, it would have contributed to the variability of results. The problem is avoided in our design because the cables are stretched only by the weight of the solenoid plunger at the beginning of the weak pull. The initial strength of the weak pull is thus constant, and both pipette carriers begin moving at the same time. Provisions are also made to prevent the solenoid plunger from rotating around its own axis, thus preserving the integrity of these adjustments. If required, the outboard pulleys may readily be readjusted by the investigator, but this should be done with due attention to the principles just described.

When the pipette carriers reach the backward limit of their motion, they encounter heavy rubber shock absorbers. Because the fast pull occurs at high velocity and over a short distance, the rubber bumpers are provided to prevent sharp shocks from breaking the tips or from bending the tips before they fully harden. After striking the rubber bumpers, the pipette carriers are caught by one-way catches that prevent them from moving forward. Without this provision the tips reenter the region of the heating filament so quickly that they are bent by the residual heat. The rubber bumpers and one-way catches are not shown in the diagram of Figure 11 but they may be seen in Figure 10. The one-way catch is a simple leaf spring that engages a groove on the back of the pipette carrier, and it may be released by pressing lightly upon the spring.

As shown in Figure 12(A), the glass capillary is mounted near the bottom of the rectangular trough of the heating filament, and a single airjet is mounted below the center of the trough. The evolution of this configuration proved especially instructive. Hence, a later portion of this chapter will describe the details of this configuration and the underlying principles that were learned during its development.

The metal heating filament in a micropipette puller must be mounted between binding posts that support the filament and serve as electrical contacts for passing current through the filament. If electrical contact is made with only a small area of the filament, of course all the heating current will flow through that small area. This intense current corrodes the contact area of certain metals (such as tungsten), or melts the metal at the contact area (as with platinum–iridium), either of which will alter the heating current and the heat output of the filament. At the binding posts, therefore, it is important to make contact with the heating filament over a relatively large surface area. In our puller the filament ends are cut long enough for each end to have a considerable area clamped at the binding posts. The binding posts and airjet are then mounted on a block which can be adjusted relative to the main axis of the glass capillary. Thus the filament-airjet system can be positioned as a unit. The heating element is powered through a heavy duty AC transformer that regulates the line voltage. Then a Variac is provided to adjust the voltage, which is reduced by a step-down transformer to a maximum value of 2.5 V. The voltage across the heating filament is normally set at about 1.25 V, and a digital readout of filament current is provided on the front panel of the puller.

In the airjet system a small bottle of compressed nitrogen provides the 'air'. In this book we shall refer consistently to the airjet system in our puller and to the resulting airjet effects, even though air is not actually employed. This terminology is used for convenience and historical continuity, and it is further justified by the lack of evidence that the gas used to produce the rapid cooling is critical. In our puller the bottle of compressed nitrogen makes it unnecessary to have a laboratory source of clean compressed air at a regulated pressure, and this nitrogen supply will last several years unless there is accidental leakage. The nitrogen is clean and also constant in its moisture content. The output pressure from the nitrogen bottle has been kept constant at 50 psi. The 'air' pulse is formed by a rapidly acting electrical valve. Flow during this pulse is controlled by a needle valve set by a micrometer, which may be seen in Figure 10. The orifice from which the air is emitted near the heating filament has a diameter of about 1.0 mm.

II.3 Operation of the Instrument and its Pulling Cycle

When pulling micropipettes, the controls and digital readout on the front panel are first used to set pull strength and current through the heating filament. The reading for pull strength is always 25% of the voltage across the pulling solenoid. So pull strength is normally set at 12.5 to provide the standard 50 V across the pulling solenoid. For special purposes, however, the voltage across the pulling solenoid may be increased to the range of 75–80 V. With a rectangular trough filament of standard dimensions, ultrafine tips will be formed on Standard Tubing when the digital reading of filament current is set at 200, which provides a filament current of about 20.0 A. The melting point of the heating filament will not be reached until the reading of filament current has been increased about 20 more units (adding 2.0 A). For definitions of standard filament dimensions and Standard Tubing, see Section III.7 of this chapter.

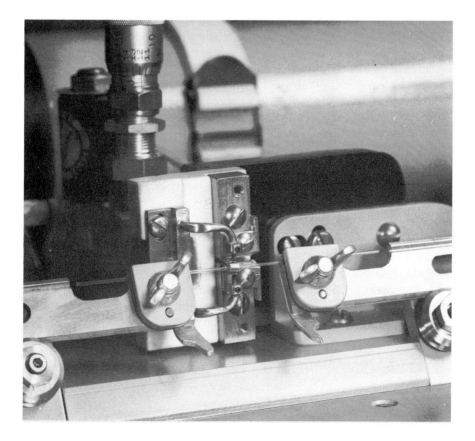

Figure 13. The original design of the heating filament and airjets. (From Brown and Flaming, (1977a), reproduced by permission of Pergamon Press, Oxford, England)

Upon pressing the 'start' button the heating circuit is activated, and the remainder of the pulling cycle is controlled automatically. When the glass capillary has been softened and drawn over a preset distance by the weak pull, a precision optical switch is activated. The length of the slow pull can be set by a micrometer with a non-rotating spindle, upon which the optical switch is mounted. The length normally used for the slow pull is 0.050 in., since this value has proved to minimize tip size when other settings of the puller are also in their usual ranges. Activation of the optical switch turns off the heating circuit, initiates the air pulse, and starts a delay circuit, at the end of which the pull solenoid is activated. It was found necessary to initiate the air pulse about 40 msec before the strong pull, due to the delay between opening the air valve and the actual delivery of air from the airjet. Though Chowdhury (1969) initiated the air pulse 4.0 msec after onset of the strong pull, the more rapid pull of our stronger solenoid required the air pulse to be triggered sooner. By employing optical switches and an oscilloscope, it has been determined that the time occupied by the strong pull can vary from about 5–100 msec, or even longer when thick-walled tubing is used without increasing the heating current. The duration of the strong pull depends upon a variety of factors such as wall thickness of the glass tubing, heating current, pull strength, and tip length as determined by airflow during the air pulse. The duration of the air pulse has been set arbitrarily at 300 msec; it thus lasts from 40 msec before the strong pull until after the micropipette tip has been formed, aside from extreme conditions that result in exceptionally long durations of the strong pull. The pull solenoid is activated for 1.0 sec and then turned off automatically.

PART III   THE HEATING FILAMENT AND AIRJET: PRINCIPLES UNDERLYING THEIR FUNCTION, DESIGN AND USE

III.1   Introduction

The heating element and its associated airjet have evolved considerably since the original description of this puller (Brown and Flaming, 1977a). A closeup of the original configuration is shown in Figure 13, which may be compared with the closeup of our current design illustrated by Figure 12(A). In addition, Figure 14 shows the early experimental filament forms that were tested, while Figure 15 shows the final filament forms that were adopted.

III.2   The Original Loop Filament and Twin Airjets

Our heating elements have been formed from flat ribbons of 90% platinum–10% iridium. The thickness has remained constant at 0.002 in., and for most purposes the filament width has been 2.0–3.0 mm. Following the design of several other pullers, we originally assumed that the most uniform heat delivery would be supplied by a 'loop' form of filament. As shown in Figure 13 and the upper half of Figure 14, our first heating element was thus of the loop type

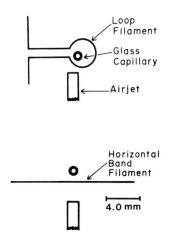

Figure 14. Scale drawings of the original loop filament, and the experimental horizontal band filament, that were tested in the Brown–Flaming puller. (Redrawn from Flaming and Brown (1982), reproduced by permission of Elsevier Biomedical Press B.V., Amsterdam)

with the 'legs' supporting the loop oriented horizontally. Of course this type of filament can sag at high filament temperatures if the legs are too long, so the leg length did not exceed 4.5 mm. Our attempt to copy the Chowdhury design had incorporated a wire coil filament, but we soon learned that the cooling air from the airjets did not have to contact the micropipette tip to be effective in shortening the tip. Indeed, the airjets proved equally effective with a band type of filament, which protects the forming tip from being bent by the puff of air. From this observation we assumed that the airjets were producing their effects by rapidly cooling the heating filament itself, thus reducing the time during which heat was delivered to the forming tip. It seemed likely that rapid cooling of the filament would be enhanced, while maintaining a uniform delivery of heat to the forming tip, if air were symmetrically directed to the heating filament from two separate airjets. So our original design featured airjets both above and below the loop filament, as shown in Figure 13.

III.3   Why One Airjet Proved as Good as Two

In the original airjet system the air tube leading from a small micrometer-controlled orifice was divided by a Y-junction to form the two airjets. In later work, at a time when the heating filament was removed, we held a strip of paper between the airjets and noted that puffs of air deflected the paper in one direction or the other. When airflow engineers were consulted about this observation, we learned that it must be expected when an orifice limiting a rather high pressure airflow precedes a Y-junction. Under these conditions a given puff of air does not divide about equally between the two arms of the Y-junction but flows mainly through one arm or the other. Since each puff of air was passing through only one airjet, a second airjet seemed unnecessary. Also, if the two airjets were exerting subtly different effects, the reliability of micropipette formation might be slightly but significantly reduced. We thus retained only the lower airjet, as shown in Figure 12(A). This simplification of the airjet system proved quite satisfactory, and no difference has been noted between micropipettes formed with one airjet instead of the original two (Flaming and Brown, 1982).

III.4 Observations Requiring a Revised View of How the Airjet Produces its Effects

Our understanding of how the airjet functions has now progressed further. If its effects resulted entirely from cooling the heating filament, it seemed surprising that the filament could be cooled so quickly, and it was similarly surprising that a single airjet directed toward a small area of the filament could cool it so effectively. These points were later clarified through a chance observation. When micropipette tips are fire-polished for patch clamping experiments, platinum has been reported to sublime off the heating filament and deposit upon the micropipette tip, where it tends to poison a membrane that is patch clamped. This has been prevented by covering the fire-polishing platinum filament with molten glass (Hamill *et al.*, 1981). While experimenting with patch clamp electrodes, we thus brought a soft glass capillary into contact with a rectangular trough heating filament to form a complete coating of molten glass over both sides of the filament. If the airjet acted mainly by cooling the heating filament itself, of course the glass coating would greatly slow the cooling of the filament, partly because of the additional mass and partly because glass cools more slowly than a metal filament. Yet this procedure did not significantly alter the effects of the airjet upon tip formation. This observation indicates that cooling of the heating filament itself is of negligible or minor importance. Thus, by the process of elimination, it now appears that the airjet acts mainly by removing heated air from the immediate vicinity of the forming glass tip. With the normal location of the airjet below the center of the heating filament, the filament deflects the puff of air from the tips, and the deflected air must flow rather rapidly past both sides of the heating filament; this would suck heated air away from the forming micropipette tip, thus reducing heat transfer to the tip. This can explain why a single airjet is so effective and how the airjet can act rapidly enough to influence tip formation.

III.5 Limitations of the Original Loop Filament

The design of the heating filament is particularly important in any micropipette puller. The loop filament shown in Figure 14 proved satisfactory in most respects, but it exhibited significant limitations when we wished to interchange filaments of varying width to extend the range of tip lengths that could be formed (Flaming and Brown, 1982). Though an original goal of our puller was to provide ultrafine short tips, for intracellular work in small cells that are readily accessible, the shortest tips are not ideal or even feasible for small cells that are deeply buried in tissues. For example, when the retina is penetrated from its vitreal side, a distance of 75–200 μm must be traversed to reach photoreceptors and most cells of the inner nuclear layer. A rapidly tapering short tip is not suitable for intracellular work under these conditions because the rapid taper, combined with the adhesion of nerve tissue to glass, makes it difficult or impossible to reach the target cell. Even if the target cell is reached, undesirable pressures can distort the tissue, with resulting functional abnormalities in either the target cell or in cells that have synaptic inputs to the target cell. In addition, in a circulated preparation the distorting pressures can cause local ischemia that impairs the functioning of all cells in the vicinity of the micropipette tip. The traditional and perhaps best solution to such problems is a rather gradual taper in relatively long tips, but of course the tip should not be any longer than required. The Livingston puller can provide long ultrafine tips, but for many cases they are longer than necessary or desirable. For the retinal work cited above, we have found tip lengths of about 15 mm to be sufficient for most cases, but in our experience the Livingston puller cannot provide ultrafine tips shorter than about 25 mm. We thus wished to extend the versatility and usefulness of our puller by modifying it to provide tips of any desired length over a relatively long range.

A simple method of lengthening micropipette tips is to widen the heating filament so that a longer segment of the glass capillary is softened before the tips are formed. Interchangeable filaments of various widths could thus provide a large range of tip lengths. The interchanging of loop filaments, however, was quite inconvenient. Equally important, when the rather long band forming the loop filament was widened appreciably, its voltage requirements exceeded the design of our power supply. Two minor problems had also become evident. One was a residual tendency of the loop filament to sag, even with the short 'legs', especially if accidentally overheated. The other was that adjustment of this filament to avoid tip bending had proved rather critical. While we had expected tip bending to be minimized by orienting the glass capillary in the center of the loop, this proved not to be the case. Instead, tip bending was empirically minimized when the glass capillary was located eccentrically in the loop, and when the airjet was also off-center, as shown in Figure 14.

III.6   Evaluation of a Horizontal Band Filament

In determining the feasibility of using simpler filament forms, we first tried the ultimate simplicity of a straight horizontal band, as illustrated in Figure 14. Of course filaments of this form are easy to interchange, require relatively low voltage because the length of filament between the binding posts can be kept quite short, and are well enough supported not to sag when heated. This band was placed below the glass capillary, rather than over it, for ease of inserting the glass tubing. In addition, this takes advantage of convective heat rise and thus improves heat delivery to the glass. With this type of filament the positioning of the airjet to avoid tip bending proved less critical, and it was usually placed about 2.0 mm below the center of the horizontal band.

Micropipettes pulled with filaments of this form did not exhibit significant tip bending, even when the filament was widened to 5.0 mm to provide tips as long as 23 mm (Flaming and Brown, 1982). Indeed, this filament form proved superior to the loop from the standpoint of tip bending. Several factors probably contribute to this result. When the glass capillary is centered in a loop filament, even the shortest tips are significantly bent. If the airjet is then turned off, at least the first 12 mm of the tip is quite straight, but a slender filament extends well beyond this initial segment of the tip and makes the micropipette unusable. This indicates that a minimal amount of air cooling is required to form usable tips, and it also shows that with the loop filament this air causes tip bending. Since the airjet is placed farther below the horizontal band filament, the velocity of airflow in the vicinity of the tip is reduced, which should decrease tip bending. In addition, there may be complex air currents within the loop that are avoided with the horizontal band. Two other factors seem especially important. First, it might be thought that asymmetric heating of the glass from a filament placed below it would always cause tip bending. But this asymmetric heating is probably significant only while the capillary diameter remains fairly large during the early stages of tip formation. The crucial stage for tip bending is after the capillary has become small enough to be bent quite easily, but at this stage the tubing is so small that the temperature gradient between the lower and upper portions of the tubing has probably become insignificant. Second, it is often assumed that in a horizontal puller the tips will be bent by gravity, especially if they are rather long. When short tips are formed in our puller under normal conditions, the fast pull is completed in only 5–8 msec (Brown and Flaming, 1977a). Though more time is required to form long tips, it appears that the rapidity of our fast pull allows insufficient time for significant tip bending by gravity.

III.7   Advantages of the Rectangular Trough Filament

The major limitation of a straight horizontal filament is its inability to deliver as much heat to a glass capillary as a loop filament, owing to so little of the horizontal filament being close to the glass. The horizontal band is thus inadequate for multi-barrel tubing or for single-barrel tubing that is either thick-walled or large in diameter. Also, since the filament is firmly attached at both ends, the lengthening of a horizontal filament during heating will cause either an upward or downward bending; this alters the distance between the filament and the glass capillary, which is a critical variable determining heat delivery to the capillary. Both of these problems are eliminated by the 'rectangular trough' form shown in Figure 15. The bottom of this 'trough' functions much like the horizontal filament, but the sides of the trough add considerably to the total heat delivered to the capillary. When the filament lengthens during heating, the

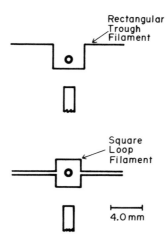

Figure 15. Scale drawings of the 'rectangular trough' and 'square loop' filaments adopted in the Brown–Flaming puller. For purposes of clarity the two metal bands making up the square loop are shown slightly separate; in practice, they are clamped together at the binding posts. (Upper half of this figure from Flaming and Brown (1982), reproduced by permission of Elsevier Biomedical Press B.V., Amsterdam)

sides of the trough take up most of this effect by tilting. This tilting is probably accompanied by a slight downward movement of the bottom of the trough, but this movement should be consistent in both direction and amount and should not affect the reliability with which micropipettes are formed.

Following some experimentation, dimensions adopted for our 'standard' trough filament were 4.0 mm for the length of the bottom segment, 3.0 mm for the height of the sides, and 2.5 mm for the filament width. These values are suitable for most purposes, and of course they may readily be altered for special purposes.

Our standard trough filament has proved quite adequate for the tubing we call *Standard Tubing* because of its common use in neurophysiology. It is made from Corning No. 7740 borosilicate glass, with outer and inner diameters of 1.0 and 0.5 mm, respectively, and a solid fiber 0.1 mm in diameter is fused along the entire length of the inner bore for convenience in filling micropipette tips (see Section I.3b of Chapter 10). Our standard trough filament will also handle borosilicate tubing up to at least 2.0 mm in outer diameter and 0.5 mm in wall thickness, as well as aluminosilicate tubing with outer and inner diameters of 1.0 and 0.58 mm, respectively. Trough filaments appreciably narrower than 2.5 mm cannot handle heavy borosilicate or aluminosilicate tubing, because heat delivery becomes inadequate. With Standard Tubing, however, filament width can be varied from 1.5–6.0 mm for the control of tip length, as reported in Part V of Chapter 5. Over this entire range of filament width, tip bending may be prevented from becoming a problem. And even with a filament width of 6.0 mm, our power supply can heat the trough filament to its melting point.

In summary, a rectangular trough filament has several advantages over the loop filament shown in Figure 14. It is easier to make and to mount in the puller, and filaments of various widths are more readily interchanged to alter tip length. It is also less likely to be damaged when inserting a glass capillary, since the capillary need not be threaded through it.

III.8   Non-uniformity of Filament Temperature

Since current must flow through the entire heating filament, temperature would be uniform along the filament's length if it were influenced only by this current. Though uniformity of filament temperature is sometimes assumed, this assumption is not valid. If a filament is observed closely, especially at relatively low heating currents, its color temperature is highest at the midpoint and falls off symmetrically toward the binding posts. If the heating current is then increased to a filament's melting point, it consistently burns out midway between the binding posts, regardless of the filament's form. These results are due to the rather large binding posts acting as heat sinks that draw off heat from both ends of the filament. Thus, the temperature of a heating filament is highest at the midpoint and falls gradually in both directions toward the binding posts, with consequences that depend upon the geometry of the filament.

A wire coil filament, which is used in many pullers, is an interesting case in point. If the coil consists of three turns, for example, the central turn will be midway between the binding posts. As a result, it will be much hotter than the two turns at the ends of the coil. So heat delivery is not uniform along the long axis of a wire coil but is greatest in the center and falls markedly toward both ends. Though we are not aware of a good example, this pattern of heat delivery may be advantageous in certain cases.

In the case of the loop filament shown in Figure 14, heat is not delivered uniformly at all points around the loop. Instead, maximum heat delivery is from the filament's midpoint at the right side of the loop. This is undoubtedly one reason why the best position of a glass capillary to avoid tip bending proved not to be the center of the loop, as originally expected, but the position shown.

In the case of a rectangular trough filament, the glass capillary is directly over the hottest portion of the filament. Thus, an important feature of this filament is that its hottest portion is ideally located for delivering heat to the glass capillary by both radiation and convection. For especially heavy tubings, or some multi-barrel tubings, even greater heat delivery may be required. Significant increases may be attained by narrowing the bottom of the rectangular trough and/or lengthening its sides. The filament may also be widened to increase heat delivery, providing that the accompanying increase of tip length is suitable to the research being conducted.

In theory the non-uniformity of filament temperature could be reduced by using relatively small metal strips to contact the heating filament, the main bulk of the binding posts being a material of low conductivity for both electricity and heat. With appropriate filament design, however, especially as described in the next section of this chapter, non-uniformity of filament temperature has not proved to be a significant problem. Furthermore, binding posts that provide effective heat sinks serve useful functions by cooling the filament rapidly. Without this rapid cooling, residual heat in the filament would increase the filament temperature when forming the next pair of micropipettes. Unless the time between successive pulls were deliberately prolonged, the reliability of tip size would thus be reduced. In addition, the life expectancy of the heating filament would be reduced, since each pull would require the filament to be at high temperatures for a longer period of time. We thus retained the heavy metal binding posts to avoid these problems.

III.9 The Square Loop (or Box) Filament

Rectangular trough filaments have long been used in micropipette pullers. In fact, a deep trough filament has always been a feature of the Livingston design. It appears, however, that the advantages of this filament form have not been well understood. It also occurred to us that this filament form could be used in a new and useful variation shown in the bottom half of Figure 15. Two rectangular trough filaments are placed one over the other to form a 'square loop' (or 'box') measuring 3.0 mm on all four sides. When a loop filament is formed in the conventional way from a single ribbon of metal, as shown in Figure 14, only one zone of the filament may be heated to just below its melting point. But the square loop in Figure 15 is formed from two filaments that are electrically in parallel, so both draw the same current and produce the same amount of heat. This provides two zones of the square loop that can be heated to just below the melting point, so heat delivery to the glass capillary is appreciably increased. Furthermore, the two midway points of maximum filament temperature are directly above and below the glass capillary, which improves the symmetry of heat delivery. In fact, heat delivery to the top and bottom of the glass capillary should be entirely symmetrical, aside from convective heat rise. Fortunately, the square loop requires no alteration of the filament holder. For any given filament temperature, of course the square loop draws twice the current of only one of the trough filaments that make up the square loop. For this reason our power supply cannot handle square loops appreciably wider than 3.0 mm, but this width has proved adequate for most purposes.

In summary, the square loop can significantly increase both the amount and symmetry of heat delivered to the glass capillary. It is thus helpful for handling particularly heavy tubing or multi-barrel tubing, and it makes tip bending easier to avoid.

III.10 Considerations in Choosing Platinum–Iridium for Making Heating Filaments

Though other metals have been considered for the heating filament, 90% platinum–10% iridium has proved difficult to improve upon. The high platinum content confers high resistance to oxidation, while the iridium makes the filament stiffer than pure platinum, and the melting point of this alloy is 1815 °C (*Chemical Engineer's Handbook*, 1973). The borosilicate glass we have used almost exclusively has been Corning No. 7740 (Pyrex®). The Corning Glass Works states that its 'softening point' (the lowest temperature at which a glass fiber elongates under its own weight under standard conditions) is 821 °C. The 'working point' is always higher, in this case 1252 °C. Since the working point is the lowest temperature at which glass may be readily molded or 'worked', it is a useful indication of the glass temperature that must be attained to form fine micropipette tips. Other formulations of borosilicate glass supplied by the Corning Glass Works have somewhat lower working points, and the two formulations of aluminosilicate glass that they supply have respective working points of 1202 °C and 1168 °C. Thus, the melting point of 90% platinum–10% iridium is well above the glass temperatures that must be achieved to form fine micropipettes from either borosilicate or aluminosilicate tubing.

While tungsten has a considerably higher melting point of 3410 ± 20°C (*Handbook of Chemistry and Physics*, 1972–1973), tungsten begins to oxidize rapidly at a temperature of 700 °C, and by a temperature of 1200 °C the oxidation of tungsten in air can be 'catastrophic' (*McGraw-Hill Encyclopedia of Science & Technology*, 1982). The oxidation of tungsten, at temperatures required to form micropipettes, is thus too rapid unless the filament is quite heavy. Alloys of nickel and chromium (Nichrome®) likewise oxidize rapidly at the temperatures required by this application. In addition, hard metals such as tungsten and Nichrome® would probably be difficult to shape into filaments of the desired form. In view of these problems, thin ribbons of platinum–iridium still offer the most satisfactory material for general-purpose heating filaments in micropipette pullers.

A minor problem is that sheets of platinum–iridium are available from only a few suppliers, and these sheets are made only on special order. As a result, different batches show slight variations from the specified thickness, and these small differences in thickness alter the filament temperature resulting from a given filament current. For this reason, it is not possible to specify a filament current that will provide an entirely consistent result. At a number of points in this book, filament currents are specified that we found to yield a certain result. These values should be useful guides, but each investigator may need to refine the filament current to satisfy any given requirement.

III.11   The Life of a Heating Filament and When it Should be Replaced

Like other metal heating filaments, platinum–iridium deteriorates with use, but fortunately at a relatively slow rate. Since deterioration becomes more rapid at higher temperatures, it is good practice to keep the heating current as low as possible, consistent with forming tips of the desired size and configuration. Significant deterioration of the filament is indicated by the appearance of small holes, which may be seen by the naked eye but are better visualized with a hand magnifier. This deterioration raises the electrical resistance of the filament, and at constant voltage causes the heating current to decrease, as indicated by the digital reading for heating current on the front panel of the instrument. Thus, if the heating current starts to decrease gradually without being altered deliberately, this also indicates filament deterioration. If a heating filament is not replaced when significant deterioration is first noted, deterioration will accelerate during the remainder of the filament's life. This occurs because loss of metal from the filament requires more current through the remaining metal to maintain total heat output at a constant level; this causes the remaining metal to be operated at a higher temperature and to deteriorate even more rapidly. During this final stage of accelerated filament deterioration, it is difficult to avoid changes of heat output and a diminished reliability of tip formation. Thus the filament should be replaced when significant filament deterioration is first noted.

Of course filament life will vary with several factors, mainly operating temperature, frequency of use, and the amount of care taken to avoid damage. We have used a single filament for as long as a year, during which there were alternating periods of heavy and light use. But the average filament life is considerably less than this, and the filament may need frequent replacement if it is operated at relatively high temperatures.

CHAPTER 4

Techniques for Examining and Measuring Micropipette Tips by Scanning Electron Microscopy

PART I   BACKGROUND

For many years the difficulties of adequately preparing micropipette tips for electron microscopy were serious obstacles to studying the principles that govern tip formation. These difficulties increase as tip size decreases, so they are especially severe with ultrafine tips. Though transmission electron microscopy (TEM) has been used for many published photographs of micropipette tips (Alexander and Nastuk, 1953; Byzov and Chernyshov, 1961; Chowdhury, 1969; Frank and Becker, 1964; Nastuk and Hodgkin, 1950), our initial efforts with that mode were not promising. We then tried scanning electron microscopy (SEM) with more encouraging results, so that mode was pursued. The limitations of TEM for this type of work have now become better defined and will be discussed at the end of this chapter. The instrument used for most of our SEM work was a Cambridge Stereoscan S150, but the recent work for Chapters 15 and 18 was conducted with an ISI model 30-E.

PART II   SPECIFIC PROBLEMS THAT MUST BE AVOIDED

II.1   Liquid Contamination from Mounting Media

The most critical problem in observing micropipettes by SEM (or TEM) is how to mount the micropipette tips. Mounting materials that are acceptable from the standpoint of outgassing in an electron microscope include silver paint, Duco ® cement, and certain epoxies. All of these were tried in our early work, including many epoxies. Though tips were occasionally clean enough for examination and measurement (Brown and Flaming, 1974, 1977a, 1979a), the yield was low and variable. The problem resulted from volatile components in all of these mounting media. As the mounting media cured, these components vaporized and then condensed upon the micropipette tips. With any given mounting medium, this problem varied greatly and unpredictably from one batch of tips to the next. When severe, this type of contamination was readily identified by a droplet of liquid at the very tip of a micropipette. Even when liquid contamination was not obvious, the measured tip sizes in some batches of micropipettes were quite variable. When volatile contaminants were later eliminated, the measured tip sizes became so consistent that this earlier high variability probably resulted mainly from liquid contamination. Hence volatile components can probably result in spuriously large measured tip sizes, even when this type of contamination is not clearly evident. This problem may be minimized by measuring only tips that appear clean and by placing greatest confidence in the smallest tip sizes that are measured under a given set of conditions. When performing experiments by SEM, however, these precautions are often insufficient. For example, determination of the reliability of a micropipette puller requires that all tips in a given group be measured. In addition, some experiments require so many tip measurements that the results cannot be obtained if a tip can be measured only occasionally. Some of the experiments in Chapter 6 required measurement of several hundred tips, and many thousands of tips have been examined during the work reported in this book.

II.2   Tip Charging

Since the tip of any sharply pointed non-conductor tends to accumulate static surface charges, the tips of glass micropipettes exhibit this phenomenon in an extreme form. In electron microscopy this problem is usually handled by coating the specimen with a layer of gold, and we have done the same, using coatings varying in thickness from about 50–200 Å. The thin layer of gold covers the entire specimen, including the mounting stub, which is electrically grounded when inserted into the SEM. Static charges are thus led off to ground by the conductive gold coating. We normally apply this coating just before SEM observations, which are performed within a few hours after mounting the tips. The gold coating prevents any further attraction of charged particles from the air that can contaminate the tip. More important, it prevents charging of the tip by the electron beam itself. We have seen this phenomenon most clearly while trying to examine uncoated ultrafine tips by TEM. Relatively low accelerating voltages could be used to resolve relatively large tips without any significant problem of tip charging. But when the magnification and accelerating voltage were increased sufficiently to resolve ultrafine tips, they disappeared in a 'bloom' of electrons which gave them the general shape of a gas flare. This effect also occurs frequently, and has been well illustrated, in the case of relatively large beveled tips that have been left uncoated and photographed by SEM (Baldwin, 1980b).

II.3   Tip Vibration by Electron Beam

The electron beam can also cause other problems. When we tried to examine uncoated tips with SEM, they could be seen at low magnification, but they became blurred as the magnification required to resolve them was approached, and the tips were later found to have shattered. Apparently the stream of electrons impinging upon the highly charged tip set up strong vibrations, which contributed to blurring of the tip and finally caused it to shatter. Vibration by the electron beam can also impair the resolution of coated tips, especially the ultrafine ones that are most flexible and require the highest accelerating voltages for adequate resolution. Fortunately, this problem may be managed satisfactorily by keeping the unembedded portion of a tip as short as possible.

II.4   Tip Softening by Electron Beam

Coated tips have even been noted to soften and bend while being observed by SEM, apparently due to heating from the electron beam. We have seen this only with ultrafine tips during attempts to achieve optimal resolution. Fortunately, the requirements of all but the most critical SEM observations may be met by accelerating voltages in the range of 20 kV, which are high enough to require gold coatings but which do not overheat the tips.

PART III   MOUNTING MICROPIPETTE TIPS FOR EXAMINATION BY SEM

III.1   Mounting Tips in Solder Glass

III.1a   Technique

The problem of liquid contamination was first solved by mounting micropipette tips with solder glass (Corning No. 7570), thus eliminating all volatile components from the mounting medium. This method was mentioned by Brown and Flaming (1977a) but has not been described previously.

The working point of solder glass is 558 °C, while the softening point of Corning No. 7740 borosilicate glass is 821 °C, so solder glass flows at 263 °C below the softening point of Pyrex ®. A heavy-duty soldering gun was clamped in a vise and operated from a Variac at a temperature just sufficient to melt solder glass. A small piece of sheet brass was placed on the tip of the soldering gun; then a small mound of solder glass, which comes in powder form, was placed on the piece of brass and melted. Using a dissecting microscope and micromanipulator, a horizontally oriented micropipette was lowered into this molten solder glass and adjusted so that the tip protruded as little as possible. The soldering gun was then turned off to cool the solder glass, after which the piece of brass was lifted by tweezers, breaking the mounted portion of the tip away from the remaining pipette. The piece of brass was then clamped under the head of a screw that was tapped into a standard SEM stub, upon which three tips were thus mounted. Figure 16(A) is a low power SEM photograph of a micropipette tip mounted as described and viewed from directly above the mounting stub, while Figure 16(B) illustrates two mounted tips at a higher magnification that shows both the embedded and unembedded portions of the tips. The lengths of the unembedded portions of these tips are 75 and 105 μm, respectively; these are typical values for our tips mounted in solder glass, and they permitted adequate resolution of ultrafine tips as shown, for example, in Figures 18, 22 and 30.

Prior to mounting the micropipette tips, it proved necessary to clean the pieces of brass thoroughly. Otherwise, heating of the brass released oily surface contaminants that condensed upon the micropipette tips. The sheet brass was 0.025 in. thick, hence quite stiff, which proved advantageous. It was first cut into long strips about 2.0 mm wide, which were cleaned on both sides and both edges by vigorous abrasion with 400 grit silicon carbide paper, followed by wiping off the abrasion products with clean laboratory tissue. After cleaning, the brass was not touched by hand. The strips were then cut into pieces about 4 mm long that were ready for use. Cleaning the brass by abrasion is quick and easy and has the additional advantage that scoring its surface probably improves the bond with the solder glass. The SEM mounting stubs were cleaned by sonication in xylene, followed by sonication in ethyl alcohol, then dried in an oven.

III.1b   Advantages and Limitations

This mounting method was employed in earlier work (Flaming and Brown, 1982), in which it permitted accurate measurements on an average of 14.4 micropipette tips per day. The occasional tips that cannot be measured result mainly from tip breakage while mounting, inadvertent embedding of the entire tip in the solder glass, or failure of the hardened solder glass to maintain its bond with the brass chip. Instances of tip contamination are quite rare and result from readily identified particles of dirt. Since the failures are for obvious reasons, the remaining tips (about 90%), may be measured accurately and with considerable confidence. This high yield of accurately measured tips expedited the large number of measurements required for experimental work on micropipette tips, as described especially in Chapter 6.

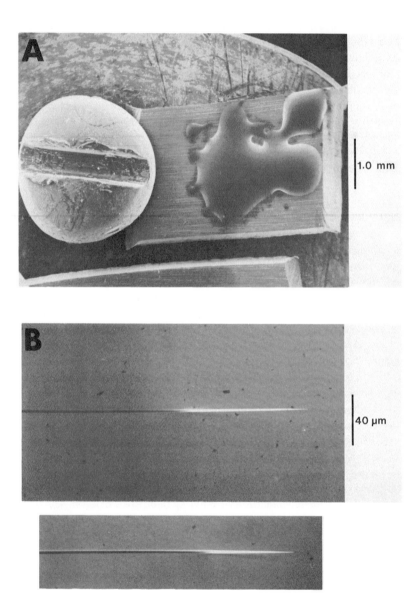

Figure 16. Micropipettes mounted in solder glass for examination by SEM. (A) Low power view of the surface of a mounting stub. A screw is used to secure a brass chip, upon which solder glass is used as the medium for mounting the micropipette tip. At this magnification the tip, which is pointing upward in the photograph, can scarcely be seen. (B) Photographs, at higher magnification, of two micropipette tips mounted in solder glass. Portions of the micropipettes that are embedded in solder glass are relatively dark, while the unembedded segments that include the tips themselves are much lighter. The respective lengths of the illustrated unembedded tip segments are 105 and 75 μm.

While solder glass offers the special advantage of completely avoiding out-gassing from the mounting medium, it has three limitations. First, this method is somewhat laborious and time consuming. Second, when the tip is drawn back into the molten solder glass until less than about 75 μm are protruding, the solder glass will suddenly cover the remainder of the tip. This apparently results from surface tension in the molten solder glass, and it limits how closely the mounting medium can support the tip. Third, since solder glass is below the tip and is electron-opaque, this mounting method cannot be adapted to transmission electron microscopy (TEM).

III.2　Mounting Tips with Double-sided Tape

III.2a　Technique

We next followed a suggestion of Kyoji Tasaki (Department of Physiology, Tohoku University School of Medicine, Sendai, Japan), who had successfully used double-sided adhesive tape to mount tips for TEM (personal communication). Following some experimentation, we adopted a procedure in which double-sided tapes made by the 3M Co. (St. Paul, MN 55144, USA) gave very satisfactory results for mounting tips to be examined by SEM.

As shown in Figure 17(A), a piece of tape was applied to the surface of an SEM mounting stub. Since tips must overhang an edge of the tape, that edge was cut by sharp scissors, and any adhesive remaining on the scissors was removed before the next cut. Micropipettes were held by a 3-dimensional micromanipulator and positioned under a dissecting microscope at a magnification of 16$\times$, the viewing axis having been adjusted to coincide with the vertical axis of the micromanipulator. The micropipette holder on the manipulator was slightly tilted so that the tips were pointed downward at an angle of about 5° from the surface of the SEM stub. The tip was first positioned close to the adhesive surface and only overhanging the cut edge enough to be sure there was an overhang. When the micropipette was then lowered, initial contact was at the cut edge of the tape, and with further lowering the flexible tip came into contact with the adhesive over most of its length. A spearpoint scalpel was then used to crush the glass well away from the edge of the tape, thus separating the tip from the remainder of the micropipette. At least 20 ultrafine tips may thus be mounted on each stub. The main limitation in minimizing overhang is how well the tip may be resolved. We direct light toward the tip at an angle of 90° from its long axis, as shown in Figure 17(A), since light at that angle is well reflected from the tip into the microscope. With a binocular dissecting microscope, careful adjustment of the light source will illuminate the tip best for only one eye, and it is the viewing axis of that eye which should coincide with the vertical axis of the micromanipulator. After mounting tips, we usually coat them with about 100 Å of gold.

Since the 3M Co. makes many double-sided tapes, we compared some of those that seemed most promising for this application. Three of the most suitable are

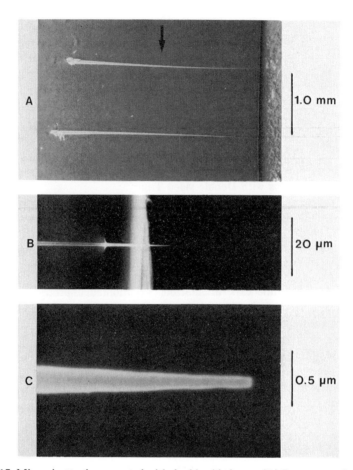

Figure 17. Micropipette tips mounted with double-sided tape. (A) Low power photograph of two complete tips. The cut edge of the mounting tape may be seen at the right, beyond which the background is the surface of the mounting stub. Near the left margin of this photograph, a sharp knife has been used to cut the tips from the parent micropipettes. The vertical arrow indicates the direction of light for optimal resolution of the tip by a dissecting microscope, in order to minimize the distance that the tip overhangs the cut edge of the tape. (B) A tip at higher magnification to show the typical overhang from the adhesive, which in this case was 22 μm. (C) A tip at still higher magnification to show the resolution obtained with this mounting method. After subtracting the 100 Å gold coating, the outer diameter of the illustrated tip measured 0.086 μm.

identified in 3M brochures as Numbers 410, 415, and 665. Number 410 is a paper tape with a rubber adhesive, and it is covered by a liner to minimize exposure to air prior to use. Numbers 415 and 665 are both film tapes coated with acrylic adhesives, and No. 415 is covered by a liner whereas No. 665 is not. In using No. 665, we thus took the precaution of always removing a few turns of tape from the roll to obtain a piece of tape that had not been exposed to air. The double-sided tape most readily available from stationery stores and art supply outlets is No. 665 or a similar formulation, while Nos. 410 and 415 may be obtained from the 3M Company.

When tips were mounted and examined by SEM on the same day, all three of these tapes performed satisfactorily, but with No. 665 the resolution of tips was not quite as high as that obtained with the other two tapes. When examined again 5 days later, all three tapes were still satisfactory for observing tips directly on the SEM screen. The slow scans required to take photographs, however, revealed marked differences. With tape No. 415 the resolution of photographs was unchanged, but with No. 410 the resolution was clearly reduced, and with No. 665 the deterioration of resolution was quite severe. As observed with tape No. 665, the main problems were loss of contrast and movement of the specimen while the photographs were being taken. It is not clear why these problems develop over a period of several days. But tape No. 415, which proved the most stable, has an adhesive coating formulated for a 'long-aging bond' that is resistant to the effects of both UV and relatively high temperatures. Since specimens tend to warm in the SEM chamber, resistance to relatively high temperatures may be a crucial factor.

In mounting micropipette tips for SEM, the double-sided tape of choice is thus No. 415. The other two tapes were also satisfactory if the tips were examined immediately, or if they were examined within a few days without requiring photographs.

Though we were concerned about outgassing from the adhesive, and perhaps liquid contamination of tips, no problem of either type has been detected. In fact, tips formed under specified conditions have yielded such reliable measurements of outer tip diameter that the possibility of any significant liquid contamination seems precluded. If tips are gold coated and examined within a few hours after mounting, particulate contamination is quite rare, and instances that do occur are seldom at the tip itself.

The mounting procedure must be modified when fine or ultrafine tips are quite short. This may be handled by beveling the top edge of an SEM stub at about $45°$ from its surface, and applying a narrow strip of double-sided tape to the surface, with one edge of the tape at the beginning of the bevel. Even the shortest tips may then be mounted across the narrow strip of tape, since the beveled edge prevents the shoulder of the micropipette from contacting the stub.

The mounting method must also be modified for patch clamp pipettes, which typically have rapid tapers to tip diameters of 1.0μm or larger (see Chapter 17). In this case the rapid taper and relatively large tip reduce vibration problems and make it unnecessary to mount the tip with minimum overhang. Instead, a final segment of the shaft may be pressed upon the double-sided tape. The shaft may then be scored and broken away, at a point several mm before the taper begins, since the tips of patch clamp pipettes are sufficiently strong to tolerate this procedure.

It should be noted parenthetically that breaking the shaft will consistently break ultrafine tips, and many tips in the fine range, unless special precautions are taken. This apparently results from strong vibrations being initiated at the break and transmitted through the glass to the tip. Thus, after forming such a tip, the shaft cannot readily be shortened. If it is scored and then grasped firmly on both sides of the score while the break is made, the tip may still be lost. But tips can be saved consistently by clamping a section of the shaft in a vise while the break is made, the vise having been faced with an elastic material such as rubber.

III.2b   Advantages

The use of double-sided tape can eliminate or greatly reduce all of the limitations of solder glass. Time and labor are saved by the simpler procedure; in fact, only 1–2 min are required to pull and mount each tip. Further time is saved during SEM observations because more tips can be mounted on each stub, and tips may be found quickly by following the cut edge of the tape. Support can also be provided closer to the tip itself. With solder glass the *minimum* overhang we have attained has been about 75 μm, while double-sided tape permits an *average* overhang of 20–30 μm. Figure 17(B) shows a typical overhang in that range, and overhangs as small as 3–4 μm have been observed without any evidence of adhesive creeping out and obscuring the tip. These shortened overhangs are probably the basis for a notable improvement in the consistency with which tips may be photographed at high resolution. Figure 17(C) shows a tip mounted by this method and photographed at high magnification. Finally, double-sided tape may be used to mount tips for TEM, as well as for SEM. In brief, this mounting method provides a marked saving of time and labor, while reducing the overhang of tips from the mounting medium and improving the average level of resolution for observing or photographing tips.

Though most of the SEM work reported in this book was done by mounting tips in solder glass, we now use only double-sided tape. In addition to assisting experimental work on micropipette techniques, this method is well adapted to occasional observations by an investigator needing to determine whether the tips formed for a given type of research meet the requirements of that work.

PART IV   COMPARISON OF SEM AND TEM FOR EXAMINING MICROPIPETTE TIPS

A limitation of both SEM and TEM is that after ultrafine tips have been examined, they cannot be used for experiments. Since ultrafine tips must be coated with gold and mounted with minimum overhang, this limitation appears difficult or impossible to remove. Fortunately, however, this limitation is no longer significant because of the high reliability with which ultrafine tips can now be formed (see Chapter 5), thus eliminating the need to examine the same tips used in experiments.

For relatively large beveled tips, Baldwin (1980b) has described an instrument that can fit into an SEM mounting chamber and hold an entire micropipette, while still providing the rotational adjustments required to assess beveling. The tips were uncoated, to permit their use in experiments after SEM; as a result, about 50% of these tips could not be assessed because of charging in the electron beam. Nevertheless, this instrument may be useful for observing relatively large tips before experiments, particularly if they are formed by a method having low reliability. Such an instrument cannot be used, of course, in the much smaller specimen chambers typical of TEM.

Several TEM photographs of ultrafine tips were published in quite early work (Byzov and Chernyshov, 1961; Chowdhury, 1969; Frank and Becker, 1964). Since these photographs are of good quality, they indicate that problems of tip charging and tip vibration may be overcome in observing ultrafine tips by TEM, at least occasionally. But these publications do not mention the use of gold coatings, nor do they give any other indication of how the ultrafine tips were successfully photographed. Kyoji Tasaki (personal communication) has found that ultrafine tips mounted with double-sided 'Scotch' tape and then coated with gold may be resolved quite well with TEM.

Compared with TEM, however, SEM offers two main advantages for this type of work. The larger specimen chambers are more convenient, for example, in mounting many tips on a single stub. In addition, SEM provides a three-dimensional view that conveys more information than the two-dimensional shadow seen by TEM. Thus the tip may be observed obliquely to see the profile of the entire tip, and end-on views can show the diameter of the inner pore (see Figure 26). Also, the adequacy of tip mounting may be readily assessed (see Figures 16B and 17B), and any contamination present may be identified. In summary, SEM is preferable, but tip size and shape can also be determined by TEM.

CHAPTER 5

Evaluation of Brown–Flaming Micropipette Puller

PART I   INTRODUCTION

This chapter evaluates performance characteristics of our P-77 series of pullers. The design features that provide these performance characteristics are either unaltered or improved in our more recent P-80 series of pullers. For example, the filament system itself was not significantly changed after our Model P-77B, but the constancy of heating current was markedly improved in the P-80C. Thus the performance characteristics reported in this chapter should be at least matched by the P-80 models. This has been confirmed by extensive testing of the P-80 series of pullers, as reported in Chapter 18 and in Tables 6 and 7 of Chapter 15. The new features of the P-80 series were introduced to fulfil the additional requirements of patch clamping and to permit the convenient handling of aluminosilicate glass (see Chapters 17 and 18).

PART II   SEM PHOTOGRAPHS: TIP SIZE AND CONE ANGLE

Figure 18 shows SEM photographs of typical micropipette tips formed with the loop filament (Figure 18A) and the rectangular trough filament

(Figure 18B). In both cases the outer tip diameter, after correction for the gold coating, measured 0.045 μm. The cone angles of the illustrated tips were 6° (Figure 18A) and 5° (Figure 18B). This defines the range of cone angles representative of ultrafine tips formed on our puller under these conditions. Our cone angles are thus only about half of the 11° that Chowdhury (1969) found typical of his puller.

The cone angle of micropipette tips is conventionally defined as the angle subtended by the tapered segment just behind the tip itself. In our experience the taper almost always remains constant for at least the first micron along the main axis of the tip, and it sometimes remains constant for a considerably greater distance. We thus obtain cone angles by measuring the outer diameter of the micropipette at the very tip, and at 1.0 μm behind the tip, from which the cone angle is readily calculated.

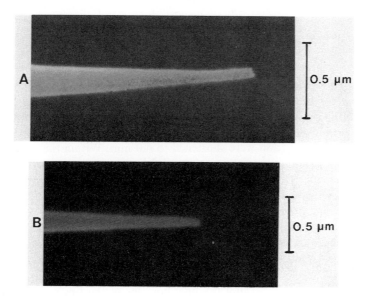

Figure 18. Scanning electron micrographs of typical ultrafine micropipette tips formed from Standard Tubing in the Brown–Flaming puller. (A) Tip formed with the original loop filament and an airflow setting of 75, which gave a tip length of about 10 mm. The cone angle of this tip was 6°, and after subtracting the 150 Å gold coating the tip's outer diameter measured 0.045 μm. Electrical resistance was measured for the other member of the pair of micropipettes formed by this pull. Of course the pair of tips should have identical tip diameters, and the value obtained for electrical resistance was 115 MΩ. (From Brown and Flaming, (1977a), reproduced by permission of Pergamon Press, Oxford, England). (B) Tip formed with the rectangular trough filament of standard dimensions, using settings of 317 for the heating current and 65 for the airflow. In this case the cone angle was 5°, and after subtracting the 120 Å gold coating the outer diameter of this tip also measured 0.045 μm.

If the cone angle is too large, micropipettes may not penetrate well through tissues that must be traversed to reach the target cells. In addition, the value of an ultrafine tip may be significantly reduced if the tip is too large at the position along its axis where it lodges in the cell membrane. If the cone angle is too small, on the other hand, tips may not be sufficiently stiff for beveling or for penetrating well through tissues. In our experience, cone angles on the order of 5–6° satisfactorily avoid all of these problems. Micropipettes with these cone angles penetrate well through retinal tissues, and they provide readily obtained and highly stable intracellular recordings from rod photoreceptors in the toad retina, as documented in Chapter 13. In addition, they are adequately stiff for beveling, as shown in Chapter 9.

PART III   AIRJET EFFECTS UPON TIP LENGTH AND ELECTRICAL RESISTANCE OF MICROPIPETTES

In evaluating the airjet effects (Brown and Flaming, 1977a), a series of micropipette tips was formed from Standard Tubing. The loop filament was still being used at that time, and puller settings were held constant except for the rate of flow during the air pulse. Airflow settings were taken directly from the airflow micrometer, which read in thousandths of an inch, with airflow increasing at the higher micrometer readings. Figure 19 shows low power light micrographs of micropipette tips formed at four representative airflows. At the lowest setting the tip length was 13.0 mm, similar to tip lengths typically provided by an Industrial Science Associates puller. As airflow increased the tips tapered more rapidly and were shortened to 6.0 mm. Within the range of airflows illustrated, tips formed at any given airflow were quite consistent in length and configuration. Tips as short as 6.0 mm proved to be near the lower limit at which such consistent results could be obtained.

For the four airflows used in Figure 19, Table 1 shows the resulting tip lengths, outer tip diameters and electrical resistances. The lengths of the tips shown in Figure 19 were measured directly under the microscope by means of a calibrated ocular micrometer. Table 1 shows that tip length decreased steadily with increased airflow. Though Figure 19 shows this general effect, it is not quantitatively accurate because the final portions of the tips were too slender for their lengths to reproduce accurately by photography. For example, Table 1 shows that the airflow setting of 100 gave a tip length halfway between the tip lengths provided by the higher and lower airflow settings, but this quantitative relationship is not evident in Figure 19.

Using the same puller settings and airflows as for the tips in Figure 19, two separate groups of tips were formed for measuring outer tip diameter and electrical resistance. Two groups were necessary because tips filled with electrolyte proved difficult to clean adequately for accurate SEM measurements. Figure 18(A) is a sample tip from the group used for SEM measurements. Tips examined by SEM were all coated with gold at a nominal thickness of 150 Å, so all measurements of outer tip diameters were corrected by subtracting 300 Å

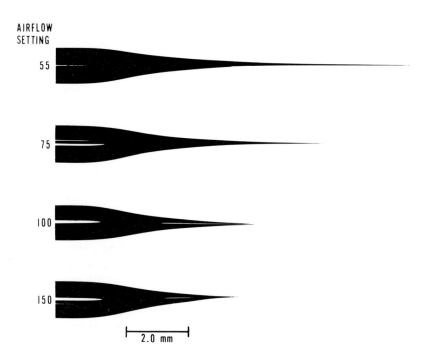

Figure 19. Low power light micrographs of micropipette tips formed on the Brown–Flaming puller, under conditions described in text, using four airflow settings. As airflow during the air pulse increased, the tip length was progressively shortened. (From Brown and Flaming, (1977a), reproduced by permission of Pergamon Press, Oxford, England)

Table 1. Tip length, tip diameter, and electrical resistance of micropipettes as a function of the airflow setting. (From Brown and Flaming (1977a), reproduced by permission of Pergamon Press, Oxford, England)

Airflow setting	Tip length (mm)	Outer tip diameter (μm)	Electrical resistance (MΩ)
55	13.0	0.052(8)	135(8)
75	10.0	0.049(8)	90(7)
100	8.0	0.063(4)	63(8)
150	6.0	0.048(5)	44(6)

or 0.03 μm. Tips used for resistance measurements were filled with 5 M K-acetate by injection from the back, then stored overnight with the tips down in a closed chamber, which contained a shallow layer of water to keep the overlying air moist. Any bubbles that appeared in the micropipettes were then removed by reinjection before DC resistances were measured the next day. For both tip size and electrical resistance, the values in Table 1 are averages, with the number of measurements contributing to each average given in brackets. At the time of this work, tips examined by SEM were still being mounted in epoxy. Hence tips clean enough for accurate measurements were difficult to obtain, and the number of tips in each group was relatively small. Within each group, however, SEM measurements of tip size were highly consistent, so it is unlikely that the obtained averages would have been significantly different if they had been based upon a larger number of measurements.

Over the range of airflows used in Table 1, there was no distinct change of outer tip diameter. From the standpoint of forming tips to meet a variety of research needs, this is a fortunate result. Since tip length is a factor influencing how well micropipettes can obtain a given type of information in a given preparation, a convenient method is needed for altering tip length independently of tip size. Table 1 shows that varying airflow can do this quite well over a large range of tip lengths. In our experience there is likewise little or no change of the cone angle when tip size is constant.

By contrast with tip size, Table 1 shows that the electrical resistance of micropipettes decreased markedly and steadily as airflow increased. Over the range of airflows used, electrical resistance dropped from 135 to 44 MΩ, a factor of about 3. Since tip size was constant, this marked reduction of resistance resulted entirely from the shorter and more rapidly tapering tips that were formed at the higher airflow settings. At the highest airflow setting in Table 1, the average tip diameter was about 0.05 μm and the average electrical resistance was only 44 MΩ. This is a very low resistance for such fine tips. By comparison, the only previous micropipette puller capable of forming ultrafine tips (the Livingston) gives much higher resistances. In our experience the shortest ultrafine tips that can be formed on the Livingston puller have a tip length of about 25 mm, and when filled with 5 M K-acetate their electrical resistance is at least 350 MΩ. Hence our puller has made it possible to reduce the electrical resistance of ultrafine tips by a factor of almost 8. Table 1 shows that increasing tip length from 6 to 13 mm (a factor of 2.2) increases electrical resistance from 44 to 135 MΩ (a factor of 3.1). Compared with the longest tips of Table 1, ultrafine tips formed on the Livingston puller increase the tip length from 13 to 25 mm (a factor of 1.9), while electrical resistance increases from 135 to about 350 MΩ (a factor of 2.6). As a rule of thumb, it thus appears that doubling the tip length approximately triples the electrical resistance of micropipettes formed by these instruments.

In summary, increased airflow can greatly decrease both tip length and a micropipette's electrical resistance without having any significant effect upon tip size.

PART IV RELIABILITY OF TIP SIZE AND ELECTRICAL RESISTANCE OF MICROPIPETTES

IV.1 Reliability of Tip Size

The importance of tip size to micropipette function is obvious and well recognized. Less emphasis has been placed upon the reliability with which tips are formed to the size required by a given research project. But this is also critically important. When micropipettes have been prepared for an experiment, they cannot be screened by SEM observation if the tip size is in the ultrafine range or only slightly above that range (see Chapter 4). This problem has been mitigated somewhat by measuring the electrical resistance of micropipettes. But this procedure can only eliminate tips that are much too large for the type of experiment being conducted, since electrical resistance is strongly affected by tip length and tip taper, as well as by tip size. Thus experiments involving intracellular work have customarily been approached with a group of micropipettes of quite variable capabilities. In fact, the experiment itself has provided the final test to determine which of the micropipettes could meet the requirements of the research. Since most biological preparations remain in good condition for only a limited period of time, this method of assessing micropipettes is wasteful of research efforts and costly in both research funds and experimental animals. These problems are particularly severe with preparations that deteriorate rapidly, are unusually costly, or are difficult to obtain. On a lucky day the first micropipette may perform well. At the other extreme, entire experiments are consumed with testing micropipettes without any notable success. Clearly this is a major problem that should be avoided if possible.

Since there is no method of measuring fine micropipette tips just before an experiment, the only apparent solution to this problem is to form micropipettes with such high reliability that little or no screening is required. In this approach it is still necessary for the experimenter to determine initially the pulling conditions that provide tips which function well in the type of research to be conducted. This can be done largely on logical grounds, as discussed in this chapter and in Chapters 6–8. Though some fine tuning by trial-and-error will still be required in many cases, it should only be necessary at the beginning of the research project, providing that given puller settings yield reliable results. This was attempted in our original puller design by providing capabilities exceeding the requirements whenever possible. In particular, electronic elements were used with specifications well above the requirements, so that their characteristics (such as resistance or capacitance) should not alter with use. While using the same puller for 7 years, we only experienced significant changes of its performance on two occasions. Both cases were traced to components that failed to have the expected durability, and they were replaced by components with even better specifications that then proved satisfactory.

The reliability with which a group of tips is formed at a given size has been assessed by direct measurements. In this work only one micropipette has been used from each pull, to determine the reliability with which micropipettes are formed on separate pulls. For the entire group of 25 tips formed with the original loop filament and measured for Table 1, the average outer tip diameter was 0.052 μm, with the largest tip measuring 0.07 μm and the smallest one measuring about 0.02 μm. These absolute values of tip size were probably slightly too low, since it later proved that our gold coatings were thinner than indicated by our coating instrument (see Chapter 6, Section III.2d). Even so, some of these tips were smaller than demonstrated with previous puller designs, and there was little variation in tip size. In a later experiment 25 more micropipettes were formed from Standard Tubing with the original loop filament, and after mounting in solder glass the outer tip diameters were measured by SEM, as reported in Table 2 of Chapter 6. That work was part of an experiment in which it was desirable to maintain the same heating filament as long as possible. To that end the heating current was set relatively low, and whereas the tips were in the ultrafine size range, they were not as small as could have been obtained with higher heating currents. Table 2 shows that the average size of these 25 tips was 0.081 μm. Only one tip was larger than the ultrafine size range (0.112 μm), and the other 24 tips ranged only from 0.068 to 0.096 μm. Thus the reliability of tip size has proved quite high. This is very helpful for physiological experiments, as documented in Chapter 13. It is also helpful for studying experimentally the factors that influence tip size, as in Chapters 6 and 7, since it reduces the number of tips that must be measured in a given experimental group of micropipettes.

IV.2   Reliability of Electrical Resistance

The reliability of electrical resistance has also been evaluated for our puller, as reported in Section II.1b of Chapter 10. Within a sample of 18 ultrafine tips, the electrical resistance varied from 70–130 MΩ. While this variability may seem high, its interpretation requires at least two considerations. First, though electrical resistance gives a crude indication of tip size, variations of electrical resistance *per se* have little significance in most experiments unless they become extreme. The importance of electrical resistance has undoubtedly been exaggerated in some cases (see Section II.2 of Chapter 10), partly in consequence of this being the only readily measured characteristic of ultrafine and fine tips. Second, the variability of electrical resistance decreases markedly as tip size increases. In fact, several investigators using our puller have reported that for tip sizes above the ultrafine range the typical variation of electrical resistance is only about ± 10%.

IV.3   Minimizing the Variability of Tip Size and Electrical Resistance

It now appears that a major source of the variability of tip size with our puller results from nonhomogeneities in the chemical composition and molecular structure of borosilicate glass. This is discussed in detail in Part IV of Chapter 15, where evidence is presented that strongly supports our interpretation. Because of the extremely small sample of glass that forms an ultrafine tip, significant variations can occur among these samples. This source of variability of tip size may be reduced if the short pieces of glass used to form ultrafine tips are all taken from a single 3-ft section of tubing, instead of being picked randomly from a large batch of short pieces of glass (see Section IV.2c of Chapter 15). Of course the effects of nonhomogeneities should be greatest with the smallest tips, and this has also been confirmed. When passing from the ultrafine to the fine range of tip sizes, the variability of tip size drops dramatically, and it then remains relatively constant over a long range of larger tip sizes (see Section IV.2b of Chapter 15).

The electrical resistance of a unit length of contained electrolyte at a micropipette's orifice is inversely proportional to tip diameter (Chowdhury, 1969). Thus the variability of tip size should result in a similar variability of electrical resistance. But other factors (notably cone angle and tip length) also contribute to electrical resistance, and these factors must also vary to some extent. So the variability of electrical resistance should be greater than that of tip size, as we have confirmed. In a typical batch of 10 or more ultrafine micropipettes formed on our puller from borosilicate tubing, the ratio of largest/smallest tip size is about 3/2, while the ratio of largest/smallest electrical resistance is about 2/1. Of course factors that reduce the variability of tip size should also decrease the variability of electrical resistance. So it is readily understood why the variability of electrical resistance is sharply reduced upon passing from the ultrafine into the fine range of tip size.

IV.4   Summary

In summary, the demonstrated variability now appears satisfactorily low for both tip size and electrical resistance. Among ultrafine tips, which exhibit the greatest variability, a major source of variability with borosilicate glass is nonhomogeneities of composition and structure among the very small samples of glass that form the tips themselves. If micropipettes are pulled in the customary manner, using pieces of glass that are randomly selected from a large amount of tubing, this source of variability is especially great. Hence variability may be reduced significantly by taking all pieces of glass from a single section of tubing several feet long. Since the effects of nonhomogeneities are greatest with the smallest tips, variability may also be reduced markedly if it is feasible to use tips larger than the ultrafine range. If significant further reductions of variability become necessary for special purposes, especially in the case of ultrafine tips, this will probably require more homogeneous glasses such as quartz (see Sections II.1 and IV.3 of Chapter 15). Though theoretically some variability must also be contributed by our puller, this has proved too small to demonstrate by present methods, and it now appears to have little significance compared with the other factors that have been isolated (see Sections IV.2 and IV.3 of Chapter 15).

PART V   EFFECTS OF FILAMENT WIDTH ON TIP LENGTH
AND SIZE

In assessing the effects of filament width upon tip length and size (Flaming and Brown, 1982), it was necessary to keep other pulling variables as constant as possible. The only variable presenting difficulties was the temperature of the heating filament. This problem was approached by deliberately increasing filament current until a filament burned out. This was done for each filament width, and the digital reading of filament current was recorded in each case, since it seems safe to assume that filaments of all widths will burn out at the same filament temperature. With filaments narrower than 3.0 mm, tip size increased as filament current was reduced from the burnout point. Hence for these filaments the filament current was reduced as little as possible below the burnout point. For filament widths of 3.0–6.0 mm, however, filament current could be reduced well below the burnout point without affecting either tip size or tip length. So for these filaments the digital reading of filament current was reduced 10 units below the burnout point. These procedures provided filament temperatures close to the maximum attainable and sufficiently constant to exert little or no influence upon tip measurements as a function of filament width.

Since the airflow required to produce usable tips increases with filament width, the airflow had to be set high enough for the widest heating filament. This was done by setting the micrometer control of the needle valve at 0.075 in. It should be noted, however, that the reading needed for this purpose might be somewhat different on another of our pullers, since the zero point on the airflow micrometer does not produce exactly the same airflow on every instrument.

Standard Tubing was used in this work. As shown in Figure 15, this tubing was located about 0.5 mm above the bottom of the rectangular trough filament, and the aperture of the airjet was about 2.0 mm below the filament. The length of the slow pull was 0.050 in., and the solenoid for the fast pull was powered by 50 V.

Six filament widths were tested covering the range from 1.5–6.0 mm. Under the described pulling conditions, this range extended from the narrowest to the widest filaments that could be used. The narrowest usable filament was determined by the amount of heat that must be delivered to the glass capillary to form useful tips, while the widest usable filament was limited by the power supply of our puller. On any given day when SEM measurements were made, all micropipettes were formed at the same filament width and then measured that same day. The minimum number of tips measured successfully in these daily filament-width groups was 12, while the average was 14.4. Data were thus obtained rapidly and easily because the tips mounted in solder glass were almost always clean. Filament widths were examined in the following order: 1.5, 3.0, 5.2, 2.25, 4.0, 6.0 and 3.0 mm. The final retesting of the 3.0 mm width was to see if results had changed between the initial test and the retest of that filament. The average test and retest values were 12.6 and 12.0 mm in the case of tip length and 0.079 and 0.073 μm for tip size. Thus conditions of

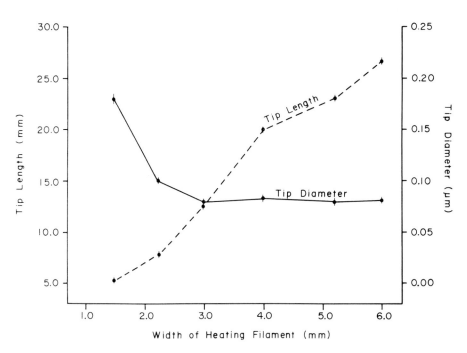

Figure 20. Tip length and tip diameter as a function of width of the rectangular trough heating filament. All tips formed from Standard Tubing. The vertical error bars indicate ± 1.0 standard error of the mean. For further details, see text. (From Flaming and Brown (1982), reproduced by permission of Elsevier Biomedical Press B.V., Amsterdam)

forming tips remained quite constant during the experiment. Figure 20 shows that varying filament width from 1.5–6.0 mm yielded tip lengths ranging from 5.4–26.8 mm. As filament width dropped from 6.0 to 3.0 mm, tip length was reduced from 26.8 to 13.0 mm, and tip diameters were all in the ultrafine range at a constant value of about 0.08 μm. Thus filament width, as well as airflow, can alter tip length conveniently and over a long range while maintaining a constant ultrafine tip size. With filament width, as with airflow, we have found cone angle to show little or no change when tip size was remaining constant.

At filament widths below 3.0 mm, tip length continued to decrease at about the same rate, but tip diameter began to increase. This is probably because narrowing the filament will eventually result in heat delivery, at the portion of the glass capillary that will form the tip, becoming insufficient to form ultrafine tips. If a smooth curve is fitted by eye to the data on tip diameter in Figure 20, it appears that tip diameter did not increase significantly until tip length had decreased to about 10.0 mm. But when filament width was decreased to 2.25 mm, the tip length was 7.0 mm and tip diameter had risen to 0.1 μm. This appears to define the lower limits of filament width and tip length at which ultrafine tips can be formed under the pulling conditions of this experiment. When filament width was further decreased to 1.5 mm, tip length fell to 5.4 mm, and tip diameter rose sharply to 0.18 μm. That rise of tip diameter is quite significant for intracellular work in small cells. As shown in Section II.1 of Chapter 14, the frequency of penetrating toad rods with 0.17 μm tips drops to only about one-third of that obtained with ultrafine tips measuring 0.08 μm.

Whereas Table 1 shows that airflow can be used to form ultrafine tips of constant size that are as short as 6.0 mm, it is noteworthy that filament width can provide ultrafine tips of constant size only down to a tip length of about 10.0 mm. This is undoubtedly because narrowing the filament eventually decreases heat delivery to the portion of the glass capillary from which the tip is formed. By contrast, when airflow is varied the glass is always thoroughly heated in the early stages of the pulling cycle, and only the rate at which the tip is cooled is altered by the airflow. Modulation of airflow can thus provide the shortest ultrafine tips, while widening the filament can provide the longest ones.

In some cases, such as preparations requiring the penetration of tough tissues en route to penetration of relatively large cells, it may be more important for the tips to be short and stiff than to have diameters in the ultrafine range. Figure 20 also shows a method of obtaining combinations of tip length and diameter that assist in meeting such requirements.

With wide filaments our puller can form ultrafine tips somewhat longer than the shortest ones we have obtained with the Livingston puller. In one research project in our laboratory, relatively long ultrafine tips formed by our puller were compared directly with micropipettes provided by the Livingston puller (Charlton and Leeper, 1985; Leeper and Charlton, 1986). This work involved intracellular recording from retinal cells in an isolated and perfused eyecup preparation of the Eastern grey squirrel. Since the retina was always covered by a thin layer of vitreous humor that was quite viscous and variable in depth, relatively long tips were required to penetrate to the target cells. The micropipettes formed on our puller were found to have five advantages. First, ultrafine Livingston tips could not be made shorter than about 25 mm, but in this preparation it proved possible to use considerably shorter tips (about 15–17 mm). By adjusting filament width on our puller, ultrafine tips could be made as long as necessary for adequate penetration of tissue without becoming undesirably long and flimsy. Second, there was appreciably less problem with tips becoming bent as they were formed. Third, cell penetration was significantly improved in this mammalian retina, in which cells are typically smaller than those of lower vertebrates. Fourth, when tips were filled with 16 mg/ml of horseradish peroxidase (HRP) in 0.5 M KCl, electrode resistances were only 500–1000 MΩ compared with 2000–3000 MΩ for electrodes formed on the Livingston puller. This assisted the injection of HRP into cells, and the shorter tips were less susceptible to clogging. Fifth, micropipettes performed more consistently, which saved valuable experimental time, an important consideration in a perfused mammalian preparation.

It should be noted that widening the heating filament has long been known to increase tip length (Frank and Becker, 1964). In addition, several investigators learned in the early 1960s that widening the filament of a Livingston puller could provide sufficiently small tips for intracellular work in vertebrate photoreceptors. Apparently that observation used the principle illustrated in Figure 20, namely, that if one starts from a sufficiently narrow filament, widening the filament can reduce tip size. Our puller was helpful in obtaining the results of Figure 20, because of the high reliability of tip size; it seems safe to assume, however, that the illustrated principles also apply to other micropipette pullers.

PART VI   SUMMARIZED ADVANTAGES OF THE BROWN–FLAMING MICROPIPETTE PULLER

When compared with previous designs, this micropipette puller exhibits the following advantages. Points 1–7 pertain to all models, while points 8–10 depend upon the improved filament design in the P-77B and all subsequent models.

1. Smaller tips can be formed than demonstrated with previous pullers.
2. The advantages of short tips can be obtained, even in combination with the very smallest tips.
3. Tips of given size and form are provided with high reliability.
4. Lowered electrical resistance of the short tips decreases the noise level of electrical recordings and shortens a microelectrode's time constant.
5. The shorter tips decrease resistance to the flow of material from the tip, thus facilitating injections into cells or tissues.
6. The greater stiffness of the short tips is an aid in beveling. It should also be helpful in penetrating cells and in reaching target cells that are overlaid with tough tissues.
7. Tip length can be conveniently modulated over a long range by the airjet, to meet varied requirements of tip length, without altering tip size.
8. Heating filaments are readily interchangeable, permitting the use of filaments of varying width and shape.
9. By using filament widths up to 6.0 mm, tip length can be greatly extended (up to about 27 mm) without altering tip size.
10. A novel double filament that forms a 'square loop' improves the radial symmetry of heat delivery and increases the amount of heat that can be delivered.

CHAPTER 6

A Theory of Micropipette Tip Formation: Quantitative Prediction and Validation of the Effects of Capillary Wall Thickness upon Tip Size

PART I   THEORY

I.1   Introduction

In view of the extent to which micropipettes are used in cell physiology, it is particularly important to understand how the tips are formed. We approached this problem by developing an explicit theory, from which quantitative predictions were made; when tested experimentally, these predictions were closely confirmed. Since our results strongly support the basic theory, it now provides a basis for understanding many factors that influence the functional characteristics of micropipettes. This work has revealed a method for further decreasing the outer tip diameter to improve the penetration of small cells with minimal damage. It has also revealed a practical strategy for increasing the inner tip diameter as much as possible, for improved ease of injecting material into cells, while minimizing the adverse effects of this procedure upon cell penetration. Thus the theory and findings of this work should permit capillary tubing to be designed and used more predictably in making micropipettes that better satisfy the varying requirements of intracellular research.

Since the early work of Byzov and Chernyshov (1961) it has been thought that the wall thickness of capillary tubing (when expressed as the ratio of outer/inner diameter of the tubing) is a factor influencing tip size. But even the *direction* of the presumed effect has remained in doubt, as discussed in Section IV.1 of this chapter. In dealing with this subject, we shall use the terms OD and ID to refer to the outer and inner diameters, respectively, of capillary tubings from which tips are formed. Though these terms are somewhat awkward in equations, they seem preferable to introducing less familiar terms for more convenient mathematical notation. In developing our theory a crucial step was to devise a method for predicting accurately the effects of OD/ID upon tip size. This prediction involved two simplifying assumptions.

I.2   Assumptions

Assumption 1 was that the ratio of outer/inner diameter at any point along the main axis of a micropipette, including the tip itself, is the same as OD/ID. This principle is widely used in the glass industry, and in previous work we had found it to hold approximately when micropipette tips were examined by SEM. This has been illustrated for single-barrel tips down to about 2.0 μm in outer diameter (Brown and Flaming, 1979a) and for thick-septum theta tips down to about 0.4 μm in outer diameter (Brown and Flaming, 1977a).

Assumption 2 was that the absolute thickness of the glass wall at the tip will be constant and independent of the OD/ID ratio, providing that the type of glass and the pulling conditions at the tip remain constant. This assumption is based upon considering the formation of a micropipette tip as a problem of viscous flow (Purves, 1980), with the viscosity of the glass at any point in space and time determined only by its chemical composition and temperature. Thus, for the case of the tip, $\eta_t = f(G, T_t)$. In this expression η_t represents the viscosity (η) of the glass at the tip (t) at the moment of tip formation (hereafter called the *tip viscosity*. This is a function (f) of G (symbolizing the chemical composition of the glass) and T_t, the temperature (T) of glass at the tip at the moment of its formation (hereafter called the *tip temperature*. It follows that if OD/ID were varied for a given type of glass, keeping tip temperature constant, the tip viscosity should also remain constant. In forming fine or ultrafine tips on our puller, the pull strength is greatly in excess of that required to separate the two tips. So a pair of tips should form when the thickness of the glass wall has become reduced to where it cannot be further attenuated at the prevailing viscosity, which becomes the tip viscosity by definition. Thus, with tip viscosity constant, the wall thickness at the tip should also be constant and independent of OD/ID.

Of course this treatment assumes that the tips separate while the glass is still in a fluid phase, which we believe the case, partly because of the appearance of micropipette tips under high resolution SEM. The tips are almost always formed at right angles to the long axis of the micropipette, and without major irregularities, as shown in Figures 18, 22, and 26. This result may be expected if the two tips separate while still in the fluid phase and then harden shortly afterward. If the tips were not formed until after the glass became sufficiently cooled and hardened that the tips could separate only by fracture, the orientation of the fracture should be inconsistent and the edges jagged and irregular, as seen in deliberately broken tips. Though deviations from the described result have been observed (see Figure 28), they are relatively rare. Also, most of these deviations follow simple patterns that appear to result from one or more assignable causes (see Sections I.2 and II.3 of Chapter 7), in contrast to the random and less patterned results that may be expected when breaking hardened tips.

I.3   Graphic Depiction of Predicted Effects of OD/ID upon Tip Size

As a micropipette tip is formed, it is lengthened by thinning of the glass wall. As this occurs the tubing also becomes smaller because surface tensions at both the outer circumference of the tubing, and at the glass–air interface around the lumen, will act to minimize the exposed surface area (see Sears, 1950).

Based upon the two assumptions described in the preceding section, Figure 21 depicts graphically the effects of altering OD/ID upon tip size. Two micropipette tips are shown in longitudinal section. The upper tip is formed from Standard Tubing, which has an OD of 1.0 mm and an ID of 0.5 mm. By comparison, the lower tip is formed from a thin-walled tubing used increasingly in recent years; it has an OD of 1.0 mm and an ID of 0.75 mm. Thus, the respective OD/ID values of these tubings are 2.0 and 1.33. At the left margin of the drawing, both pipettes are shown at the same outside diameter. This only involves starting from appropriately chosen points along their tapering portions. Also, both pipettes are outlined by construction lines that converge to a point on the right side of the drawing. This assures that the ratio of outer/inner diameter remains constant along the length of each pipette. For simplicity of illustration the distance to the convergence point is the same for both pipettes, which thus taper at the same rate. The lower pipette is shown to terminate and form a tip where the wall is assumed to have become sufficiently thin that the cohesive forces associated with viscosity of the glass will not permit further thinning. At that point along the longitudinal axis of the drawing the upper pipette has the same outer diameter as the lower pipette, but the wall thickness of the upper pipette is twice as great, so a tip will not yet be formed. Instead, the upper pipette must be further attenuated until its wall thickness becomes identical to that at the tip of the lower pipette. In the illustrated case that will occur at half the remaining distance to the convergence point. Of course the tip formed there will have only half the outer diameter of the tip formed on the lower pipette. Thus, Figure 21 predicts that as OD/ID decreases from 2.0 to 1.33, the outer tip diameter will increase sharply by a factor of 2.0. As that occurs, the inner tip diameter will increase even more dramatically. If thin-walled and Standard Tubings had equal outer tip diameters, the inner tip diameter would be 1.5 times greater in the thin-walled tubing. Since the outer tip diameter of thin-walled tubing is twice that of Standard Tubing, the inner tip diameter of thin-walled tubing is thus greater than in Standard Tubing by a factor of 3.0 (1.5 × 2.0), as shown in Figure 21.

I.4   Equations for Effects of OD/ID upon Tip Size

Figure 21 is presented mainly for its value in visualizing how our assumptions lead to predictable effects of OD/ID upon outer and inner tip diameters. Algebraic methods are more convenient for calculating effects of OD/ID upon tip size, so three useful equations were derived. The following list of definitions covers terms used in these equations, as well as additional terms that have proved helpful in discussing issues in this chapter.

OD = outside diameter of capillary tubing
ID = inside diameter of capillary tubing
OD_t = outside diameter of tip
OD_{ts} = outside diameter of tip, Standard Tubing
F_o = factor by which outside tip diameter is changed relative to that of Standard Tubing, i.e., $F_o = OD_t/OD_{ts}$
ID_t = inside diameter of tip
ID_{ts} = inside diameter of tip, Standard Tubing
F_i = factor by which inside tip diameter is changed relative to that of Standard Tubing, i.e., $F_i = ID_t/ID_{ts}$
u = twice the wall thickness of tubing
u_t = the value of u at the tip, assumed constant as OD/ID varies

Our three basic equations, the derivations of which are given in Appendix II, are as follows:

$$F_o = \frac{OD}{2(OD - ID)} \qquad \text{(EQUATION 1)}$$

$$F_i = \frac{ID}{OD - ID} \qquad \text{(EQUATION 2)}$$

$$F_i = 2F_o - 1 \qquad \text{(EQUATION 3)}$$

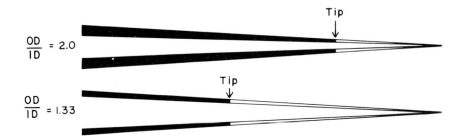

Figure 21. Graphic illustration of predicted effects upon tip size when altering the OD/ID ratio of glass tubing. For explanation, see text.

In short, knowing only the OD and ID of any given capillary tubing, Equations 1 and 2 give the values of F_o and F_i (the tip size factors relative to Standard Tubing) predicted for that tubing. These equations may also be used to design tubing with specific predicted values of F_o and F_i. For example, if any given F_o is desired, it is only necessary to set a value for OD, and Equation 1 can be solved for the requisite value of ID. As shown by Equation 3, there is also a simple relationship between F_o and F_i that can be useful in calculations.

PART II   EXPERIMENTAL METHODS

We next performed experiments using custom-made tubings, with variable values of OD/ID, to determine how closely the experimental results would fit the predicted theoretical values of F_o.

Experimental tubings used in this work and in Chapter 7 were all supplied by the Glass Company of America, Inc. (Oakland and Ridge Avenues, Bargaintown, NJ 08232, USA). These tubings were made of borosilicate glass (Corning No. 7740) and contained an 'Omega Dot' (see Part I of Chapter 7). At the time of this work the original loop filament was still in use; its inner diameter measured 3.5 mm and its width was 2.0 mm. But by this time we had converted to a single airjet. Only one micropipette was used from each pair that was formed, so each micropipette represented the result of a different pull. When tip size was plotted as a function of length of the slow pull, it was found to pass through a minimum at a value of about 0.050 in., so that setting was used for length of the slow pull. The digital readout for strength of the fast pull was 1250 (providing 50 V across the pulling solenoid), and the micrometer controlling airflow was set at 0.080 in.

Since tip size decreased progressively as heating current increased over a considerable range, the constant value of heating current for this experiment was somewhat arbitrary, and it was set as high as judged compatible with long life of the filament (13.3 A). This is well below the 20.0 A normally employed to form ultrafine tips with the rectangular trough filament (see Section II.3 of Chapter 3). Smaller tips could have been obtained at higher heating currents, but in this experiment it seemed more important to form and measure a great many micropipettes without changing the heating filament.

In determining the effects of OD/ID upon OD_t, it was particularly important to hold tip temperature constant. In our puller, as in most others, the capillary tubing is not pulled apart until the glass has reached a temperature at which it can be attenuated by the strength of the slow pull. Because of this feature the temperature of the segment of glass heated by the filament, at the beginning of the slow pull, may be assumed to remain constant and independent of OD/ID. The distance of the slow pull was constant, and during the slow pull heat continued to be delivered by the filament. Under these conditions, thin-walled tubing would be expected to heat more rapidly and thus have a somewhat higher temperature at the end of the slow pull. On the other hand, thin-walled tubing should cool more rapidly after turning off the heating filament and initiating airflow. The duration of the slow pull varied with several factors but was never less than about 3 sec, which was much longer than the time available for cooling. The delay between activating the air pulse and onset of the fast pull was 40 msec, and the air had no effect unless the delay exceeded 20 msec. Thus, with a delay of 40 msec the first 20 msec was consumed before the air began to take effect, and only 20 msec remained for an actual cooling effect, followed by a fast pull that was completed in 5–8 msec (Brown and Flaming, 1977a). So the total duration of the cooling effect was only 25–28 msec. As OD/ID is lowered and the wall becomes thinner, the more rapid heating and cooling effects would tend to be compensatory. The more rapid heating would be expected to dominate by occurring over a longer time. On the other hand, the capillary tubing has become much attenuated before the cooling phase, which would greatly increase the effectiveness of the brief cooling period. The net effect upon relative tip temperatures of tubings with varying OD/ID is not known. The length of the tips formed during the fast pull may also vary somewhat with the OD/ID ratio, but the rapidity of the fast pull should minimize any alterations of tip temperature resulting from different lengths of the fast pull. In summary, it seems likely that with the described pulling conditions the assumption of tip temperature being independent of OD/ID was approximated but not fully met.

Table 2 summarizes measurements of the tubings used in the first experiment and the results obtained. In addition to Standard Tubing, experimental tubings numbered 1–5 were used. For each tubing the OD and ID were measured with a dissecting microscope and used to calculate the predicted F_o, and these values were entered in Table 2. By comparison with Standard Tubing, Tubing 1 had a higher OD/ID and a lower predicted F_o. It is evident from Equation 1 that decreasing ID to zero would reduce the predicted F_o to 0.5; since this would convert the tubing to a solid rod, 0.5 is the theoretical lower limit of F_o. In practice the absolute value of ID cannot be less than about 0.4 mm, which was the design value for Tubing 1. This lower limit of ID results from the standard Omega Dot having a diameter of 0.1 mm, while the smallest stainless steel tubing that is readily available for injecting solutions into pipettes is about 0.2 mm in outer diameter (see Section I.3c of Chapter 10), and this injection tubing requires a clearance of about 0.1 mm. To maximize the OD/ID of Tubing 1, its OD was set at 1.65 mm. This gave a predicted F_o of 0.67, which was close to the practical lower limit, because a significant further decrease of F_o would require OD to be increased so markedly that the glass tubing would be too heavy for the heat capacity of existing micropipette pullers. Tubings 2–5 had predicted values of F_o that ranged upward from 1.17 to 2.52, which is close to the practical upper limit. The upper limit results mainly from difficulties in making thin-walled capillary tubings, which tend to collapse and become oblong in cross-section when the wall is thinned too severely.

In each session of SEM measurements, samples of Standard Tubing were included with experimental tubing, to determine whether any inadvertent change occurred in the pulling conditions during the experiment. All tips were mounted in solder glass, as described in Chapter 4. The few tips that showed contamination were rejected, and outer diameters of all the other tips were measured from high resolution SEM photographs similar to those shown in Figures 18 and 22. These measurements were then corrected by subtracting twice the nominal thickness of the gold coating.

PART III   RESULTS

III.1   Effects of OD/ID upon Tip Size (OD_t): First Experiment

Figure 22 shows SEM photographs of four sample micropipette tips from this series of measurements. In order of increasing tip size, they were formed

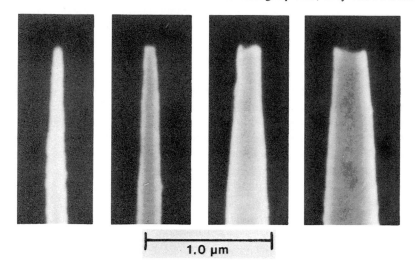

Figure 22. Sample SEM photomicrographs of micropipette tips formed from four of the capillary tubings represented in the data of Table 2. From left to right, in the order of increasing tip size resulting from a decreasing OD/ID ratio, these tips were formed from tubings designated in Table 2 as No. 1, Standard Tubing, No. 3 and No. 5.

Table 2. Data of first experiment showing effects of OD/ID upon outer diameter of tip (OD$_t$) and obtained values of F_o. For details, see text

Designation of tubing	OD (mm)	ID (mm)	OD/ID	Wall thickness (mm)	Omega Dot diameter (mm)	N (number of tips measured)	Mean OD$_t$ (μm)	S.E.M. (standard error of mean)	F_o (predicted)	F_o (obtained)
No. 1	1.65	0.42	3.93	0.61	0.10	11	0.062	0.002	0.67	0.77
Standard	0.98	0.49	2.00	0.24	0.10	25	0.081	0.002	1.00	1.00
2	1.05	0.60	1.75	0.22	0.10	10	0.100	0.006	1.17	1.23
3	1.02	0.74	1.38	0.14	0.10	10	0.174	0.007	1.82	2.15
4	1.51	1.12	1.35	0.19	0.10	11	0.182	0.007	1.94	2.25
5	1.51	1.21	1.25	0.15	0.10	11	0.242	0.009	2.52	2.99

from Tubing 1, Standard Tubing, and Tubings 3 and 4. Throughout this series of measurements there was no significant change in the tip size of Standard Tubing. Hence all measurements of Standard Tubing were combined. For each type of tubing, Table 2 gives the number of tips measured (N), the mean outer tip diameter (OD_t), and the standard error of the mean (S.E.M.). In no case was N less than 10, and for Standard Tubing it was 25. The reliability of these measurements is indicated by the low standard errors.

The results in Figure 22 and Table 2 confirm our prediction that as the wall is thinned and OD/ID decreases, micropipettes formed from the tubing will have progressively larger tips. As OD/ID decreased from 3.93 to 1.25, the mean OD_t increased from 0.062 μm to 0.242 μm. Hence OD/ID can be used in practice to alter tip size by a factor of at least 3.9.

In Figure 23 the average values of OD_t are plotted as a function of OD/ID, and a curve has been fitted by eye that passes through all the obtained points. For comparison, the tip size of Standard Tubing (OD_{ts}) was multiplied by the predicted F_o of each experimental tubing, and these theoretical values of OD_t are plotted as solid points. Based upon the assumptions of our theory, it is readily shown that

$$OD_t = u_t + \frac{u_t}{\dfrac{OD}{ID} - 1}$$

This is the equation for the curve that would fit the theoretical points of Figure 23, and it predicts that OD_t will be related to OD/ID by a hyperbolic function. This is borne out by the form of the experimental curve, which closely fits the theoretical points. In consequence, at values of OD/ID above 2.0 the OD/ID must increase greatly to achieve a significant further reduction of tip size, but

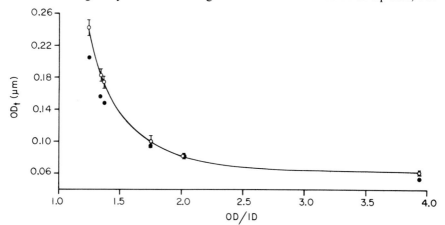

Figure 23. Mean outer diameter of tip (OD_t) as a function of the OD/ID ratio, plotted from data of Table 2. Curve fitted by eye to obtained points. Error bars indicate ± 1.0 standard error of the mean. Filled circles indicate theoretical tip sizes obtained by calculating the F_o of each tubing from Equation 1 and multiplying it by the measured tip size of Standard Tubing.

tip size rises with increasing rapidity as the practical lower limit of OD/ID is approached.

Obtained values of F_o were calculated by dividing the measured OD_t of each tubing by the measured tip size of Standard Tubing (OD_{ts}). In Figure 24 these values of F_o (obtained) are plotted against the F_o (predicted), using data from the final two columns of Table 2. A perfect fit to our theory would be the illustrated straight line at a slope of $45°$. For predicted values of F_o ranging from 1.0 to 2.52, a straight line closely fits all the data points, but the slope of this experimental line is somewhat greater than that of the theoretical line. For Tubing 1 the predicted F_o was 0.67 and the experimental value was 0.77; hence the measured F_o of this tubing was less than that of Standard Tubing but not as low as predicted by our theory.

III.2   Effects of OD/ID upon Tip Size (OD_t): Second Experiment

III.2a   Possibilities for resolving minor discrepancies between experimental and theoretical effects of OD/ID upon OD_t in first experiment

At this point in the work, we identified three potential causes of the differences between experimental and theoretical results in Figure 23, from which results were expressed in terms of F_o in Figure 24.

First, it will be demonstrated in Chapter 7 that when wall thickness of the capillary tubing is held constant, and the diameter of the Omega Dot is increased, the outer tip diameter can be reduced markedly. This effect is discussed in Chapter 7, and it may result in part from the *relation* of the Omega Dot diameter to the thickness of the capillary wall. In our first experiment relating OD/ID to OD_t, Table 2 shows that the diameter of the Omega Dot remained constant at 0.1 mm, but it was necessary to allow the absolute wall thickness to decrease considerably as OD/ID was reduced. Thus, as OD/ID fell, the diameter of the Omega Dot increased *relative to* thickness of the capillary wall, and this may have influenced the value of OD_t. But any effect of this type should have been minor because of the small absolute size of all the Omega Dots in that experiment.

A second and potentially more important factor was the slower heating of thick-walled tubing than of thin-walled tubing during the slow pull, which may have resulted in a lower tip temperature and larger tip size with thick-walled tubing. This factor could have been important for Tubing 1, which had an OD/ID almost twice that of Standard Tubing, and which gave measured values of OD_t and F_o that were higher than the theoretical values. The slower heating of thick-walled tubing would be expected to be especially significant if the filament temperature were too low to handle this tubing with the highest OD/ID. In the experiment of Figures 23 and 24, the filament temperature was deliberately kept relatively low to complete the entire experiment with a single heating filament. More efficient heat delivery for all tubings was anticipated to reduce this problem.

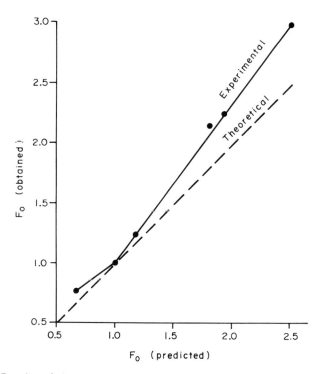

Figure 24. Results of first experiment to determine the relation between F_o (obtained) and F_o (predicted), plotted from data of Table 2. The theoretical result is given by the dashed line, while the SEM measurements are given by the solid line drawn through the obtained points.

Third, we questioned whether the actual thickness of the gold coatings was as great as the nominal values indicated by the coating device. If the amount subtracted in measuring electrode tips were greater than the actual thickness of the coating, the slope of the experimental line in Figure 24 would be too great, as was the case for all values of F_o greater than 1.0.

III.2b   Removal of Omega Dots

For our second experiment we used only Standard Tubing and Tubings 1 and 4. Standard Tubing was available without an Omega Dot, and the Omega Dots were removed from Tubings 1 and 4 by running through them stiff wires that were only slightly smaller than the ID of each tubing.

III.2c   Use of improved heating filament

As described in Section III.9 of Chapter 3, the square loop filament can greatly increase heat delivery to the capillary tubing, while also improving the symmetry of heat delivery. Hence this filament form was used so that the thick-walled Tubing 1 could be heated more adequately relative to the other tubings in this experiment.

III.2d   Corrected thickness of gold coating

In this second experiment the gold coatings were applied by a Hummer Model 5 sputter coater, (Technics, Inc., 80 N. Gordon St., Alexandria, VA 22304, USA). This instrument measures thickness of the applied coating but does not indicate the accuracy of those nominal values. In assessing the actual thickness of the coating a nominal 50 Å of gold was first applied to a group of 16 micropipettes, the tips of which were photographed and measured. The 50 Å was chosen as a baseline coating because it proved about the minimum at which high-resolution photographs were possible. A nominal 100 Å additional coating was then applied to the same micropipettes, and the values of OD_t were again measured. If a full 100 Å of additional gold had been applied, OD_t should have been increased by 200 Å, but the mean increment of OD_t was only 124 $\pm$ 13 Å (S.E.M.). Thus, the measured increment of tip diameter was only 62% of the nominal increment. This cannot be applied as a correction to the experiment shown in Figures 23 and 24 because the coating device used at that time was a Hummer Model 1 sputter coater. This correction was applied, however, to the new results.

III.2e   Experimental design and results

A reduced version of the first OD/ID experiment was conducted with Tubing 1, Standard Tubing and Tubing 4, which had respective theoretical F_o values of 0.67, 1.0 and 1.94. While only one point was represented in the range above an F_o of 1.0, this point was near the upper end of that range, and the reduced number of points made it easier to conduct the experiment during the life of a heating filament.

Tips were measured from all three types of tubing in each of two SEM sessions. In one session the nominal gold coating was 100 Å, while in the other it was 150 Å; for each session the correction applied was 62% of twice the nominal thickness of gold. The square loop filament was 3.0 mm on all sides and also 3.0 mm in width along the main axis of the glass capillaries. Puller settings were altered in only two respects from those used in the first experiment. The digital reading for heating current was increased to 360 (39.5 A), to provide a heat delivery near the maximum obtainable from the square loop filament, and the reading of the air micrometer was reduced from 0.080 to 0.075 in. to slightly reduce airflow. The new filament design and these adjustments were expected to deliver more heat to the capillary tubing than in the first experiment. Though heat delivery could not be measured directly, the success of these procedures may be inferred with considerable confidence from the smaller tip sizes that were obtained in this experiment, by comparison with tip sizes obtained in the first experiment from the same tubings that contained Omega Dots.

Results are tabulated in Table 3 and plotted in Figure 25. If the full nominal thickness of gold had been subtracted, the respective values of OD_t for Tubing 1, Standard Tubing and Tubing 4 would have been 0.039, 0.065 and 0.142 μm. When compared with values of OD_t obtained from these same tubings in the earlier experiment, OD_t was reduced 37% for Tubing 1, 20% for Standard Tubing and 22% for Tubing 4. Thus, the improved heat delivery decreased all values of OD_t, but the greatest percentage decrease was for the thick-walled Tubing 1, as had been anticipated

At the right of Table 3, four numbered columns give values of F_o under various conditions. Columns 1 and 2 compare theoretical predicted values of F_o with the experimental values of F_o obtained in this experiment when 62% of the nominal thickness of the gold coating was subtracted. For Tubing 1 the theoretical value of 0.67 compares with an obtained value of 0.65, while

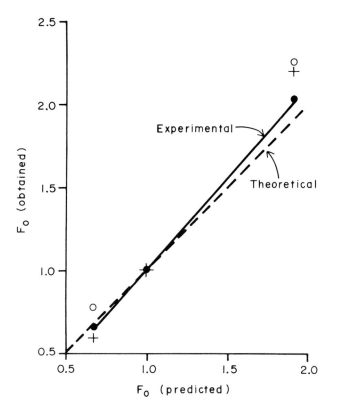

Figure 25. Results of second experiment to determine more accurately the relation between F_o (obtained) and F_o (predicted). Unfilled circles are values obtained from the first experiment of this type. Crosses are values from second experiment when full nominal thickness of gold was subtracted. Filled circles are values from second experiment when 62% of the nominal thickness of gold was subtracted. For further explanation, see text.

Table 3. Data of second experiment showing effects of OD/ID upon outer diameter of tip (OD_t) and obtained values of F_o. As described in text, several changes were made from procedures in the first experiment. These changes provide a more accurate comparison of theoretical and obtained values of F_o (Columns 1 and 2), and the effects of those changes are analyzed in Columns 2–4

Designation of tubing	OD/ID	N (number of tips measured)	Mean OD_t (μm)	S.E.M. (standard error of mean)	Column 1 F_o (predicted)	Column 2 F_o (subtracting 62% of nominal thickness of gold coating)	Column 3 F_o (subtracting full nominal thickness of gold coating)	Column 4 F_o (obtained in previous experiment shown in Table 2)
No.1	3.93	12	0.048	0.003	0.67	0.65	0.60	0.77
Standard	2.00	10	0.074	0.006	1.00	1.00	1.00	1.00
No.4	1.35	11	0.151	0.005	1.94	2.04	2.20	2.25

for Tubing 4 the theoretical value of 1.94 compares with an obtained value of 2.04. Thus the improved conditions of comparison in this experiment yielded closer agreement. The effects of factors yielding this more accurate comparison may be seen better by starting with Column 4, which gives the values of F_0 obtained for these same tubings in the earlier experiment, and then working to the left. Columns 2–4 are also plotted graphically in Figure 25, in which both of the unfilled circles representing experimental tubings of Column 4 are well above the theoretical line. Since the point representing Standard Tubing must always lie on the theoretical line, of course Column 4 does not plot as a straight line. Column 3 gives values of F_0 in the second experiment when the full nominal thickness of the gold coating was subtracted. It thus shows the effects of only the improved heat delivery and removal of the Omega Dots. When plotted in Figure 25, all three of the crosses representing Column 3 lie on an approximately straight line. This is because the obtained F_0 of Tubing 1 dropped more than that of Tubing 4, as expected from improving heat delivery to the thick-walled tubing. Column 2 shows the further correction of subtracting only 62% of the nominal thickness of the gold coating. Figure 25 shows that this further correction caused the line representing Column 3 to be rotated clockwise around the point plotted for Standard Tubing. A straight line through the filled circles representing Column 2 then almost coincided with the theoretical straight line. Comparison of Columns 2 and 3, especially as plotted in Figure 25, shows the nature and magnitude of effects upon experimental values of F_0 when incorrect values are used for the gold coating. This is clearly a critical factor in comparing experimental and theoretical values of F_0.

In summary, the main reasons for minor discrepancies between experimental and theoretical values of F_0 in Figure 24 appear to have been identified. When the two main factors that appeared responsible for the earlier discrepancies were corrected separately, each had the predicted type of effect upon experimental values of F_0, and the experimental values of F_0 then fitted very closely to the theoretical ones.

III.3 The Relation of OD/ID to OD_t/ID_t

III.3a Experimental findings

The simplifying assumption that $OD/ID = OD_t/ID_t$ is amenable to experimental testing. Initial attempts were inconclusive because of inability to form large enough tips to provide accurate measurements of ID_t. That problem was solved by using a rectangular trough filament only 1.0 mm wide (see Figure 20), combined with appropriate settings of heating current and airflow. Standard Tubing was used without an Omega Dot, to avoid any influence the Omega Dot might have. The measured OD/ID of this batch of Standard Tubing was 1.90. When the ratio of outer/inner diameter was measured at the back ends of tips mounted for SEM, where the tips were broken away from the parent

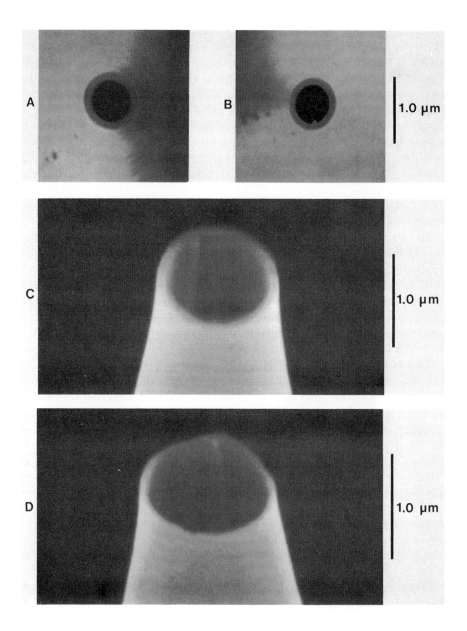

Figure 26. End-on and oblique views of micropipette tips photographed by SEM. (A) End-on view of Standard Tubing without an Omega Dot. (B) Similar view of Standard Tubing with Omega Dot oriented downward toward the heating fila- ment. The tips in (A) and (B) were formed by a rectangular trough filament only 1.0 mm wide and with identical puller settings chosen to give relatively large tips. (C and D) Oblique views of tips formed from tubings No. 3(C) and No. 5 (D). Both of these tips were formed with a rectangular trough filament 1.5 mm wide.

micropipettes, 11 cases gave a range of 1.53–1.76 with a mean of 1.66 ± 0.034 (S.E.M.). The value of OD_t/ID_t for 10 tips ranged from 1.30–1.91 with a mean of 1.51 ± 0.069. A sample tip picture from which these values were measured is shown in Figure 26(A). In summary, the ratio of outer/inner diameter dropped from 1.90 in the original tubing to 1.66 at the broken back ends of the tips and then to 1.51 at the tips themselves. While the reduction of this ratio from the original tubing to the broken back ends of the tips is clearly significant, the further reduction of this ratio at the tips themselves was also statistically significant ($p < 0.05$). Our assumption that $OD/ID = OD_t/ID_t$ is thus incorrect. Since the measured value of OD_t/ID_t is less than OD/ID, this would make the absolute values of all tips somewhat larger than if our simplifying assumption were correct.

We have since learned of a considerably earlier study that yielded a similar result, though the methods employed were quite different (Ujek *et al.*, 1973). In that work the ratio of outer/inner diameter was 1.834 at a distance of 350 μm behind the tip, and this ratio was reported to decrease steadily to 1.415 at the tip itself.

It would be of interest to obtain similar measurements on tubing with an Omega Dot, to see whether the Omega Dot contributes to the altered diameter ratio from tubing to tip (see Section II.4 of Chapter 7). Figure 26(A) and (B) shows micropipette tips formed under similar conditions from Standard Tubing with and without an Omega Dot. The tip containing the Omega Dot is slightly oblong in form, an effect that will be examined in Chapter 7. The tip without the Omega Dot (Figure 26A) had an OD_t/ID_t of 1.38, while the tip with the Omega Dot (Figure 26B) had values of OD_t/ID_t that measured 1.35 for the longer axis and 1.40 for the shorter axis. Thus, there was no clear effect of the Omega Dot upon OD_t/ID_t. Since the Omega Dot was the small one used in Standard Tubing, this result does not preclude the possibility that larger Omega Dots can influence the value of OD_t/ID_t (see Section II.4 of Chapter 7). On the other hand, large Omega Dots that might alter OD_t/ID_t distort the tip shape considerably (see Figure 29) and make accurate measurements more difficult.

Figure 26 also shows tips formed from Tubings 3 and 5. Though these are oblique views of the tips, values of OD_t/ID_t could be measured accurately along the horizontal axis of these illustrations. For Tubing 3 the OD/ID was 1.38 and the tip in Figure 26(C) had an OD_t/ID_t of 1.16. For Tubing 5 the OD/ID was 1.25 and the tip in Figure 26(D) had an OD_t/ID_t of 1.06. Hence for these thin-walled tubings, as with Standard Tubing, OD_t/ID_t proved less than OD/ID. Viewed from another standpoint, Figure 26 shows that the value of OD_t/ID_t dropped from 1.38 for Standard Tubing to 1.16 for Tubing 3, and then to 1.06 for Tubing 5. As expected, this indicates that in thin-walled tubing the value of ID_t becomes a larger fraction of OD_t than in Standard Tubing. This yields a clear advantage of thin-walled tubing for any application where it is desirable to minimize electrical resistance of the tip, or where materials must be injected through the tip.

III.3b Theoretical explanation for OD_t/ID_t being somewhat smaller than OD/ID

This finding may have a simple explanation. When capillary tubing is initially heated, air temperature rises inside the tubing but probably does not raise the internal pressure because the heated air can escape readily through the relatively large lumen. As the tip is formed, however, this heated air cannot escape so readily through the highly attenuated lumen. Hence heating of the contained air probably results in a significant rise of pressure in the tip region during the brief period while the tip is being formed. In addition, narrowing of the lumen as the tip is formed would tend to squeeze the contained air and cause a further brief increase of pressure within the region of the tip. An elevation of internal pressure will increase both outside and inside diameters of the tubing, while also thinning the walls, so OD_t/ID_t will be decreased. The internal pressure may be expected to increase steadily toward the ultimate tip, as the lumen narrows and air can escape less readily. Also, the thinner wall toward the ultimate tip will offer less resistance to the effects of this increased internal pressure. Hence these considerations seem to provide a satisfactory explanation for the ratio of outer/inner diameters decreasing progressively toward the tip of a micropipette.

PART IV   DISCUSSION

IV.1   Effects of OD/ID Upon Tip Size (OD_t)

Previous work on this subject has been scanty and difficult to interpret. Byzov and Chernyshov (1961) illustrated tips labeled to indicate that a lowered OD/ID decreased tip size, which is contrary to our findings. But their text stated that with a lowered OD/ID the tips were 'thicker', which implies they were larger. So their report is ambiguous concerning which type of result was obtained. In addition, our analysis indicates that considerable care is required in making this type of comparison, and it is not clear from their brief report whether the necessary precautions were taken. Frank and Becker (1964) stated that '... a thinner wall yields a pipette with larger lumen and hence lower resistance.' This conclusion is in accord with ours, but it seems to have received little attention, probably because they did not present any supporting data.

More recently Frederick Haer & Co. advertised a borosilicate thin-walled tubing with an OD of 1.0 mm and an ID of 0.75 mm as 'Ultra-tip capillaries', described as 'a new Omega Dot tubing configuration which gives ultra-small tips...' (Frederick Haer & Co., Bulletin L1-1, 1979). In support of this claim, a later bulletin (L1-2, 1979) referred to an unpublished report. When published, however, the referenced report did not support the claim, stating instead that Standard Tubing and thin-walled 'Ultra-tip' tubing both gave outer tip diameters of 0.20 μm (Jacobson and Mealing, 1980). Tip sizes were given in that report only for Standard Tubing pulled on an *unmodified* Industrial Science Associates puller and thin-walled tubing pulled by a *modified* version of that instrument, the main modification being an increased pull strength. As pointed out in Section III.4 of Chapter 2, the unmodified version of that instrument has a relatively weak pull, so increasing its pull strength should decrease tip size. Hence modification of the puller probably masked the increase of tip size that we have demonstrated with thin-walled tubing. In any event, the effect of wall thickness cannot be evaluated when the pulling conditions are significantly different, and Jacobson and Mealing appropriately drew no conclusion about the relationship of wall thickness to tip size. Unfortunately, however, the advertised claims for 'Ultra-tip' tubing have been widely thought to be well supported by their report. For example, the recent 1984/85 catalog of WPI (World Precision Instruments) states that 'The significant features of thin wall electrodes are their fine tip,...'.

In fact, when pulling conditions were held as constant as possible in our work, and various thin-walled tubings were compared with Standard Tubing, the 'Ultra-tip' configuration (Tubing 3 in Table 2) more than doubled tip size, while the frequency of penetrating toad rods dropped by a factor of about 3, and after penetration the cells usually deteriorated much more rapidly (see Section II.1 of Chapter 14). Thus, the advantage of thin-walled tubing is not in smaller tips, but in larger tips that increase ID_t, thus lowering electrode resistance and facilitating injections into cells. But this advantage may be used only in cells that are large enough to tolerate the enlarged tips without significant damage.

IV.2   The Basic Theory of Tip Formation

The basic theory was tested primarily by determining the effects of OD/ID upon OD_t. The assumptions of testing the theory in this way may now be restated as follows: (1) that with varying OD/ID, the absolute wall thickness at which the tip is formed will be constant, providing that tip temperature is held constant, (2) that tip temperature was, in fact, held constant, (3) that OD/ID = OD_t/ID_t, or that any discrepancy between these ratios will not significantly alter the function relating OD_t to OD/ID. Assumption 1 cannot be tested directly because tip temperature cannot be held rigorously constant. Since this assumption is so critical to our theory, however, it seems quite unlikely that our results would have fitted the theoretical prediction so closely unless this assumption is substantially correct. Stringent attempts were made to satisfy Assumption 2, and logically it should have been better met in the second OD/ID experiment, which gave an improved fit of obtained to theoretical results. But this assumption was probably not fully met in either experiment, and this remains the most difficult condition to meet in testing the theory accurately. Assumption 3 was tested directly, and OD_t/ID_t proved less than OD/ID. For any given tubing this would increase the absolute value of OD_t. The close fit of our results to the theory, however, suggests that the difference between OD/ID and OD_t/ID_t has little if any effect upon the function relating OD/ID to OD_t. In summary, our results provide strong support for the assumptions of the theory. It thus appears that the theory itself has been validated to the extent permitted by the inherent limitations of this type of experiment.

If our theory is correct, OD_t is governed by only three basic factors. These are (1) OD_t/ID_t, (2) tip temperature, and (3) chemical composition of the glass tubing. Other aspects of tubing design, and pulling conditions that affect tip size, appear to exert their influence through these three factors. For example, OD/ID affects tip size by strongly influencing OD_t/ID_t, while settings of micropipette pullers that influence OD_t seem to exert their effects mainly through tip temperature. Since tip temperature can be affected by a variety of puller settings, it is readily understood why OD_t often varies so complexly with puller settings. Effects of chemical composition of the glass upon OD_t are less well understood, but this subject is discussed in later chapters (See Part II of Chapter 8, Parts II and IV of Chapter 15, and Section VII.4 of Chapter 18).

CHAPTER 7

Effects of a Fused Internal Fiber (Omega Dot) upon Micropipette Tips

PART I EXPERIMENTAL FINDINGS

A glass fiber is commonly fused along the inner bore of capillary tubing to facilitate the filling of micropipette tips with conducting solutions (see Section I.3b of Chapter 10). The Glass Company of America, which supplied our experimental tubing, refers to this internal fiber as an 'Omega Dot'. The term is convenient and widely used, so we shall also use it here.

In seeking improved strategies for intracellular work in small cells, by altering the design of capillary tubing, we examined the effects of an Omega Dot upon tip size and shape.

I.1 Effects of Omega Dot upon Tip Size

Preliminary work suggested that increasing the size of the Omega Dot decreases OD_t. So this was investigated by an experiment using custom-made experimental tubings numbered 3, 6, 7 and 8, the dimensions of which are given in Table 4. These tubings were as constant as possible in both OD and ID. The value of ID was set large enough to permit the Omega Dot to vary from 0.10 to 0.40 mm in diameter, and the relatively low OD/ID of 1.38 provided

Table 4. Data of experiment showing effects of Omega Dot diameter upon outer diameter of tip (OD_t)

Designation of tubing	OD (mm)	ID (mm)	OD/ID	Wall thickness (mm)	Omega Dot diameter (mm)	N (number of tips measured)	Mean OD_t (μm)	S.E.M. (standard error of mean)
3	1.02	0.74	1.38	0.14	0.10	16	0.213	0.008
6	1.05	0.77	1.36	0.14	0.20	14	0.194	0.009
7	1.02	0.74	1.38	0.14	0.30	13	0.175	0.011
8	1.02	0.74	1.38	0.14	0.40	18	0.133	0.009

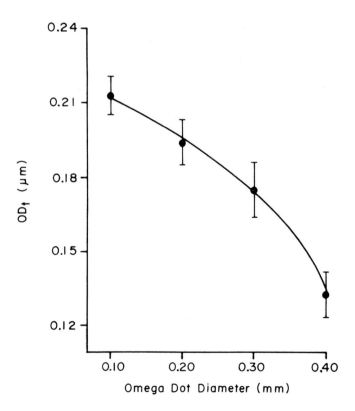

Figure 27. The effect of Omega Dot diameter upon outer diameter of the tip (OD_t) plotted from data of Table 4. Curve fitted by eye to obtained points. Error bars indicate ± 1.0 standard error of the mean.

large enough tips to facilitate their examination by SEM. The upper limit of Omega Dot diameter was determined by the clearance required for injecting solution into the back of the micropipette. In the absence of that limit, the Omega Dot could not have been made much larger, because the asymmetry of a micropipette's cross-section causes bending of the tip when the Omega Dot becomes too large in relation to thickness of the capillary wall. But that effect did not occur over the range of Omega Dot sizes in this experiment. Tips were formed under the same conditions described for our first experiment on effects of OD/ID upon OD_t (see Part II of Chapter 6). The results of Tables 2 and 4 were thus obtained with the same pulling conditions, with one exception. Tubing 3 was used for the experiments of both Table 2 and Table 4, yielding a mean tip diameter of 0.174 μm in the former case and 0.213 μm in the latter one. This difference resulted from replacing and repositioning the loop heating filament between the two experiments. During the Omega Dot experiment, samples of all four experimental tubings were included in each SEM session, and there was no indication that tips formed from any of these tubings changed significantly in size during the experiment.

Table 4 shows that with OD/ID almost constant, increasing the Omega Dot diameter from 0.10 to 0.40 mm caused the average value of OD_t to drop from 0.213 to 0.133 μm, a 38% reduction of outer tip diameter. This result is plotted in Figure 27, which shows that the reduction of tip size was progressive and significant, being especially marked when the Omega Dot diameter was increased from 0.30 to 0.40 mm. Thus, tip size may be influenced markedly by varying the diameter of the Omega Dot, as well as by varying OD/ID.

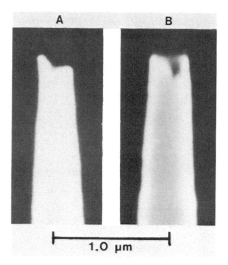

Figure 28. Two variants from the typical squared-off tips shown in Figure 22. (A) Tip formed from Tubing 3. (B) Tip formed from Tubing 5. Both types of tubing described in Table 2. Puller settings chosen to form relatively large tips for resolution of details.

I.2   Can the Omega Dot Form a Spear?

We also considered the possibility that cell penetration may be improved by using a large Omega Dot to form a fine spear on the tip of the micropipette. As the glass capillary is attenuated during the pulling process, it was reasoned that after the wall has terminated, the Omega Dot might continue to be drawn out over an additional distance and thus form the desired spear. If the Omega Dot were large in relation to the wall thickness, it seemed particularly likely that such a spear would be formed.

In experimenting with the effects of OD/ID upon tip size, Table 2 shows that as OD/ID decreased, absolute wall thickness decreased markedly while the Omega Dot diameter remained constant. Nevertheless, Figure 22 shows that the typical tips formed in that experiment did not exhibit a spear.

Though most of our micropipette tips are formed at right angles to the main axis and without any distinctive features, two variants from that description have been identified and are illustrated in Figure 28. The tubings used were Nos. 3 and 5, described in Table 2, both of which had sufficiently low OD/ID ratios to form relatively large tips. In addition, puller settings were chosen to enlarge the tips further for revealing details. The tip in Figure 28(A) shows an extension on one side, while the tip in Figure 28(B) shows a distinct notch. The extension and notch have both been seen often enough that they must be significant features of tip formation rather than mere artifacts. The short protrusion from the tip in Figure 28(A) is a spade-like spear that is occasionally formed in association with the Omega Dot, as also shown in Figure 26(D). Our failure to find the expected stiletto-like point is now understood, and possible explanations have become evident for the occasional spade-like protrusion that is seen instead. This subject, along with our explanation of the occasional notch, will be discussed in Section II.3 of this chapter, following presentation of the evidence underlying these explanations.

I.3   Effects of Omega Dot upon Micropipette Cross-sections

In seeking to understand effects of the Omega Dot upon tip size and form, we next looked at cross-sections of micropipettes. For this work we used a rectangular trough filament only 1.0 mm wide, in order to form tips that were large enough to permit accurate cross-sectional views of the lumen (see Figure 20). It seemed likely that orientation of the Omega Dot would be significant with a rectangular trough filament, which delivers heat mainly from below, so that the downward part of the capillary tubing is softened more than the upward part when pulling begins. Thus, Figure 29 shows cross-sections of micropipettes formed with the Omega Dot either down toward the filament or upward away from it. In each case, cross-sections are shown at four different locations. These are (A) the capillary tubing prior to pulling, (B) the tubing softened by heat and attenuated only by the weak pull, the strong pull having been inactivated, (C) the broken back end of the tip mounted for SEM observations, and (D)

Omega Dot Down   Omega Dot Up

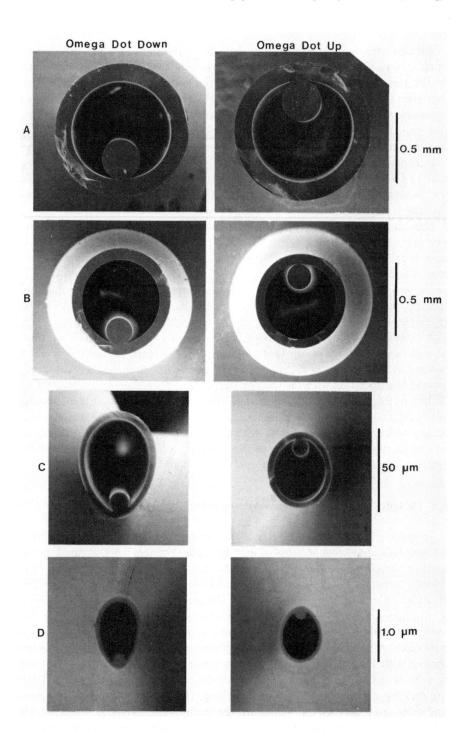

A

0.5 mm

B

0.5 mm

C

50 µm

D

1.0 µm

the tip itself. The tubing used was No. 7, as described in Table 4. In addition to having a low enough OD/ID to form relatively large tips, the diameter of its Omega Dot was about twice the wall thickness, so this tubing was favorable for illustrating effects of the Omega Dot.

Let us look first at the form of the Omega Dot itself, which in the capillary tubing is round and fused to the tubing wall by only a narrow line. This remains essentially unchanged until the broken back ends of the tips, where the junction of the Omega Dot with the tubing wall broadens, and more so with the Omega Dot down rather than up. But dramatic changes occur at the tip with either orientation of the Omega Dot. Instead of standing out from the tubing wall as a distinct glass rod, the Omega Dot has fused much more completely with the tubing wall and appears only as a semicircular intrusion into the lumen of the tip.

Let us look next at the form of the outer wall of the micropipette, which is almost perfectly round in the original tubing (Figure 29A). With the Omega Dot down, the lower portion of the tubing has already begun to sag slightly when the tubing has been softened and slightly attenuated (Figure 29B). At the broken back end of the tip, this sagging has become so marked that the cross-sectional form is like an inverted teardrop (Figure 29C), and this form becomes further accentuated at the tip (Figure 29D). By contrast, with the Omega Dot up, the cross-sectional form remains almost perfectly round until the broken back end of the tip (Figure 29C), where the form has become elliptical with the long axis vertical. Then, at the tip itself, the form becomes similar to a hanging teardrop (Figure 29D).

PART II   DISCUSSION

II.1   Altered Form of the Omega Dot During Tip Formation

Alteration of the Omega Dot, from a round rod to a flattened semicircular intrusion into the lumen of the tip, probably results from surface tension while the Omega Dot is in the molten state. If the Omega Dot were a free glass rod, its surface tensions would be radially symmetrical and in equilibrium. But an Omega Dot is always fused along a line to the inner wall of the glass tubing.

Figure 29. Cross sections of micropipettes formed from Tubing 7 (see Table 4). The Omega Dot was oriented either downward toward the heating filament or upward away from the filament. All photomicrographs taken by SEM. Illustrated for both Omega Dot orientations are: (A) the capillary tubing before heating, (B) the tubing attenuated only by the weak pull, (C) the broken back end of a tip mounted for SEM observations, (D) an end-on view of the tip itself. At each stage of tip formation the same magnification was used with the Omega Dot both up and down, and scale markers are given for each stage. In breaking tubing for cross-sections the cleanest breaks were obtained by using a 'glass knife' to make a small nick in the vicinity of the Omega Dot, and these nicks may be seen at stages (A) and (B). The micropipette tips in (C) and (D) were formed with a rectangular trough filament only 1.0 mm wide and with puller settings chosen to give relatively large tips.

When the Omega Dot becomes molten, the surface tensions around most of its circumference tend to squeeze it, being directed inward, and these tensions are not in equilibrium because molten glass can escape through the line of fusion with the capillary wall. So glass flows from the Omega Dot into the capillary wall.

As shown in Figure 29, this process is hardly noticeable at the end of the weak pull, but it accelerates as the tip is formed. Two main reasons are apparent for the acceleration of this process during tip formation. First, as the Omega Dot becomes smaller and its radius of curvature decreases, surface tension will squeeze glass out of the Omega Dot with increasing pressure (see Sears, 1950). Second, as the line of fusion with the capillary wall is widened, resistance to flow of glass from the Omega Dot will be reduced. Taken together, these factors will cause glass to flow from the Omega Dot more rapidly as it becomes smaller and fuses more completely with the capillary wall. In addition, the loss of any given volume of glass from the Omega Dot will become more apparent as the Omega Dot becomes smaller.

It has previously been assumed that the form of the Omega Dot does not change during tip formation and that the Omega Dot thus occludes a significant portion of the lumen at the tip. In fact, Figure 29 shows cases where about 1/2 of the Omega Dot flowed into the capillary wall during tip formation, and Figure 31 of Chapter 8 shows a case where only about 1/3 of the Omega Dot remained in the lumen of the tip. Thus adverse effects of the Omega Dot partially occluding the tip, including increased electrode resistance and increased difficulty of injecting material from a micropipette, are not nearly so great as previously assumed.

II.2   Effects of Omega Dot Upon Cross-sectional Form of Micropipette

It appears that effects of the Omega Dot upon the form of the micropipette's outer wall, as illustrated in Figure 29, result from two factors. First, the Omega Dot adds to the local weight of glass and sags under the influence of gravity. Figure 29 shows that this process begins early in tip formation and is marked when the Omega Dot is downward toward the heating filament. This effect has also been noted to increase when the Omega Dot is enlarged, or when wider filaments are used to soften the tubing more thoroughly at the beginning of the slow pull.

A second factor, temperature gradients across the capillary tubing, can either amplify or counter the effects of gravity upon the Omega Dot. When the Omega Dot is oriented downward, as in the left column of Figure 29, heat delivery from below will cause glass in the region of the Omega Dot to be warmer than upward portions of the tubing. Under these conditions the temperature gradient will exaggerate gravitational effects upon the Omega Dot. But with heat delivery mainly from below and the Omega Dot oriented upward, as in the right column of Figure 29, the Omega Dot should be cooler than other regions of the capillary tubing. Under these conditions the Omega Dot should act as a relatively stiff backbone, from which the hotter glass in lower regions of the tip sags downward, an effect well illustrated by the two bottom pictures in the right column of Figure 29.

II.3   The Spade-like Spear and the Notch

Our original expectation of a consistent stiletto-like spear was based upon the assumption that the cross-sectional form of the pipette would not change as the tip was formed, an assumption shown incorrect by Figure 29. Since the Omega Dot merges with the tubing and forms a thickening of the tubing wall at the tip, it should instead form an occasional spade-like extension of the wall similar to that shown in Figures 26 and 28. There are at least two ways in which this may occur.

Let us consider how the Omega Dot might affect the profile view of a tip, under the simplifying assumption that there is radially symmetrical heat delivery to the capillary tubing. At the beginning of the slow pull the Omega Dot and its adjoining portion of the tubing wall will have just reached a sufficient temperature for the pull to begin, whereas all thinner regions of the capillary wall will have reached a higher temperature. This temperature differential will become accentuated during the slow pull because of continued heat delivery throughout that period. After the airflow is activated, the glass will have a maximum of 28 msec to cool before the tip is formed (See Chapter 6, Part II). During this period the Omega Dot and its adjoining part of the tubing wall will cool less rapidly than other portions of the tubing, and this will tend to counteract the temperature differential established at the end of the slow pull. The net effect cannot be predicted with certainty. But the cooling period is very short. Also, since the pipette is quite small throughout the period of cooling, the difference between the rate of cooling in the Omega Dot and in the remainder of the tubing is probably small. At the time of tip formation, we would thus expect the Omega Dot and its adjoining portion of the tubing to remain at a lower temperature than the thinner portions of the tubing wall.

As previously discussed (Sections III.8 and III.9 of Chapter 3), the assumption of radially symmetrical heat delivery is far from satisfied with some heating filaments, and it can only be approximated in special cases such as the square loop. When heat delivery is not radially symmetrical, any temperature gradient resulting from the Omega Dot itself will be strongly modulated if the orientation of the Omega Dot is allowed to vary in relation to the heating filament. Aside from the experiment of Figure 29, we have not controlled how the Omega Dot is oriented during the pulling of micropipettes. At the time of tip formation we would thus expect a temperature gradient across the tip in most cases. But in some cases the warmer glass may be expected in the capillary wall opposite the Omega Dot, while in other cases it will probably be in the region of the Omega Dot. As indicated by the results of Figure 29, this would depend upon the orientation of the Omega Dot to the heating filament.

When the two micropipette tips separate, this separation must be initiated by breaking the surface tension of the molten glass at some point around the circumference of the tip. With non-uniform glass temperature at the tip, separation would tend to begin where the glass is coolest. When the coolest glass is opposite the Omega Dot, of course tip separation should begin in that region, where the wall is also relatively thin. When the coolest glass is in the Omega Dot and its adjoining part of the wall, this is where mergence of the Omega Dot with the wall causes it to be especially thick. In that case it is not clear whether tip separation would begin at the cooler but thicker region of the Omega Dot or at some other location in the hotter but thinner glass at the other regions of the tubing.

Wherever tip separation begins, breaking of the surface tension at that point should result in an 'unzipping' that passes rapidly around the tip in both directions. Let us first consider the consequences if tip separation began opposite the Omega Dot. Because the tips are being pulled apart very rapidly, while the line of separation passes around the tips in both directions from the starting point, a notch may be formed at the starting point and this may account for the type of notch shown in Figure 28(B). In that event the ensuing rapid 'unzipping' may sometimes pass through the Omega Dot and prevent formation of a spear, but an occasional spade-like spear may be formed at the Omega Dot. Alternatively, if tip separation begins at the Omega Dot, this separation may not always be clean, and a short spear may sometimes be formed on one tip while a notch may be left on the other tip. Present evidence does not discriminate between these alternatives, but it may be significant that thus far both a notch and a spear have not been seen on the same tip.

II.4   Reduction of Tip Size by the Omega Dot

As the Omega Dot merges with the wall of the tubing, it adds glass to the capillary wall. This added glass could increase the outer diameter of the tubing or decrease the inner diameter, or some combination of these effects. The increase of outer diameter should be small because it is opposed by surface tension, while the decrease of inner diameter is facilitated by surface tension and hence should dominate. In any event, these changes of outer and inner diameter will act in concert to increase OD_t/ID_t. Tip size should thus be decreased, as shown in Part III of Chapter 6. The volume of glass available to run into the tubing wall from the Omega Dot should vary as the square of its radius. As the diameter of the Omega Dot increases, the effect of a given increment of its diameter upon tip size should thus become progressively more prominent. Figure 27 suggests such a relationship, since the decrease of tip size was particularly great when the Omega Dot diameter was increased from 0.3 to 0.4 mm.

As reported in Section III.3a of Chapter 6, we have not yet demonstrated an effect of the Omega Dot upon OD_t/ID_t. But our most direct test was done with an Omega Dot of 0.1 mm diameter in Standard Tubing, for which the wall thickness is 0.25 mm, so the Omega Dot could not significantly affect wall thickness under these conditions. On the other hand, a large Omega Dot in thin-walled tubing tends to distort the shape of the tip, as shown in Figure 29, rendering OD_t/ID_t difficult to measure.

In short, we favor the above explanation of the reduction of tip size by an Omega Dot, because it accounts for observed facts in terms of well established principles. But this explanation is difficult to subject to a critical experimental test.

II.5   Summary

In summary, though the Omega Dot was originally used to facilitate filling of electrode tips, it has other important advantages. While slightly stiffening tips, it can also decrease tip size, and it may form an occasional spade-like spear on the tip, effects that would all facilitate penetration of small cells without significant damage. Also, disadvantages from the Omega Dot partially occluding the tip have proved much less significant than was previously believed to be the case.

CHAPTER 8

Minimizing Tip Size with Borosilicate Tubing

PART I NEW STRATEGIES TESTED

I.1 Introduction

The results presented in Chapters 6 and 7 provide effective strategies for forming even smaller micropipette tips than previously available, and our theoretical explanations of those results suggest further possibilities. Since minimal tip size is of paramount importance for much intracellular work in small cells, these new possibilities were explored and our findings are presented in this chapter.

I.2 Thick-walled Tubing

We first assessed the value of thick-walled tubing from the standpoint of minimizing tip size. Though Chapter 6 demonstrates that an increase of OD/ID decreases tip size, it was necessary to determine whether this principle still holds at the extreme lower limit of tip size. For this test we used Tubing No. 1, since its OD/ID of 3.93 is near the practical upper limit. The heating filament was a square loop measuring 3 by 3 mm, and the width of the filament was also 3 mm. The digital readout of heating current was set at 360 (39.5 A), a value close to the maximum the filament could withstand. If the airflow through the

96

airjet system were unnecessarily great, this might reduce tip temperature and thus increase OD_t. On the other hand, turning off the airjet entirely results in such long filamentous tips that they are unusable (see Section III.6 of Chapter 3). For this experiment the airflow was set just high enough to form tips of usable length. The setting for pull strength was kept at its usual value of 1250, and the length of the slow pull was kept at 0.05 in.

The resolution of SEM photographs is a factor in measuring tip size, since poor resolution will increase the apparent tip size. Compared with previous SEM work, it proved possible during this experiment to improve resolution significantly by special attention to several factors of SEM operation. During this work, however, tips were still being mounted in solder glass, which limited the consistency with which high resolution was attained. Since the goal of this experiment was to determine the minimum tip size attainable, tips measured were only those that could be photographed with a resolution at or near the optimum. Resolution was judged by the sharpness of the border between the micropipette and the darker background of the photograph, and tips that could not be photographed with near-optimal resolution were rejected without regard for their size. All tips were coated with a nominal 100 Å of gold, and 62% of 200 Å was subtracted in measuring OD_t (see Section III.2d of Chapter 6).

For the 13 tips that yielded the highest resolution, tip length varied from 11–15 mm and averaged 12.9 mm, while OD_t varied from 0.029–0.047 μm and averaged 0.039 μm. A photograph of one of the smallest tips obtained in this work is shown in Figure 30.

In much earlier work with Standard Tubing and the original loop filament, we reported tips with an average length of 13.0 mm and an average OD_t of 0.052 μm (Brown and Flaming, 1977a). In that work, however, 150 Å of gold was applied and the full 300 Å was subtracted to obtain the stated values. It is not certain whether 62% of the gold coating would have been accurate with

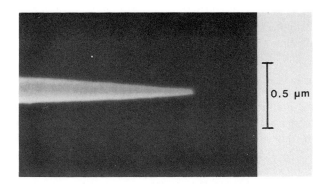

Figure 30. One of the smallest tips formed as described in text from the thick-walled Tubing No.1, using a square loop filament that measured 3 mm in all three dimensions. After subtracting 62% of the gold coating (see Section III.2d of Chapter 6), the outer diameter of this tip measured 0.029 μm.

the coating instrument used in earlier work, but based upon that assumption the corrected average value of OD_t should have been 0.063 μm. When that value for Standard Tubing is multiplied by 0.67 (the calculated F_0 of Tubing 1; see Section III.1 of Chapter 6), the predicted average tip size for Tubing 1 is 0.042 μm. This compares favorably with the average value of 0.039 μm obtained with Tubing 1 in this experiment. In the earlier work with Standard Tubing, we also reported occasional tips as small as 0.020 μm. But if only 62% of the gold coating had been subtracted, the value would have been 0.031 μm, which is probably more accurate. When that value is multiplied by the F_0 of Tubing 1, the minimal tip size with Tubing 1 is predicted to be 0.021 μm, which compares rather well with the occasional tips as small as 0.029 μm in this work with Tubing 1.

In brief, when the thick-walled Tubing 1 was used with pulling conditions chosen to minimize tip size, tips were formed that were about one-third smaller than the finest tips previously obtained from Standard Tubing. This comparison cannot be exact because the original loop filament was used for Standard Tubing, whereas our square loop filament was used for Tubing No. 1. Even if the same filament had been used, it is difficult or impossible to adjust puller settings to provide the same tip temperature for capillary tubings of significantly different design, as discussed in Part II of Chapter 6. Nevertheless, our results suggest that thick-walled tubing provides a practical strategy for pushing the minimum tip size further downward.

I.3   Use of a Smaller Heating Filament

In our early work with the square loop filament, it was never smaller than 3 $\times$ 3 mm. For minimum tip size, however, a smaller filament seemed likely to provide higher tip temperatures and smaller tips. We thus experimented with a square loop filament measuring 2 $\times$ 2 mm, the width likewise being 2 mm. Though the smallest tips previously obtained with Standard Tubing measured about 0.04 μm, the smaller filament provided occasional tips measuring only 0.03 μm. A smaller filament is thus helpful for minimizing tip size, probably because of its closer proximity to the capillary tubing.

I.4   Use of a Large Omega Dot

As demonstrated in Chapter 7, enlarging the Omega Dot is another effective method of decreasing tip size. We thus designed and obtained experimental tubings to utilize this effect, and the one designed to take maximum advantage of the Omega Dot was designated Tubing 9. When we compared the effectiveness of various tubing designs for penetrating toad rods and providing large light-evoked responses (see Section II.2 of Chapter 14), the tubing that proved most effective was Tubing 9. As described in Table 5 of Chapter 14, Tubing 9 has an OD of 1.85 mm, an ID of 0.81 mm, and an Omega Dot 0.56 mm in diameter. The relatively large ID provides room for a large Omega Dot, plus a clearance of 0.25 mm for the 0.20 mm tubing used to inject filling solutions (see Section I.3c of Chapter 10). When effects of enlarging the Omega Dot upon tip size were studied in Chapter 7, thin-walled tubing was used to keep the OD from exceeding 1.05 mm. From the standpoint of minimizing tip size, however, thin-walled tubing probably negates much of the advantage of an enlarged Omega Dot. In Tubing No. 9, therefore, the OD was increased to 1.85 mm to provide an OD/ID of 2.28. Since this value is somewhat higher than the OD/ID of Standard Tubing, it should provide some decrease of tip size to reinforce the effects of an enlarged Omega Dot. Yet the OD of 1.85 mm is small enough to be readily handled by our puller, and the resulting wall thickness of 0.52 mm is slightly less than the diameter of the Omega Dot (0.56 mm).

In Figure 31, (A) is a cross-sectional view of Tubing 9, while (B) is an end-on SEM photograph of a tip formed from this tubing. Though the Omega Dot fills much of the tubing, it appears only as a crescent intruding into the lumen of the tip. In fact, the Omega Dot occupies about 48 percent of the total area

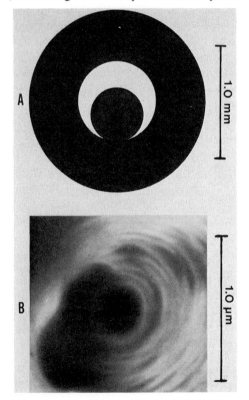

Figure 31. Cross-sectional views of Tubing No. 9. (A) Diagram of the capillary tubing. The relative values are all the same as in Table 5, but the OD has been decreased to 1.6 mm, for reasons described in text. (B) SEM photograph of a tip to show the marked alteration in the form of the lumen at the tip, compared with the original capillary tubing. The outer diameter of this tip measured 0.32 μm; it was deliberately pulled to this relatively large size to permit resolution of the lumen at the tip.

of the lumen in the tubing but only about 15 percent of the lumen at the tip. Thus Figure 31 shows that the large Omega Dot of Tubing 9 flowed into the capillary wall to an even greater extent than the smaller Omega Dots illustrated in Figure 29.

We compared tips that were formed from either Standard Tubing or Tubing 9, using a heating filament measuring $2 \times 2 \times 2$ mm. Though the clearance inside this filament is adequate for Standard Tubing, it is very small for Tubing 9, a problem that was handled in two ways. First, a batch of Tubing 9 was obtained with the relative dimensions unchanged, but with the OD reduced to 1.6 mm. This is the lowest value of the OD which provides sufficient room to fill the micropipette by injection from the back. Second, the filament was slightly enlarged by altering it to a more circular form which better accommodated the large tubing. The resulting clearance was adequate but minimal, as desired to maximize tip temperature and minimize tip size. Puller settings were employed that gave control tips on Standard Tubing in the upper part of the ultrafine size range. For this comparison, and all subsequent work on minimum tip size, the tips were mounted for SEM observations with double-sided tape. This greatly improved the consistency with which high resolution was obtained, so that only a few tips had to be rejected because of inadequate resolution.

The 11 tips formed from Standard Tubing yielded an average outer tip diameter of 0.091 μm $\pm$ 0.001 μm (S.E.M.), whereas the 10 tips formed from Tubing 9 had an average outer tip diameter of 0.051 μm $\pm$ 0.001 μm. This difference between means was significant at a p-value of 0.00006, and the average tip size was decreased 44 percent when using Tubing 9. Most of this reduction of tip size probably results from the design of Tubing 9, but some was undoubtedly because Tubing 9 more closely fitted the square loop filament. This is another example of the great difficulty in providing identical pulling conditions for widely differing tubing designs.

I.5 Filling the Glass Capillary with Helium

If our explanation is correct for why OD_t/ID_t is less than OD/ID in the general case, it results from trapping air inside the forming tip (see Section III.3b of Chapter 6). Because this trapped air is heated, and also squeezed as the tip is formed, its relatively high pressure will expand the tip, thus decreasing OD_t/ID_t and increasing tip size. If the trapped air could be released, smaller tips should be formed. Filling the capillary lumen with helium instead of air seemed a simple possibility for doing this. Since the helium atom has a smaller size and higher mobility than either nitrogen or oxygen, it can escape much more readily through a small pore.

This approach was tested by attaching a polyethylene tube to a piece of glass capillary tubing mounted for pulling. Helium was then flushed through the glass capillary at a slow rate, and the flow of helium was stopped just before activating the pulling cycle. The glass capillary was thus filled with helium when pulling began, but there was no flow of helium during tip formation, since this would have introduced undesirable cooling effects that might have obscured effects of filling the tip with helium. Control tips contained room air and were formed in the usual manner. For this test we used Standard Tubing and a 3 × 3 × 3 mm square loop filament. Puller settings were chosen to form tip sizes in the upper portion of the ultrafine range; these puller settings were held constant, and experimental and control tips were alternated in the pulling sequence.

For the 15 control tips the average outer tip diameter was 0.082 μm, and for 19 helium-filled tips the average value was 0.080 μm. The standard error of the mean was 0.0007 μm in both cases, and a t-test failed to reveal any statistically significant difference between the two means, the p-value being about 0.4. In any event, the difference between means is so small that this approach does not have any practical value under present conditions of forming tips. Apparently the long slender lumen behind the tip is such an effective barrier to the outflow of trapped gas that even helium cannot escape through it within the very short time required to form the tip.

I.6   Reduction of Air Pressure in the Glass Capillary

In glass working, an elevation of pressure within a closed vessel is routinely used to expand the vessel. It occurred to us that a reduced pressure within the glass capillary should have the opposite effect, since the higher outside pressure should provide an additional force causing tip size to decrease as the tip is formed. We thus experimented with the effects of either elevating or lowering the air pressure within capillary tubing during the period of tip formation.

For this purpose one end of a glass capillary was sealed by heating it in a flame. A polyethylene tube was force-fitted to the other end of the capillary, which was then mounted in the puller. Controlled elevations of pressure were provided from a bottle of compressed nitrogen, while decreases of pressure were provided by a vacuum pump and measured with a mercury manometer.

Initial tests were performed with Standard Tubing and a square loop filament measuring 2 × 2 × 2 mm. When the internal pressure was raised by 20 psi, tip size increased about 35 percent. On the other hand, reducing the internal pressure to 450 mm of Hg below the external air pressure resulted in a 20 percent reduction of tip size. Thus, raising or lowering the pressure within a glass capillary is another method of controlling tip size.

From the standpoint of minimizing tip size, the crucial question is how effective a reduced internal pressure can be. This question was approached by using Tubing 9 in conjunction with a square loop filament measuring 2 × 2 × 2 mm. Pulling conditions were set for ultrafine tips, but not the smallest that could be formed, since the smallest tips would make the effects of a reduced internal pressure more difficult to measure. As measured by our manometer, the internal pressure was reduced by 680 mm of Hg below the prevailing external air pressure, this being the strongest vacuum obtainable with our equipment.

Following correction for the gold coating, the outer tip diameter of 8 control tips averaged 0.071 μm, while the 8 tips formed with reduced internal pressure averaged 0.049 μm. Thus the outer tip diameter was reduced about 31 percent, and the difference between means was statistically significant at a p-value of 0.005.

I.7   Adjustment of Puller Settings

As summarized in Section IV.2 of Chapter 6, there are compelling reasons to believe that puller settings influence tip size mainly through their influence upon tip temperature. Though Table 1 shows that airflow settings have little or no effect upon tip size over a considerable range, an extreme reduction of airflow may increase tip temperature and thus decrease tip size. But airflow cannot be reduced indefinitely because of the unusually long tips that finally result. Thus airflow settings have little if any value for further reducing tip size within the ultrafine range. Filament temperature is critical, however, and its upper limit is determined by the temperature that the filament material can withstand. Filament width is likewise critical, especially within the range of 1.5–3.0 mm, as shown by Figure 20.

Our digital readout of pull strength was normally set at 1250, and this could be increased to a maximum of about 1975, which decreased tip size about 10 percent. The increased pull strength probably increases tip temperature by reducing the time during which the tip is formed. At a setting of 1250 the tips are already formed in a very short time, and this is probably why increasing pull strength to its maximum value has only a small effect.

Under our initial conditions employing a loop filament, the optimal length of the slow pull for providing minimum tip size was 0.050 in., and that value had been used in all previous work. In view of the altered filament design, we determined the effects of changing length of the slow pull in the range from 0.020–0.050 in. When Standard Tubing was used in a rectangular trough filament measuring 3 $\times$ 3 mm, and 2 mm in width, there was little or no effect upon tip size when length of the slow pull was varied over the described range. When the filament was changed to a square loop measuring 2 $\times$ 2 $\times$ 2 mm, however, tip size was minimized when the length of the slow pull was in the range of 0.030–0.040 in. This result was first obtained with Standard Tubing and then found to hold true also for Tubing 9. For minimizing tip size, therefore, we shortened the length of the slow pull to 0.035 in.

I.8   Combined Effects of All Strategies to Minimize Tip Size

We next assessed the results when all strategies that had proven effective for the reduction of tip size were applied simultaneously. For this test we used Tubing 1 (thick-walled) and Tubing 9 (containing the large Omega Dot), both of which were pulled under the same conditions. The heating filament was 2 $\times$ 2 mm in cross-section and 2.5 mm in width. Thus the heating filament was as small as could be used with these tubings, and its width was as great as possible without unduly increasing the tip length. The length of the slow pull was 0.035 in., and the setting of pull strength was 1975, as discussed in the preceding section of this chapter. Filament current was set as high as possible, and the airflow was set as low as possible without the tips becoming too long to be useful. One end of each piece of capillary tubing was sealed, and a vacuum of 680 mm of Hg relative to the external air was applied while the tip was formed. Tips were coated with a nominal 100 Å of gold, and 62% of 200 Å was subtracted when measuring tip size.

For the thick-walled Tubing 1, the average OD_t of 7 tips was 0.044 μm and the range was 0.029–0.059 μm. When tips were formed on Tubing 1 in Section I.2 of this chapter, without applying the various factors shown to reduce tip size in later sections of this chapter, the average OD_t was 0.039 μm and the range was 0.029–0.047 μm. Since results of the two tests were not significantly different, it appears that tip sizes obtained in Section I.2 were very close to the minimum obtainable with Tubing 1. Though additional strategies have been found to reduce tip size, compared with tips in the upper end of the ultrafine size range, these strategies become ineffective when tip size is in the range of 0.040–0.050 μm.

Similar results were obtained for Tubing 9 with the large Omega Dot. In Section I.4 of this chapter, this tubing yielded an average OD_t of 0.051 μm and a range of 0.041–0.074 μm, whereas application of the additional strategies for minimizing tip size yielded an average OD_t for 10 tips of 0.052 μm and a range of 0.032–0.069 μm. Here also, the minimum tip size appears to have been obtained earlier, so that the additional strategies could not further reduce tip size.

This interpretation was tested further by obtaining results when all strategies for minimizing tip size were applied simultaneously, compared with results when filament current and pull strength were reduced. For this comparison the setting of filament current was reduced from 202 to 197, which increases tip size significantly when one is working in the upper end of the ultrafine range of tip size, and pull strength was reduced from a setting of 1975 to 1250 (see Section I.7 of this chapter). The number of tips in each group varied from 7-10. With Tubing 1 the use of all strategies to minimize tip size gave an average OD_t of 0.044 μm, while the lower heat setting and reduced pull strength gave an average value of 0.048 μm. With Tubing 9 the average values of OD_t were 0.052 μm in both cases. Hence the altered puller settings, which influenced tip size when working in the upper portion of the ultrafine range of tip size, became ineffective when the tip size of each tubing was at or very near the minimum value.

PART II SUMMARY AND INTERPRETATION

When pulling conditions are used which form tips on Standard Tubing that are in the upper part of the ultrafine size range, Tubing 9 with the large Omega Dot can reduce tip size by about 44 percent, and the thick-walled Tubing 1 can reduce tip size by almost as much. The question remains whether Tubings 1 and 9 could be equally effective when compared with the very finest tips that can be formed on Standard Tubing. While it would be desirable to test this point experimentally, this has not been attempted because it seems beyond the capabilities of our present techniques. At the lower limit of tip size using Standard Tubing, it is not yet feasible to measure accurately the effect of a factor that would theoretically alter tip size by only 30–40% This is partly because of the limited resolution of SEM pictures. In addition, uncertainties in measuring the gold coating become critical with very small tips, since the measured thickness of the gold will strongly influence the percentage change of tip size associated with any measured change of tip size. Finally, in comparing tips formed by Standard Tubing with those formed by Tubings 1 or 9, it is not possible to assure identical tip temperatures, and tip temperature must be quite critical with such small tips. Theoretically, however, effects of an elevated OD/ID ratio and an enlarged Omega Dot should operate as effectively at the lower limit of tips formed on Standard Tubing as in higher ranges of tip size. Since theory strongly indicates that Tubings 1 and 9 should reduce the lower limit of tip size by 30–40%, it seems best to proceed on that assumption.

Capillary tubings with either a thick wall (Tubing 1) or a large Omega Dot (Tubing 9) appear about equally useful for minimizing tip size. Among six groups of tips (three groups from each type of tubing), the average value of OD_t varied only from 0.039–0.052 μm, while the smallest tips obtained occasionally measured 0.029 μm for Tubing 1 and 0.032 μm for Tubing 9. These special tubings are available from either the Glass Company of America or the Sutter Instrument Company.

Several additional strategies have been found effective for reducing the tip size of Standard Tubing from values in the upper end of the ultrafine range. These strategies include (1) reduction of pressure in the capillary tubing, (2) reducing the size of a square loop filament to fit the capillary tubing as closely as possible, and (3) adjustment of a variety of puller settings to further increase tip temperature. But the use of all these factors combined, in the case of Tubings 1 and 9, did not further reduce tip size from the values given above. Hence these factors all appear to become ineffective when the lower limit of tip size has been reached because of some other factor. We thus conclude that the tip sizes in the preceding paragraph closely define the lower limit of tip size that can be attained with tubings formed from Corning No. 7740 borosilicate glass. It likewise seems clear that this lower limit of tip size does not result from any remaining limitations in the pulling conditions, but from the molecular structure of this type of glass.

Throughout the process of tip formation, one may visualize the two forming tips as being in contact at the center of the zone of molten glass. This contact area is annular in form, and initially this annulus will have the thickness of the original capillary wall. At that time the contact area will be large and strong, and pulling will attenuate the thickness of the glass instead of tearing the molten glass apart. At the moment of tip formation, however, the contact area has become so small that cohesive molecular forces within the contact area can no longer attenuate the tip by further thinning of the molten glass. So the two tips separate. For any given tip temperature and tip viscosity, the tip size at which this occurs must depend largely upon the strength of molecular bonds within the glass. Thus the molecular structure of the glass itself may be expected to place an ultimate limit upon the minimum tip size that may be attained. If this analysis is correct, still finer tips would require other types of glass. The properties of available glasses are discussed in Chapter 15, and in Section VII.1 of Chapter 18 we show that a significant further reduction of tip size can be obtained by using aluminosilicate glass.

CHAPTER 9

Beveling Micropipette Tips:
Techniques and Applications

PART I BACKGROUND

I.1 The Need for Beveling

Most of the critical characteristics of micropipette tips are determined by the type of glass, design of the capillary tubing, and how the tips are formed. After tips are formed, however, they may be modified significantly by beveling, and some of the potential advantages of this procedure were recognized early in micropipette work. For example, beveling should improve the penetration of micropipettes through tissues and into cells. But a variety of problems had to be solved before beveling could be done with reasonable ease and reliability, particularly in the case of fine tips.

I.2 Terminology for Measuring Beveled Tips

In measuring beveled tips it is necessary to adopt a consistent terminology. As shown in Figure 32, beveled tips may be described by three measurements. The *bevel angle* is the angle between the long axis of the micropipette and the beveled surface, a definition that has been followed consistently in the literature. The size of beveled tips has usually been reported as the outer diameter at the base of the bevel (Brown and Flaming, 1974, 1975, 1979a; Tauchi and Kikuchi, 1977; Baldwin, 1980a). But tip size has also been given as the 'diameter of the extreme point' (Barrett, 1973), while Ogden *et al.*, (1978) appear to use this term for the thickness of the cutting edge. In our terminology the *tip size* refers to the micropipette's diameter at the base of the bevel, while *thickness of the cutting edge* refers to the distance across the sharpened leading edge of the beveled tip. For any given bevel angle, these two latter factors determine how easily and cleanly a beveled tip will penetrate through tissues and cell membranes. Of course, tip size also indicates the diameter of a beveled tip that must be inserted through a cell membrane before the tip can be sealed into the cell.

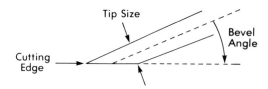

Figure 32. Definition of terms for beveled micropipette tips.

I.3   Early Beveling Methods

I.3a   Breaking micropipette tips

The crudest early method of approximating beveling was deliberately breaking the tips. The angle of such breaks is sometimes different from 90°, thus providing a tip form similar to that resulting from beveling, and the edges of broken tips are usually jagged and sharp. But in most cases the tip size is increased considerably when the tip is broken, and it is quite difficult to obtain bevel angles less than about 45° (Burke and ten Bruggencate, 1971), which is greater than desired for optimal penetrating capabilities. Thus, these tips are not satisfactory for work in small cells. For example, Van Essen and Kelly (1973) tried this technique for intracellular work in the cat's visual cortex, where diameters of the cell somata do not exceed about 25 μm. Though the broken tips occasionally penetrated these cells, and were helpful for passing sufficient current to stain the cells with Procion yellow, there were frequent signs of cell injury, and the intracellular recordings were too brief to yield much useful information. By contrast, Burke and ten Bruggencate (1971) found that tips broken to a diameter of 1–3 μm performed better than unbroken tips for intracellular work in alpha motoneurons of the cat spinal cord. Significantly, these are among the largest cells in the mammalian central nervous system, their somata having typical diameters of about 50 μm (Barrett, 1973). Thus, the usefulness of broken tips is limited to types of research in which relatively large tips are tolerated by the cells or tissues that must be penetrated. Of course broken tips also vary greatly in size and form.

I.3b   Beveling with abrasive stones and diamond dust

It was apparent for many years that the main disadvantages of breaking tips would be avoided if tips could be beveled by an abrasive surface. In retrospect one might wonder why this was not done sooner. The delay appears to have resulted mainly from persistent doubt about the feasibility of beveling such highly flexible glass tips. Initial attempts were rather tentative, and beveling techniques developed by several steps, each of which provided the requisite confidence to undertake further improvements.

To our knowledge the first published beveling technique was that of Barrett and Graubard (1970), who used a hard Arkansas stone as the abrasive material. This type of abrasive stone is formed naturally and is used extensively for the fine honing of metal edges. The stone was rotated at 600 rpm or less and was pretreated by holding the edge of a microscope slide against it for about 10 minutes, which presumably 'dressed' the surface by removing some of the irregularities. Tips beveled on such a stone had elliptical openings measuring about 1 by 3 μm, so the tip size in our terminology must have been about 2 μm. These beveled tips were employed for intracellular work in cat motoneurons, where they proved helpful for penetrating cells without significant damage, while providing sufficiently large tip openings to stain the cells with Procion yellow (Barrett and Graubard, 1970). Tips beveled by this method were also used by Van Essen and Kelly (1973) for intracellular work in cells of the visual cortex, where they likewise provided both adequate cell penetration and successful cell marking with Procion yellow. Since broken tips proved unsatisfactory in that study of the visual cortex, the beveling of tips using an Arkansas stone was a distinct advance in technique that permitted the use of beveled tips for intracellular work in smaller cells.

The next advance was the use of diamond dust as the abrasive (Barrett and Whitlock, 1973; Shaw and Lee, 1973). Because of its greater hardness and sharp cutting edges, diamond dust offered the advantage of faster and more effective beveling. When applied on a smooth surface, it also promised less wobble of the abrasive surface and thus less damage to the cutting edge of a beveled tip after the cutting edge was formed.

The method of Barrett and Whitlock (1973) is shown in Figure 33. A quartz rod 3.0 mm in diameter was rotated at 10–100 rpm by a motor that was mounted on a separate block to minimize the transmission of vibrations. A fine sable brush was used to paint the spinning quartz rod with a thin layer of dry 0.25 μm diamond particles, which adhered strongly to the rod, presumably by electrostatic attraction. Micropipette tips were then lowered into contact with this abrasive surface and beveled at an angle of about 30°. Of course the initial contact had to be made carefully, and it was controlled visually by means of a spotlight and dissecting microscope. This beveling method was also used to fabricate tips with elliptical openings measuring about 1 by 3 μm, and these tips were employed for intracellular work in cat motoneurons (Barrett, 1973). Electrodes beveled with diamond dust, rather than an Arkansas stone, were not mentioned to have specific advantages during intracellular experiments. But Barrett (1973) preferred the diamond dust. One may infer this was partly because of more rapid beveling, which required only 10 sec to several minutes (Barrett and Whitlock, 1973), and the diamond dust probably formed sharper cutting edges.

Shaw and Lee (1973) obtained similar results by brushing dry 0.25 μm diamond dust upon the flat side of an unspecified type of abrasive wheel rotated at about 50 rpm. Control of beveling was improved by using an audio readout to detect vibrations of the tip when it contacted the abrasive surface. In addition, air pressure was applied through the micropipette tip, and the progress of beveling was monitored by watching the velocity of movement of a droplet

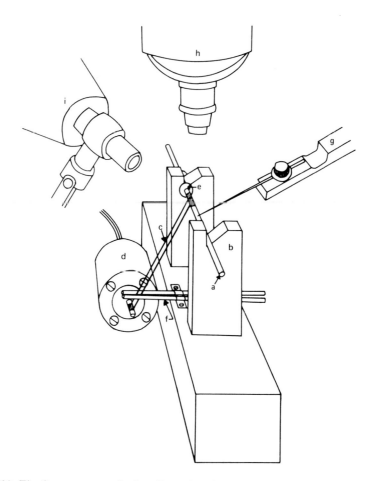

Figure 33. The first apparatus for beveling micropipettes with diamond dust. Elements are as follows: (a) quartz rod; (b) stainless steel supports; (c) thread belt; (d) motor; (e) guide rings; (f) thread guides; (g) electrode holder and manipulator; (h) 50× microscope; (i) spotlight. For details see text. (From Barrett and Whitlock (1973), reproduced by permission of Springer-Verlag, New York, N.Y.)

of fluid in the transparent air hose. This method provided 'tip diameters' as small as about 1.5 μm, and these tips proved useful for penetrating small blood vessels to measure blood pressure and inject vital dyes.

I.3c   Beveling fine tips with 0.05 μm alumina particles

For beveling tips smaller than about 1.5–2.0 μm, and for optimally sharp cutting edges, more delicate beveling techniques were required. Kripke and Ogden (1974) made several advances toward that goal. First, the abrasive used was 0.05 μm particles of alumina (Al_2O_3). On the Mohs scale of hardness the index of diamond is 10, while alumina is 8, and Pyrex ® glass is only 5. So alumina is an effective abrasive for Pyrex ®, and it can be obtained in smaller particles than diamond dust. Second, the alumina was suspended in a conductive salt solution and beveling was performed wet, thus reducing contamination of the tip by adherent particles of abrasive. Third, the micropipette's impedance was measured continuously and used to monitor the progress of beveling. Fourth, the alumina solution was laid upon a glass plate, which was rotated upon a wobble-free bearing formed by a thin film of oil between the glass plate and a lower stationary glass surface. Fifth, a differential micrometer provided the necessary fine control for advancing the micropipette tip against the abrasive surface.

Some of the main features of the Kripke and Ogden beveling technique are shown in Figure 34. The success of this method was evaluated by SEM, and well beveled tips were illustrated with tip sizes as small as about 0.3 μm.

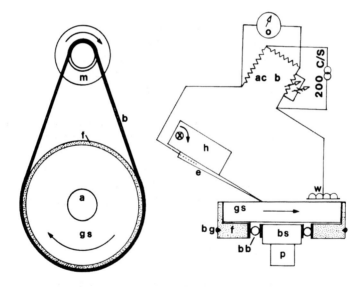

Figure 34. The first apparatus for beveling micropipettes with 0.05 μm alumina. On the left is a diagram of the apparatus from above, and on the right is a cutaway side view. Elements are as follows: (m) motor; (b) drive belt; (gs) glass surface supporting abrasive suspended in saline; (f) flange of ring holding gs; (a) optional Arkansas stone in center of glass disc for rapid beveling of relatively large micropipettes; (bg) belt groove; (bb) ball bearing; (bs) glass bearing surface upon which gs rotates in a film of oil; (p) stationary pedestal; (e) micropipette; (h) micropipette holder that rotates around the point X; (ac b) an ac bridge system for measuring micropipette impedance at 200 Hz; (w) moistened wick completing the circuit for measuring micropipette impedance. For further details, see text. (From Kripke and Ogden (1974), reproduced by permission of Elsevier Biomedical Press B.V., Amsterdam)

PART II   THE BROWN–FLAMING MICROPIPETTE BEVELER

II.1   Introduction

When we began intracellular research in vertebrate photoreceptors in 1973, and found that work in these small cells was severely limited by micropipette techniques, we first undertook beveling because it appeared to offer the simplest solution to the problem. Though the other developments of technique that have been described were undertaken later, the treatment of beveling has been deferred in this book to place it more logically among the various aspects of micropipette technique.

Our original goal of beveling was to improve the penetration of small cells without significant damage, and that goal was attained. Micropipette pullers available at that time offered a choice between the ultrafine but unduly long and flexible tips of the Livingston puller, or the somewhat larger but shorter tips formed by two-stage pullers. Since neither was satisfactory for vertebrate photoreceptors, we tried beveling tips with the technique of Kripke and Ogden, which they had kindly made available to us prior to publication. But very slow grinding by the suspension of freely moving abrasive particles proved a major limitation. Kripke and Ogden reported that even the relatively short and stiff tips formed by a two-stage puller required about 10–15 min for beveling, and in our experience even longer was needed. This was a serious problem because a group of micropipettes was needed for each experiment, and these were best prepared shortly before the experiment to avoid damage by the contained electrolyte.

We thus developed a method for embedding 0.05 μm alumina particles to form an abrasive surface for rapidly beveling fine micropipette tips (Brown and Flaming, 1974). This embedding method was later extended to diamond dust of various sizes, for the beveling of relatively large tips (Brown and Flaming, 1979). These abrasive surfaces were incorporated into a device permitting the rapid, precise, and convenient beveling of micropipette tips extending from about 0.06 μm to indefinitely large sizes (Brown and Flaming, 1975).

II.2   Fabrication of Abrasive Surfaces

II.2a   An abrasive surface containing embedded 0.05 μm particles of alumina

Our method of embedding fine alumina particles has not been altered significantly since it was first described (Brown and Flaming, 1974). As embedding media we chose polyurethanes because they adhere tightly to glass, resist mechanical wear, and are unaffected by water or saline. The two we have used are Varathane (No. 90 gloss) and Humicure. These materials are made by the Flecto Company, Inc. (1000-45th St., Oakland, CA 94608, USA), and they both proved satisfactory (Brown and Flaming, 1974). But Humicure is no longer used because it is so strongly catalyzed by atmospheric moisture that it is difficult to handle and the curing is hard to control. A film of embedding medium is first laid upon a mirror surface on one side of a precision glass plate with a diameter of 2.0 in. Since Varathane is transparent, the underlying mirror surface assists in visualizing the micropipette while bringing it into contact with the abrasive surface. The glass plates are coated in pairs. Surfaces to be coated are thoroughly cleaned, 8–10 drops of Varathane are applied to the upturned mirror surface of one plate, and the mirror surface of the other plate is immediately placed upon it. Surface tension quickly forms a uniform layer of embedding medium between the two plates, which are then slid apart. This leaves a thin and uniform layer of embedding medium on both plates, which are then placed in a dust-free cabinet for initial curing.

When the powdered alumina is embedded, the Varathane must still be sticky enough for the alumina to adhere to it. Yet the Varathane must have cured to a high enough viscosity that it will not fully coat the alumina particles. This condition is usually established after an initial cure of 20–60 min, the curing time being shorter at higher atmospheric humidities and temperatures. During embedding, a pile of 0.05 μm particles of alumina (Linde alumina B) is placed upon a clean glass surface held slightly above and to one side of the partially cured Varathane surface. Gentle air puffs from an empty squirt bottle are directed toward the alumina to produce a cloud of abrasive particles, some of which settle upon the Varathane. The embedded surface is then replaced in the dust-free cabinet to harden the Varathane by 3–4 days of final curing, after which the abrasive surface is rubbed by hand under running water to remove all unattached alumina. It is then ready for use.

Kripke and Ogden (1974) noted that such small particles of alumina have a strong tendency to clump. This probably results from the high surface-to-volume ratio in conjunction with electrostatic attractions, and we have also not found a way to prevent it. Instead, the Varathane is cured to a relatively high viscosity, and the clumps of alumina contact the Varathane only by the very small force of their own weight. Under these conditions only certain particles of a clump will become embedded, and the unattached particles are easily removed by washing. An abrasive surface made in this way is quite durable and with reasonable care may be used to bevel many hundreds of micropipette tips. If it is damaged, the Varathane may be stripped off with toluene, and the glass plate may be recoated.

Figure 35 illustrates by SEM both an abrasive surface made as described (A and B) and the results of beveling a fine micropipette tip on this type of surface (C and D). Control observations of the embedding medium without any abrasive reveal an entirely featureless surface that is indistinguishable from a high quality glass surface, so it is ideally smooth for our purposes. When alumina is embedded in this surface, Figure 35(A) shows that each clump gives a patch of abrasive particles. These patches are quite similar, aside from variations in size and shape. Figure 35(A) shows that these patches are raised only slightly above the surface of the embedding medium, and Figure 35(B) shows this same patch of abrasive at higher magnification to reveal its very fine texture.

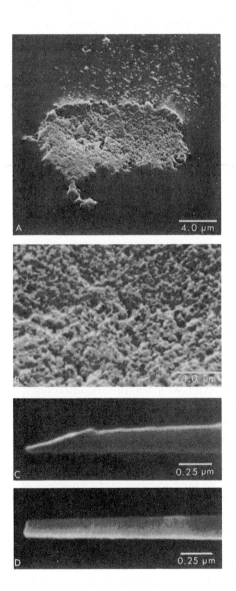

Figure 35. SEM photographs of an abrasive surface containing embedded particles of 0.05 μm alumina, a micropipette beveled with this type of abrasive surface, and a control unbeveled tip. (A) Patch of 0.05 μm alumina particles embedded in a polyurethane film on a glass surface. (B) Surface texture, at higher magnification, of the same patch of abrasive shown in A. (C) Profile view of tip beveled at an angle of 20°. (D) Micropipette tip before beveling. (From Brown and Flaming (1974), Copyright 1974 by the AAAS, which granted permission for this reproduction)

The abrasive patches are sufficiently low and flat that they may be used without further treatment to bevel micropipette tips formed by an Industrial Science Associates puller. This is illustrated in Figure 35(C), where the beveled tip has a diameter of about 0.17 μm. These tips seldom break during beveling on such an abrasive surface, apparently because their flexibility permits them to ride up and over the abrasive patches without damage. But the shorter and stiffer tips provided by our puller were later found to break rather often under these same conditions. This was handled by dressing the abrasive plates in two ways.

The abrasive surface was first scraped with a sharp glass edge. For this purpose we used the end of a microscope slide, the corners of which had been rounded off. When the slide was held at a low angle, the higher portions of the abrasive patches were readily scraped off. This was either done under running water, or the loose material was washed off later. Second, the abrasive surface was rubbed by hand, under running water, with a lapping paper consisting of 0.3 μm alumina particles embedded in a plastic film (3M Co., St Paul, MN 55144, USA).

When abrasive plates were dressed as described, beveling was improved in several respects. There was a more gradual and continuous decrease of electrical resistance, indicating a smoother abrasive action, with only an occasional sharp drop of electrical resistance suggesting chipping of the tip. As expected from this result, the best quality of beveling was obtained more reliably, as indicated by results in penetrating small cells such as vertebrate photoreceptors. More important, perhaps, the short and stiff tips formed by our puller could be beveled satisfactorily. This is particularly helpful since the combination of short tips with precision beveling seems the most effective way of minimizing tip resistance for many types of research. Abrasive plates of the type just described, as provided by the Sutter Instrument Co., are now dressed only with lapping paper, which has proved satisfactory. So the coarser initial stage of dressing can be eliminated for most (if not all) applications. In any laboratory with especially critical requirements, however, additional dressing might prove helpful.

II.2b   *Abrasive surfaces containing various grades of embedded diamond dust*

For the beveling of relatively large tips, a coarser abrasive is required because more glass must be removed. Though alumina is available in 0.3 μm particles, diamond dust is superior for beveling all but the finest tips, for reasons given in Section IV.5 of this chapter. Diamond dust had been used in earlier beveling procedures (Barrett and Whitlock, 1973; Shaw and Lee, 1973), but it had not been embedded in a durable abrasive surface suitable for precision beveling. This was accomplished by modifying our procedure for embedding 0.05 μm alumina (Brown and Flaming, 1979).

Diamond dust was obtained from Keen-Kut Products (361 Beach Road,

Burlingame, CA 94010, USA). Since diamond dust is graded by sifting, it is usually rated by the largest particles that can pass through the sieve. Of course any given grade contains particles varying considerably in size, and the finest grade available is rated as 0–0.25 µm. When diamond dust is this small, it has a strong tendency to clump, and these clumps must first be broken up. This is done by placing some diamond dust between two pieces of plate glass, which are then rubbed together. Initially the diamond dust sounds and feels gritty, and rubbing is continued until it is like a fine powder that can no longer be made finer by further rubbing. At this stage the diamond dust forms a thin layer adhering to each of the glass surfaces, and it is ready for embedding.

Varathane is applied to the precision glass plates and initially cured as already described. For embedding diamond dust the Varathane should no longer feel sticky when touched, and the curing time to reach this criterion is usually 3–8 hr, much longer than the curing time for embedding alumina. The prepared diamond dust will adhere to a finger pressed upon it, and the finger may then be used to rub the diamond dust into the Varathane. If this is done at the appropriate stage of curing, it will not damage the Varathane, yet enough curing time will remain to lock the diamond particles into the Varathane. The diamond dust gives the surface a gray color, and this is a convenient criterion for obtaining an even coating of embedded abrasive. The Varathane is then cured for an additional 30 days to attain its full hardness, so that it will be optimally resistant to the mechanical wear of beveling relatively large and stiff tips. The abrasive surface is then rubbed by hand under running water to remove particles that are not well embedded.

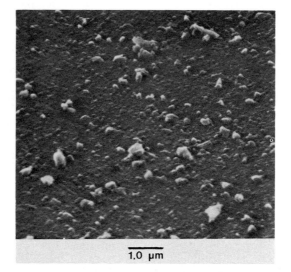

1.0 µm

Figure 36. SEM photograph of an abrasive surface consisting of 0–0.25 µm particles of diamond dust embedded in a film of Varathane laid upon a glass surface. (From Brown and Flaming (1979a), reproduced by permission of Elsevier Biomedical Press B.V., Amsterdam)

Figure 36 is an SEM photograph of 0–0.25 μm diamond dust embedded in a film of Varathane. The diamond dust is distributed rather uniformly and mainly in single particles. The uniformity of distribution probably results from rubbing the diamond dust into the surface, since any area without diamond particles remains free to accept them until the entire surface is covered, while the freedom from clumping is probably improved by the final hand washing. Almost all the particles in Figure 36 are 0.25 μm or less in size. The occasional larger particles are probably glass chips that result from scoring the glass plates used to break up the clumped diamond dust. No method has been found to prevent this contamination by glass particles, but they do not seem to compromise the quality of beveling. Since they have relatively low hardness and a very scattered distribution, they should have little abrasive effect.

When diamond abrasive surfaces are made as described, they are likewise quite durable, providing care is taken not to attempt beveling too rapidly. If a pipette tip is lowered faster than the diamond abrasive can cut it away, the abrasive surface can be scored. Though this is not a problem with the fine tips beveled by 0.05 μm alumina, it can occur with the larger and stiffer tips beveled with diamond dust, and the need for caution increases as coarser diamond dust is used to bevel even larger tips. But this is not a serious limitation because of the rapid beveling action of embedded diamond dust. For example, 0–0.25 μm diamond dust can bevel a fine pipette to a tip diameter of 2–3 μm in only 1–2 min.

II.3   Overall Design of Micropipette Beveler

Figure 37 shows our beveling instrument, which was labeled the 'K.T. Brown Micro-Pipette Beveler' when it was produced and made available by the

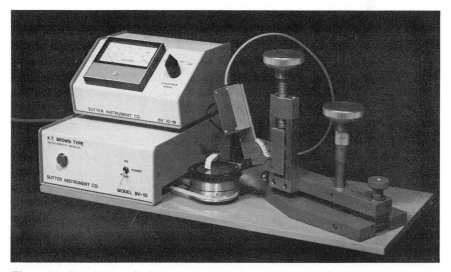

Figure 37. Our design of micropipette beveler, as produced and labeled by the Sutter Instrument Co.

Sutter Instrument Co. Since it was developed as a collaborative project, it would more appropriately be called the Brown–Flaming micropipette beveler, and that designation will be used here.

Briefly, this instrument contains a covered motor that rotates the abrasive surface, upon which a wick supplies saline for the wet grinding process, and the electrical resistance of a micropipette is monitored continuously as the micropipette is lowered by a special micromanipulator. Each of these features will now be described.

II.4   Rotation of Abrasive Surface

For beveling fine tips, especially if they are relatively short and stiff, the abrasive surface should rotate with minimal wobble and vibration. Figure 38 shows a schematic cross-section of our grinding pedestal, which uses the basic type of wobble-free bearing introduced by Kripke and Ogden (1974). The lower bearing surface (LBS) is an optical flat, upon which is placed a few drops of oil, followed by the upper bearing surface (UBS), which is the precision glass plate coated with abrasive. The interposed thin film of oil permits the upper plate to rotate freely, yet the two plates are strongly held together by surface tension in the oil. Using this type of bearing in conjunction with the flat and parallel surfaces of the abrasive plate and the uniformly thick layer of Varathane, wobble of the abrasive surface does not exceed 1.0 μm at the outer margin of the abrasive disc. Mounting screws (MS) are used to clamp the abrasive plate between upper and lower flanges (UF and LF). Inside the lower flange is a ball bearing that is fitted loosely around the base and that serves to keep UBS centered upon the base. Oil must occasionally be added to LBS, and for this purpose the surface of LBS may be exposed by sliding off UBS after removing the mounting screws.

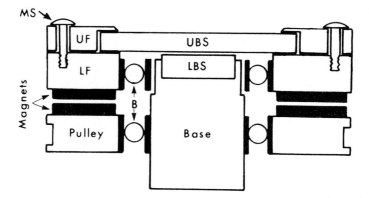

Figure 38. Schematic sectional side view of the grinding pedestal of our micropipette beveler. Elements with abbreviated labels include the lower bearing surface (LBS), upper bearing surface (UBS), lower flange (LF), upper flange (UF), ball bearings (B), and mounting screws (MS). For further details, see text. (From Brown and Flaming (1975), reproduced by permission of Elsevier Biomedical Press B.V., Amsterdam)

Kripke and Ogden used a motor and belt to drive directly the flange hold-ing their upper plate (see Figure 34). As shown in Figure 38, our instrument features a separate pulley mounted to the base by a ball bearing. Six perma-nent magnets are cemented at intervals upon the upper surface of the pulley, and a matching pattern of magnets is cemented upon the lower surface of LF. This magnetic coupling transfers the rotary motion of the pulley to LF, while greatly reducing the probability that undesirable vibrations of the pulley will be transferred to the abrasive surface. An additional advantage of this weak magnetic clutch is that the abrasive surface stops rotating when the oil in the bearing becomes too thin, thus providing a useful warning when it is time to add oil. Vibrations are further handled by using a quiet single speed motor, a very flexible fabric or Mylar drive belt, and by mounting the entire instrument on a heavy 3/8 in. steel base. With these precautions no significant vibrations of the abrasive surface have been detected. The rate of rotation of the abrasive surface proved not to be critical, and a speed of 60 rpm was adopted.

II.5   Special Micromanipulator for Beveling

Since a commercially available micromanipulator ideally adapted to the re-quirements of beveling could not be found, one was designed for this purpose, as shown in Figure 37. A micropipette is clamped to a mounting block, which may be rotated around its own axis to adjust the angle of beveling, as indicated on a scale. In our work the bevel angle has usually been about 25°, and it has seldom exceeded the range of 20–35°. The same element that holds the micropipette also carries the headstage of the device for measuring the micropipette's elec-trical resistance. This permits the lead between the micropipette and headstage to be short, which reduces interference in measuring electrical resistance.

The entire micromanipulator may be moved over the baseplate of the beveler to position a micropipette for beveling. Yet the micromanipulator is sufficiently heavy to prevent inadvertent horizontal movements as a micropipette is lowered in two stages to contact the abrasive surface. A coarse movement brings the micropipette close to the abrasive surface, followed by a much finer movement to prevent damaging the tip when it makes contact. A screw operating against a spring provides the coarse control, which is mounted on an upper plate hinged to the baseplate of the micromanipulator. The fine control acts by slightly tilt-ing this upper plate. The desired 'fineness' of the fine control varies somewhat between different beveling situations, so it was made adjustable as shown in Figure 37. A pivoted 'seesaw' is mounted in a cutout in the baseplate of the manipulator, and a micrometer rests upon one end of this seesaw, while a 'bear-ing element' rests upon the other end. The micrometer and bearing element are both fitted with ball tips, and the micrometer has a large knob to facilitate fine adjustments. As the micrometer is advanced, the other end of the seesaw lifts the bearing element, thus lifting the hinged upper plate of the manipulator and advancing the micropipette toward the abrasive surface. The bearing element may be clamped at any position in a slot in the upper plate, thus adjusting the distance between the pivot of the seesaw and the bearing element. For a given advance of the micrometer, of course the largest tilt of the upper plate will occur when the bearing element is at the end of the seesaw, and the tilt will become extremely small as the bearing element closely approaches the seesaw's pivot. Even when the bearing element is near the end of the seesaw, a micropipette will move considerably less than a given micrometer movement. This is partly because the distance from the hinge of the upper plate to the bearing element is greater than the distance from the hinge to the micropipette tip. The actual ratio depends somewhat upon how the micropipette tip is mounted, but it is never less than 2. In addition, when the micrometer and bearing element are equidistant from the seesaw's pivot, any given micrometer movement is twice the vertical distance traversed by the bearing element. Taken together, these factors provide a ratio of micrometer movement to micropipette tip movement that is never less than 4, and this ratio becomes much higher when the bearing element is set close to the pivot of the seesaw. A fine control is thus provided in which the 'fineness' of the control may be varied over a long range, which has met the requirements of all beveling situations encountered to date. If specialized applications made it desirable to alter the range covered by the fine control, this could readily be done by using a coarser or finer micrometer.

In our original description of this beveling micromanipulator, the seesaw was used for an entirely different purpose (Brown and Flaming, 1975). A standard micrometer was mounted at one end, and a differential micrometer for much finer movement was mounted at the other end. That design provided three stages of tip advancement, and the seesaw was a simple method of keeping both micrometers in control of tilting the upper plate, so that either one could be used at will. We later learned that both fine and ultrafine controls are not necessary for common applications of beveling, but this alternative use of the seesaw may be helpful to some investigators with specialized requirements.

II.6   Monitoring Micropipette Resistance

Precision beveling requires detecting when the tip contacts the abrasive surface and then monitoring the progress of beveling until a predetermined criterion is met. In cases where the tips are so fine that they cannot be seen, we adopted the continuous monitoring of micropipette resistance. A top view of the beveling plate, as it appeared in an early version of our beveler, is shown in Figure 39. A small well contains 0.9 percent (by weight) NaCl solution, which is laid by a wick as a thin ring of fluid upon the abrasive surface, and the wick is connected by a platinum wire to the reference side of the instrument measuring micropipette resistance. The abrasive surface is rotated counterclockwise, and the micropipette is lowered into the ring of fluid, which completes the electrical circuit to the wick. Since 0.9 percent NaCl approximates physiological saline, the measured electrical resistance of a micropipette should be quite similar to its value during an experiment.

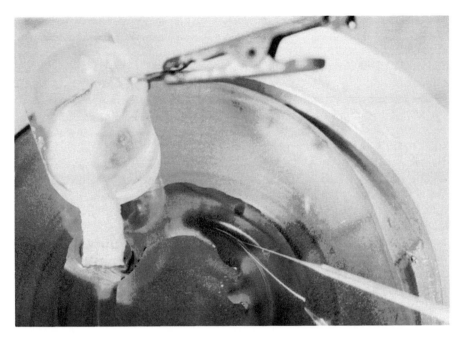

Figure 39. Top view of the beveling plate in an early version of our micropipette beveler, as described in text.

The AC impedance bridge that was used by Kripke and Ogden (1974) proved too slow for our more rapid beveling. Thus a new instrument (shown in Figure 37) was designed to measure the impedance of micropipettes at 135 Hz. In this device a high-impedance probe stage with a gain of 10 is followed by a 60 Hz notch filter and a 135 Hz peaked narrow band amplifier. An AC–DC feedback converter is also employed with a DC microammeter in the feedback loop, and the probe input follower is driven by a 135 Hz oscillator that is coupled by way of a 10^9 Ω resistor. Compensation for RC time constants at the input is provided by negative capacity feedback, and a direct reading meter is calibrated in ranges of 0–100 and 0–500 MΩ. Measurements of micropipette impedance at 135 Hz proved not to be significantly different from the DC resistance. For simplicity, therefore, we have tended to refer to the obtained values as micropipette 'resistance', though the term 'impedance' would be technically more correct.

PART III   BEVELING FINE MICROPIPETTES

III.1   Technique

Oil is lost slowly from the wobble-free bearing, even when it is not in use, so we remove the abrasive plate and add 3–4 drops of oil before each session of beveling. An SAE No. 40 motor oil is good for this purpose, being light enough for the bearing to operate freely with the magnetic clutch, yet heavy enough not to be lost too rapidly from the bearing. Also, the abrasive surface is degreased at this time by flowing a detergent over it, since this reduces the thickness of the ring of saline. The abrasive plate is then washed and remounted.

One of the most time-consuming aspects of beveling is establishing contact of the micropipette tip with the abrasive surface, because this must be done slowly enough to prevent tip damage. The mirror coating on the abrasive plate saves time because the micropipette tip and its reflection appear to meet when the tip contacts the saline. Additional time may be saved by adding to the saline a little detergent (Kodak Photo Flo at 1.0% by volume). Since this improves the ability of the saline to wet the abrasive surface, the thickness of the saline film is thus reduced. Though we originally supplied saline to the wick from a well (see Figure 39), we later draped the wick onto the abrasive plate without any fluid reservoir, as shown in Figure 37. This permits better control of the amount of fluid supplied by the wick, which also influences thickness of the saline film. Saline is fed to the wick one drop at a time, with 4–5 drops usually being enough to form a ring of saline, and this is maintained by an additional drop of saline whenever required. With these procedures the thickness of the saline film is only about 25–50 μm.

In lowering a micropipette, the coarse control is used first to quickly bring the tip just short of contact with the saline. This is done by using a reading lamp to provide a mirror image of the tip and by stopping when the tip itself does not quite meet its mirror image. The fine control is used thereafter. For beveling fine tips, positioning the bearing element about midway between the pivot and end of the seesaw is usually adequate. This gives a rapid enough advance to reach the abrasive surface within about 30 sec, providing that the thickness of the saline has been minimized. Yet the advance is not rapid enough to endanger the tip at the moment of contact, which is usually indicated by a perturbation of electrical resistance.

When the purpose of beveling is to provide the sharpest possible cutting edge, without enlarging the tip any more than necessary, an important question is how much the electrical resistance of a micropipette should be reduced. If a tip of 0.2 μm outside diameter were beveled at an angle of 20°, but only sufficiently to produce the sharpest possible cutting edge, the site of the minimum diameter of the conducting pore would be moved back along the micropipette's main axis by only 0.55 μm. Aside from very unusual conditions, fine or ultrafine tips formed by two-stage pullers taper quite gradually in the region behind the tip (see Figures 18, 22, 28 and 30). Hence minimal beveling for an optimally sharp cutting edge should reduce a micropipette's electrical resistance only slightly. When we attempt minimal beveling for this purpose, we thus bring the tip into contact with the abrasive surface and then lift it as soon as the resistance shows a distinct change *in either direction*. When this criterion is used, a tip usually contacts the abrasive surface for only a few seconds, which bevels tips adequately as indicated by their improved performance in penetrating verte-brate photoreceptors.

Minor increases of electrical resistance are not unusual during beveling, and they probably result from slight plugging of the tip by fine particles of glass and abrasive. The increased resistance sometimes disappears when the tip is lifted from the abrasive surface, as if the material plugging the tip had dropped out. In most cases the increased resistance persists, but this has not been a serious problem. Persistent plugging may be decreased by reducing the angle of beveling, or by allowing a month for full curing of the embedding medium. The latter procedure is probably effective because the abrasive particles become more securely locked into the embedding medium.

When beveling is continued beyond the minimum, to significantly decrease a micropipette's resistance, its electrical resistance drops rapidly at first and then more slowly. The rapid initial drop is partly because a micropipette's electrical resistance per unit length is greatest at the tip and falls steadily as the lumen enlarges behind the tip. In addition, the reduction of tip length per unit time is greatest at the tip itself, because of the small amount of glass removed per unit length, and this also changes rapidly with distance from the tip. During the secondary slower fall of electrical resistance, it may be well controlled by advancing a micropipette to achieve the desired final value. Since tips bend during beveling, it is advantageous to stop advancing the tip at a resistance somewhat higher than that desired. As beveling continues, the tip straightens and becomes beveled at the preset angle, while its resistance falls to a final stable value, and the tip may then be lifted. When lifted before straightening, undesirable effects occur. If a sharp cutting edge has been formed with the tip bent, this cutting edge will briefly contact the abrasive surface at an angle when the tip is lifted and will thus tend to be chipped off. If the tip has been advanced much more rapidly than material can be removed by the abrasive surface, it can become severely bent. In this case a long thread of glass is sometimes formed that extends from the tip, and if the tip is lifted prematurely this glass thread tends to break off, likewise blunting the tip. But these effects may readily be prevented by giving the tip time to straighten while the final bevel is formed. Tips may thus be beveled to predetermined values of the bevel angle and tip size, with the cutting edge remaining optimally sharp after it is lifted from the abrasive surface.

Finally, we have noted that if micropipettes are filled and allowed to stand overnight before beveling, the beveling action is improved. This is indicated by a more gradual and continuous decrease of electrical resistance, with fewer signs of small but sharp resistance drops that suggest chipping of the tip. As might be expected, the advantage of this procedure is most obvious with fine tips and it decreases as tip size increases. The basis of this observation is not clear, but glass undergoes slow hydration and its chemical composition also changes slowly in contact with H^+ or K^+ ions (Isard, 1967). Thus one possibility is that overnight changes in physical properties of the glass promote a smoother abrasive action during beveling.

III.2   Evaluation of Results by SEM

When our techniques for beveling fine tips were assessed by SEM, our own puller had not been developed, so micropipette tips were formed using an Industrial Science Associates puller. This puller had been modified by interposing a 25-sec delay between turning on the heating filament and onset of the slow pull, to increase tip temperature and decrease the tip sizes that could be obtained. All micropipettes were formed from Standard Tubing and filled with 5 M K-acetate ($KC_2H_3O_2$). Since Omega Dot tubing had not yet become available, tips were filled by the original fiber filling method that employs a bundle of glass fibers (see Section I.3a of Chapter 10). Tips were then beveled on a washed but *undressed* abrasive plate containing 0.05 μm alumina particles, as shown in Figure 35 (A and B). The final micropipette resistance was measured after completing beveling and lifting the tip slightly from the abrasive surface.

Since micropipettes had to be filled with electrolyte for the control of beveling, the electrolyte had to be removed before SEM observations. For that purpose a stainless steel tube was inserted down the shaft to where the initial taper began, in order to flush out the electrolyte. This was done three times with distilled water, with intervals of a few hours to allow diffusion of electrolyte from the tip, followed by several additional flushings with methyl alcohol and a final flush with acetone. Micropipettes were then dried in a clean laboratory oven that had never contained common contaminating substances such as paraffin. Owing to these cleaning procedures, the SEM examination of beveled tips was rather laborious.

When minimally beveled for optimally sharp tips, it was found that 10–12 micropipettes could be beveled easily within 1/2 hr. Figure 35(C) shows a tip beveled in this manner. After subtracting the gold coating, the tip size at the base of the bevel is about 0.15 μm. The bevel angle is $20°$, and the cutting edge is extremely sharp. Though the cutting edge is rounded at a diameter of slightly less than 0.03 μm (300 Å), this is the approximate amount of rounding that would result from the nominal 150 Å gold coating that was used for these SEM observations. So the sharpness of this tip, before it was coated, must have closely approached the theoretical limit. The obtained quality of beveling was quite reliable, as indicated both by SEM and by the performance of beveled tips during intracellular work in vertebrate photoreceptors. By comparison, unbeveled control tips usually had squared-off ends, as shown in Figure 35(D). Though some unbeveled tips deviated from this result, as shown in Figure 28, we have never seen an unbeveled tip that could be mistaken for a beveled one.

If micropipettes are beveled to enlarge the tip, while maintaining a very sharp cutting edge, it is desirable to know the relation between tip size and micropipette resistance. This is shown in Figure 40, where tip size after subtracting twice the nominal thickness of the gold coating is designated 'electrode tip diameter', and where micropipette resistance is designated 'electrode resistance'. Though ultrafine tips cannot be obtained reliably with the Industrial Science Associates puller, our modified puller yielded two such tips, the smaller of which measured 0.06 μm. As explained in Section I.3a of Chapter 10, these ultrafine tips probably resulted in part from the multiple glass fibers fusing with the tip and thickening its wall. Even the ultrafine tips could be minimally beveled, as revealed by SEM, and other tips were beveled to various larger tip sizes, the largest of which measured 0.54 μm. Over this range of tip size, micropipette resistance dropped from about 150 to 25 MΩ. All points in Figure 40 fitted closely to a single curve, which was drawn through the data by eye, so the tip diameter of any given micropipette can be inferred accurately from micropipette resistance. Figure 40 shows that with increasing tip size, resistance falls rapidly at first and then more slowly. This may be expected, since beveling will initially reduce micropipette resistance by a relatively large amount for a given increase of tip size, and the decrement of resistance per unit increase of tip size will fall rapidly as the tip is enlarged during beveling. In fact, the form of the experimental function in Figure 40 conforms closely to theoretical functions calculated by Frank and Becker (1964). The form of this function is of considerable interest, since most applications require that either micropipette resistance or tip size be minimized. Figure 40 shows that when either parameter is reduced to a given low value, any further reduction that can be attained is quite small and is obtained only at the expense of a large and undesirable increase of the other parameter.

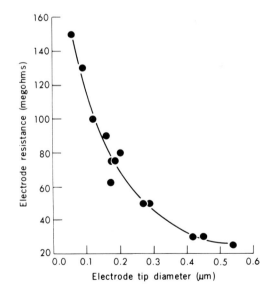

Figure 40. Electrical resistance of micropipettes as a function of tip size after beveling. Just after beveling each tip, its impedance at 130 Hz was recorded in MΩ. The tip was then evacuated and dried, as described in the text, and its diameter at the base of the bevel was measured from SEM photographs. The curve was drawn by eye through the obtained points. (From Brown and Flaming (1974), Copyright 1974 by the AAAS, which granted permission for this reproduction)

With any given micropipette puller, type of tubing, and filling solution, there should be a well defined relation between micropipette resistance and the tip size that is obtained by beveling. For tips smaller than 0.5 μm, this relation can be determined only by electron microscopy, but for tips significantly larger than 0.5 μm it can be determined by light microscopy. Once the relation is determined, tips of any desired size may be obtained by beveling to the requisite micropipette resistance. Another example of this was provided by Clementz and Grampp (1976), who used a two-stage puller to form tips from tubing with an OD/ID of 1.5; these tips were then filled with 3 M-KCl and beveled with an abrasive called 'Degussit'. As shown in Figure 41, their beveled tips were measured by SEM and ranged from 0.2–1.2 μm, thus covering a size range extending above that of Figure 40. As their tip sizes increased, micropipette resistance fell from about 13.5–1.3 MΩ. The form of their function is very similar to ours, and also to the theoretical function calculated by the methods of Frank and Becker (1964), which they included for direct comparison.

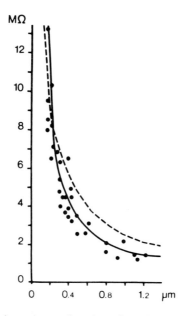

Figure 41. Electrode resistance as a function of tip diameter at the base of the bevel. The solid line was fitted to the obtained points by eye, and the interrupted line is the theoretical function according to Frank and Becker (1964). (From Clementz and Grampp (1976), reproduced by permission of *Acta Physiologica Scandinavica Stockholm*)

III.3   Advantages of Our Beveling Technique

When compared with the results of Kripke and Ogden (1974), our beveling technique has exhibited the following advantages. (1) Beveling is greatly speeded, so that an entire group of micropipettes may be beveled just before an experiment. (2) Beveling may be extended downward from tips of about 0.3 μm to tips in the ultrafine size range. (3) Based upon published SEM photographs, sharper cutting edges may be formed. (4) Ogden (personal communication) found that beveled electrodes were more fragile than unbeveled controls when they were tested in monkey retinas, and the beveled tips likewise broke more readily when they were cleaned by sonication. This problem seems avoided or minimized with our beveling technique. Many penetrations have been made through the retina of a snapping turtle, using a single beveled electrode, without any decrease in the ability of the tip to penetrate smoothly. When beveled and unbeveled tips were sonicated, with electrical resistance being used to match tip size and to detect breakage of the tip, this method likewise failed to reveal any difference in fragility. While the basis of these results is not known, the great amount of flexing of the tip during slow beveling may result in a work-hardening that renders the tip more brittle. If so, the marked reduction of this problem with our technique derives from the more rapid beveling.

III.4 Beveling of Short or Long Tips

The especially short and stiff tips formed by the Brown–Flaming puller are well adapted to beveling for two reasons. First, the stiffness of the tips permits particularly rapid beveling. Second, beveling is frequently needed to lower micropipette resistance as much as possible while maintaining a very sharp cutting edge, and short tips also reduce micropipette resistance. Hence the beveling of short tips is an effective strategy for minimizing micropipette resistance. Though especially short and stiff tips are more prone to chipping, this is readily avoided by dressing the abrasive plate as described in Section II.2a of this chapter. We have not used SEM to evaluate the beveling of tips formed from our puller, mainly because beveled tips formed by the Industrial Science Associates puller have proved so satisfactory and so close to the theoretical limit that our puller seems unlikely to improve the aspects of beveling that are revealed by SEM.

At the other extreme, the long slender tips formed by a Livingston puller present special problems for beveling. When such a flexible tip contacts the saline film, it is drawn down markedly by surface tension. If this occurs with a thin saline film, the tip may be drawn immediately against the abrasive surface, an effect that may be prevented by adding saline to thicken the saline ring. Of course this downward bending of flexible tips also causes the angle of beveling to be greater than indicated on the scale, which may be prevented by setting the scale to a smaller angle than desired. But these adjustments reduce the ease and precision of beveling. In addition, beveling of such flexible tips is unduly time consuming and the quality of results is uncertain. So especially long and flexible micropipette tips are poorly adapted to the requirements of beveling.

PART IV   BEVELING RELATIVELY LARGE MICROPIPETTES

IV.1   Prevention of Tip Plugging

The techniques described for beveling fine micropipettes with 0.05 μm alumina may be readily adapted to beveling relatively large micropipette tips with diamond dust (Brown and Flaming, 1979).

Though tip plugging is only an occasional minor problem when beveling fine tips, it becomes important when beveling relatively large tips with diamond dust. This is because the removal of more glass causes an accumulation of abrasion products (glass and diamond particles) in the tip as it enlarges. Unless steps are taken to prevent this, it occurs consistently and increases the electrical resistance of the tip. We found that increases of electrical resistance which had occurred in this manner could not be reversed by either sonicating the tip or applying a pressure as high as 100 psi to the contained electrolyte. Since material plugging the tip is difficult or impossible to remove, formation of the plug must be prevented. This may be done by applying pressure to the contained electrolyte to drive it through the tip during beveling.

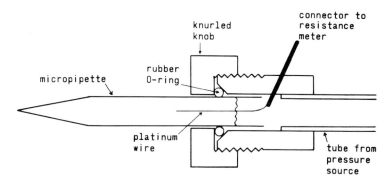

Figure 42. Schematic drawing of device for connecting micropipette with a source of pressure while monitoring the micropipette's electrical resistance. (From Brown and Flaming (1979a), reproduced by permission of Elsevier Biomedical Press B.V., Amsterdam)

In our method of doing this, a pressure of 50 psi is provided by a bottle of compressed nitrogen with a standard regulator and gauge. A valve is opened to introduce pressure to the micropipette, and after this valve is closed a leak valve releases the pressure. The device used to connect the pressure source to the micropipette is shown schematically in Figure 42. This connector is sealed by epoxy to the tube from the pressure source. When a micropipette is inserted backward into this connector, a platinum wire makes contact with the contained electrolyte to measure electrical resistance. The micropipette is then clamped firmly by tightening a knurled knob upon a rubber O-ring. This connector is sufficiently light that the micropipette may then be clamped in the beveler in the usual manner. For beveling under these conditions we fill micropipettes with

5 M K-acetate that has been passed through a Nuclepore filter with a pore size of 0.1 μm, which effectively removes contaminants that might plug the tip as the filling solution is driven through it.

IV.2 Pressure-induced Effects upon a Micropipette's Electrical Resistance

Micropipettes planned for beveling to relatively large tips have been formed from Standard Tubing by either the Brown–Flaming or the Industrial Science Associates puller. Using a bevel angle of 25–35°, the tip is lowered into the ring of saline and the pressure of 50 psi is applied to the filling solution. Application of pressure usually causes an immediate drop of micropipette resistance (Brown and Flaming, 1979). The magnitude of this effect varies between micropipettes and is sometimes as much as 30% of the original resistance, which is always restored immediately upon releasing the pressure. This pressure-induced lowering of micropipette resistance was also noted by Kelly (1975), who ascribed it to a bulk flow of electrolyte through the tip. Plamondon *et al.*, (1976) suggest that standard methods of filling micropipettes leave small bubbles in the tip, so compression of such bubbles may also contribute to this effect.

IV.3 Control of Beveling by Measuring Electrical Resistance

While applying steady pressure to the filling solution, the electrical resistance of a micropipette proved stable. If a micropipette tip is to be enlarged considerably by beveling, it may be lowered rather rapidly toward the abrasive surface, since chipping of the tip upon contact is not significant in this case. When tips were beveled with 0–0.25 μm diamond dust, and pressure was not applied to the filling solution, beveling slowed and virtually stopped when the tip had reached a diameter of 2–4 μm, at which time the resistance measured 8–10 MΩ, When pressure was used, beveling ceased in the same range of tip size, but the electrical resistance dropped more smoothly to a final value of only 2–3 MΩ, These results demonstrate the efficacy of pressure upon the filling solution for keeping the tip clear during beveling. For tips larger than 0.5 Ωm, the electrical resistance associated with any desired tip size is readily determined, since tip size may be measured with the light microscope. When the micropipette resistance during beveling approaches the desired final value, it is necessary to lift the tip from the abrasive surface and to release the pressure upon the filling solution to obtain an accurate final resistance value.

IV.4 Control of Beveling by Monitoring Bubble Size

As tip size increases, the electrical resistance of a micropipette becomes a decreasingly sensitive index of tip size and finally becomes ineffective, as shown in Figures 40 and 41. With our methods and instruments, even the more sensitive range of our resistance meter cannot overcome this problem for tip sizes greater than about 4.0 μm. But considerably larger tips are occasionally required for some types of research, such as kidney micropuncture and extracellular injections into localized brain sites.

As shown by Shaw and Lee (1973) and Anderson *et al.* (1974), air may also be driven through the tip to prevent plugging. For the beveling of tips larger than about 4.0 μm, we pass compressed nitrogen through unfilled micropipettes, and the size of the bubbles rising through the saline provides an index of tip size as beveling progresses. For applications where the filling solution during experiments is not suitable for measuring micropipette resistance, this method has the additional advantage that an electrolyte does not have to be removed from the micropipettes prior to filling with the final solution.

In applying this method we have used a 10 × dissecting microscope to monitor the bubbles. At a pressure of 50 psi, a stream of bubbles first became visible when tips were enlarged to 2–4 μm, whereas a pressure of 25 psi gave the same result when the tips were enlarged to 6–8 μm. When the pressure was 10 psi, tip sizes of 20–25 μm yielded considerably larger bubbles that could be measured with an ocular micrometer. By altering pressure and monitoring the bubbles, criteria may thus be adopted to measure tip sizes that extend upward to indefinitely large values. Since contact with the abrasive surface tends to block the flow of bubbles, this method also requires that the tip be lifted slightly to obtain an accurate estimate of tip size, particularly when an accurate measurement is desired at the termination of beveling.

IV.5   Choice of Abrasive

An abrasive surface consisting of 0.05 μm alumina particles can bevel tip sizes up to about 0.5 μm, as shown in Figure 40, and 0–0.25 μm diamond particles have proved highly satisfactory for beveling tip sizes from about 0.5–4.0 μm, as illustrated in the following section of this chapter. Tips larger than 4.0 μm require an even coarser abrasive, and various additional sizes of diamond dust are available from Keen-Kut Products. Diamond dust rated at 0–1.0 μm has proved satisfactory for beveling tips up to a diameter of at least 10 μm, and 1–5 μm diamond dust can bevel tips up to at least 25 μm. These coarser grades of diamond dust seem to reduce plugging of the micropipette tip, probably because the larger abrasive products do not become so tightly compacted. When coarser diamond dust is used to bevel larger tips, the sharpness of the cutting edge is probably reduced; the extent of this effect has not been evaluated, since it may readily be prevented. One method is to break the tip near the desired size (see Figure 50) and then bevel the broken tip with fine diamond dust. In the laboratory of M.M. Merzenich, breaking and then beveling with 0–1.0 μm diamond dust has produced tips in the size range of 20–50 μm. When introduced into the cat brain, even tips of this size penetrated the pia mater with only slight dimpling, and these micropipettes proved satisfactory for injecting a variety of markers and tracers at selected brain sites. Another method, of course, would be to bevel tips to approximate size with a coarse abrasive, followed by final beveling with a finer abrasive for optimal sharpness of the cutting edge.

We have also made abrasive plates embedded with 0.3 μm alumina parti-cles, and their performance has been compared with 0–0.25 μm diamond dust. Beveling with the alumina was slower, and the tip size could be increased to only about 2.0 μm. Tips beveled with the alumina also appeared by SEM to have slightly blunter cutting edges. These differences probably result from the less effective abrasive action of the alumina. This is partly because the hard-ness index of alumina is lower than that of diamond. In addition, the hexagonal shape of 0.3 μm alumina particles probably gives a less effective cutting action than the very jagged diamond particles (see Figure 36). The reduced abrasive action of 0.3 μm alumina probably accounts for our impression that a tip must be more firmly pressed against this abrasive surface to become beveled. Of course the additional pressure would cause more tip bending during beveling, and the tip would then tend to be chipped when lifted from the abrasive sur-face, as described in Section III.1 of this chapter. This probably accounts for the somewhat blunter cutting edges when tips were beveled with 0.3 μm alumina instead of diamond dust. Though diamond dust offers advantages over alumina particles of similar size, 0–0.25 μm diamond dust clumps so strongly that it is more difficult to embed than 0.3 μm alumina. Thus alumina of this size can be a useful alternative for beveling tips in the size range of about 0.5–2.0 μm.

IV.6 Evaluation by SEM of Tips Beveled with Diamond Dust

After beveling micropipette tips with diamond dust, abrasion products often adhere around the tip. Sonication was used to remove most or all of this ma-terial prior to SEM observations, and this may also be advisable prior to using these micropipettes in certain types of experimental work. Figure 43 shows tips beveled with 0–0.25 μm diamond dust. The tip shown in profile (Figure 43A and B) measured 3.4 μm. It was beveled at a preset angle of 25°, and the ob-tained bevel angle was 27°. The view at high magnification in Figure 43(B) shows the cutting edge to be extremely sharp. Though a little abrasive material is still clinging to the back of this tip, the cutting edge itself appears to be uncovered. The slight rounding of this cutting edge is readily accounted for by the 150 Å gold coating, as in the case of the tip beveled with 0.05 μm alumina and shown in Figure 35. This quality of beveling with 0.25 μm diamond dust was not unusual, but was obtained with a high proportion of the tips beveled in this manner. Figure 43(C) shows the beveled face of another micropipette tip that measured 2.4 μm. This tip is almost completely free of abrasive material, and an Omega Dot is visible within its lumen.

The most critical feature of a beveled tip of given size is probably the sharp-ness of the cutting edge, since this must be the main determinant of how well a tip will penetrate into cells or through tissues. When beveling with 0–0.25 μm diamond dust, the sharpness of the cutting edge has proved to be independent of tip size. Hence the sharpness illustrated in Figure 43(A and B) may readily be obtained for tip sizes ranging from 0.5–4.0 μm. If the final beveling of still larger tips is also done with 0–0.25 μm diamond dust, the sharpness illustrated in Figure 43 may be expected for tips of indefinitely large size.

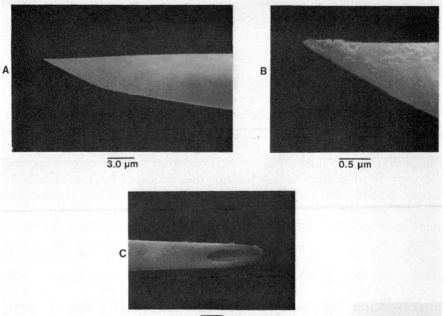

Figure 43. SEM photographs of micropipette tips beveled with 0–0.25 μm diamond dust embedded in Varathane on a glass surface. (A) Profile of tip beveled at a preset angle of about 25°, which yielded a tip beveled at an angle of 27° to an extremely sharp cutting edge and to a tip size of 3.4 μm. (B) Profile of same tip at higher magnification to reveal the sharpness of its cutting edge. (C) The beveled face of another micropipette showing the pore entirely clear of abrasive material. Inside the tip, which measured 2.4 μm, an Omega Dot may be seen. (From Brown and Flaming (1979a), reproduced by permission of Elsevier Biomedical Press B.V., Amsterdam)

PART V   ADDITIONAL BEVELING TECHNIQUES

V.1   Commercial Abrasive Films

Sheets of tough plastic film with a self-adhesive backing, and with 0.3 μm particles of alumina embedded in the surface, are available from Thomas Scientific (P.O. Box 779, Philadelphia, PA 19105-0779, USA). A similar abrasive film without the adhesive backing is made by the 3M Co. under the trade name of 'Imperial Lapping Film'. Thus far, these appear to be the finest abrasives commercially available in sheet form.

The Thomas Scientific product was first used by Anderson *et al.* (1974) to bevel dual-channel micropipettes with tip sizes (measured along the minor axis) that ranged upward from about 0.33 μm. The abrasive film was rotated at 60 rpm by an aluminum disc fitted to a motor, and micropipettes were lowered by a Narishige micromanipulator under direct view of a 30 × dissecting microscope. Though the EM photographs show that the tips were sometimes beveled, breakage was a significant problem and the authors describe the cutting edges as 'somewhat ragged'. These deficiencies probably resulted from the beveling equipment, rather than the abrasive surface, because Baldwin (1980a) also used the Thomas Scientific film and obtained better results. Baldwin's equipment included a precision device similar to our own for rotating the abrasive surface, and the micropipette was advanced by a precision hydraulic micropipette advancer. Following Shaw and Lee (1973), an audio method was used to detect contact of the tip with the abrasive surface. This was done by bringing a piezoelectric crystal into contact with the micropipette shaft, and an amplified audio signal was then led to earphones worn by the operator. It was also reported that the frequency spectrum of this audio signal changed with tip size and that with practice this could be used to monitor the approximate tip size during beveling. In agreement with our own results with 0.3 μm alumina (see Section IV.5 of this chapter), Figure 44 shows that Baldwin obtained beveled tips with reasonably sharp cutting edges. When it is undesirable to fill tips with electrolyte during beveling, the audio method of monitoring tip size may be a useful alternative to our bubble method described in Section IV.4 of this chapter. The lower limit of tip size to which the bubble method may be adapted has not been determined, but the audio method appears useful for tips at least as small as 0.25 μm.

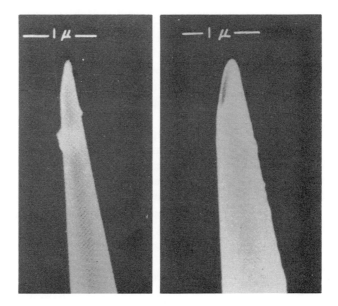

Figure 44. SEM photographs of tips beveled dry. Right: Tip beveled with 0.05 μm alumina particles embedded in Varathane. Left: Tip beveled with 0.3 μm alumina particles embedded in surface of a film, as supplied by Thomas Scientific. (From Baldwin (1980a), reproduced by permission of Elsevier Biomedical Press B.V., Amsterdam)

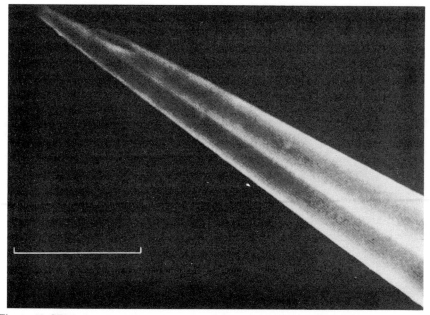

Figure 45. SEM photograph of a dual-channel micropipette beveled dry upon an abrasive surface consisting of 0.3 μm alumina particles embedded in film ('Imperial Lapping Film' made by the 3M Co.). Calibration marker is 1.0 μm. Note that only one barrel is beveled, thus separating the tips of the two channels by about 0.5 μm. (From Werblin (1975), reproduced by permission of The Physiological Society, Cambridge, England)

'Imperial Lapping Film' was first used by Werblin (1975) to separate the tips of dual-channel micropipettes, thus decreasing electrical interaction between the two channels. The dual-channel micropipette was oriented so that only one of the tips made initial contact with the abrasive surface. The bevel angle was set at about 30°, but bending of the tip upon contact made the effective bevel angle much smaller. As shown in Figure 45, this procedure resulted in beveling only one of the two barrels. In the case illustrated, the unbeveled barrel has an outer diameter of about 0.1 μm, and the beveled barrel is displaced backward by about 0.5 μm. Similar results were reportedly obtained with more than 40 dual-channel micropipettes. The extended barrel was not beveled, and the tip of the beveled barrel was displaced from it by 0.5–1.5 μm. This method of separating the tips should improve the performance of dual-channel micropipettes in many research applications. Since this type of beveling does not require the formation of sharp cutting edges, it should not require precision beveling equipment, and this was confirmed by Werblin (1975). In fact, this procedure appears to take advantage of the less efficient abrasive action of 0.3 μm alumina, compared with 0–0.25 μm diamond dust, as discussed in Section IV.5 of this chapter. This feature of 0.3 μm alumina probably permits the tip to make contact and become markedly bent before beveling begins, thus beveling only the lower barrel and sparing the upper one.

Electrical interaction between the two channels of a dual-channel micropipette may be assessed conveniently by measuring the coupling resistance. This is done by passing a known current through one channel and measuring the voltage across the other channel. The coupling resistance is then defined and given by $R_c = E_2/I_1$, where R_c is the coupling resistance, I_1 is the current passed through one channel, and E_2 is the voltage measured across the other channel. One would expect interaction between the two channels to be minimized by a high resistance between the channels, and of course this is true. But coupling resistance is so defined that a lower coupling resistance indicates less interaction between the tips. If the two tips were perfectly coupled, then the voltage (E_2) recorded across the second channel would be identical to the voltage (E_1) used for passing current (I_1) through the other channel. As the two tips are separated to become less coupled, E_2 will fall and the value of R_c will likewise decrease. When Werblin's electrodes were formed by a Livingston puller and filled with 4 M K-acetate, typical resistances were 500 MΩ for the unbeveled barrel and 50 MΩ for the beveled barrel. The typical coupling resistance was about 100 kΩ, which is very low for such fine tips.

V.2 Simplified Beveling Methods

Some recent efforts have been directed toward beveling techniques that require particularly simple and inexpensive instruments and a minimum of experience to operate, while providing satisfactory results for certain applications.

V.2a *Ceric oxide in agar*

Tauchi and Kikuchi (1977) mixed ceric oxide into agar and rotated this abrasive material with a phonograph turntable. The ceric oxide, a polishing compound, was obtained from Buehler Ltd. (2120 Greenwood St., Evanston, IL 60204, USA). The size of the ceric oxide particles was not specified, but it was noted that the lighter and smaller particles remained near the surface of the agar disc, while the larger particles sank toward the bottom. Micropipettes were lowered under visual microscopic control, and beveling was usually accomplished within 3 min. when the turntable was operated at 33 rpm. The softness of the agar apparently protected the tip from damage resulting from either contact with the abrasive medium or wobble during rotation of the abrasive material. The progress of beveling was monitored by measuring micropipette resistance, and final tip sizes ranged from 0.1–0.5 μm. As shown in Figure 46, this procedure yielded beveled tips with sharp cutting edges on single channel micropipettes, and good results were also obtained in beveling only one barrel of a dual-channel micropipette. The single barrel tips were formed by a Livingston puller from borosilicate tubing with an OD/ID of 1.33. In view of the length and flexibility of these tips, the quality of beveling shown in Figure 46 is surprisingly good. It would be helpful to know how reliably this quality of beveling was obtained, but information was not provided on that point. The authors

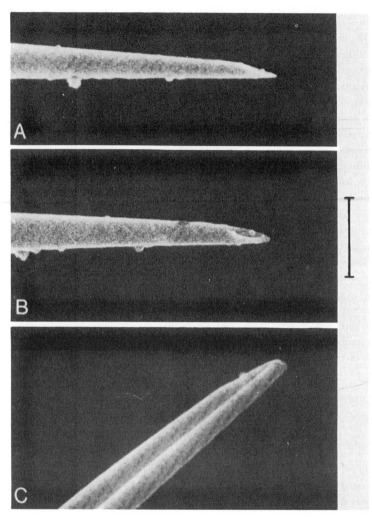

Figure 46. SEM photographs of micropipette tips beveled with ceric oxide in agar. (A and B) Single-channel tip viewed from two different angles. (C) A dual-channel micropipette. Calibration marker is 1.0 μm. (From Tauchi and Kikuchi (1977), reproduced by permission of Springer-Verlag, New York, N.Y.)

found that this beveling technique did not improve the penetration of frog photoreceptors, but it significantly reduced electrode resistance and tip potentials, while also reducing the coupling resistance of dual-channel micropipettes.

V.2b   The jet stream microbeveler

A still simpler beveling device has been described by Ogden *et al.* (1978). As shown in Figure 47, a container of abrasive material was placed upon a magnetic stirrer. The abrasive was Buehler Micropolish (obtained from Buehler Ltd.), which consists of 0.05 μm particles of gamma-alumina suspended in water. This was mixed with saline to render it more conductive, and the abrasive solution was ejected by pressure through a 20-gauge hypodermic needle. A micropipette tip was then lowered into the ejected stream by a 'micromanipulator of mundane design'. The micropipette's electrical impedance was monitored to detect its entry into the stream of abrasive material and to follow the progress of beveling. As shown in Figure 48, evaluation of this method was limited by the quality of the authors' SEM photographs. Reference to their calibration mark indicates that the cutting edge of the illustrated beveled tip was not very sharp and that the tip size in our terminology was at least 0.5 μm. Nevertheless, they report that tips beveled in this manner permitted stable intracellular recordings and adequate injections of HRP during intracellular work in ganglion cells of the frog retina. Hence this beveling technique is probably useful for certain applications, but further testing is required to assess its capabilities and limitations.

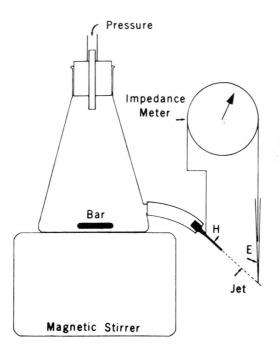

Figure 47. Diagram of jet stream microbeveler. A suspension of 0.05 μm particles of alumina is prevented from settling by a magnetic stirrer, and this abrasive material is ejected by pressure through a 20-gauge hypodermic needle (H). The tip of a micropipette (E) is held in the jet stream by a micromanipulator, while micropipette impedance is monitored by a meter. (From Ogden *et al.* (1978), Copyright 1978 by the AAAS, which granted permission for this reproduction)

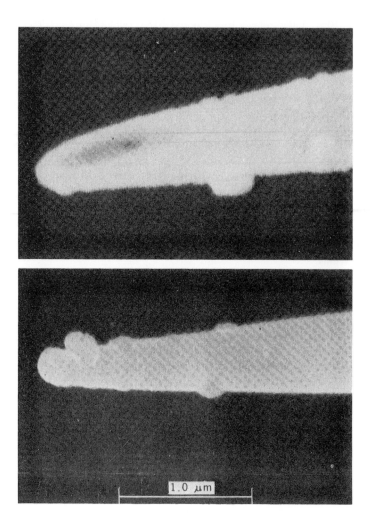

Figure 48. (Top) SEM photograph of micropipette filled with 0.2 M KCl and beveled by the jet stream microbeveler from 300 to 100 MΩ. (Bottom) SEM photograph of unbeveled micropipette with an impedance of 300 MΩ. (From Ogden *et al.* (1978), Copyright 1978 by the AAAS, which granted permission for this reproduction)

V.2c Thick slurry beveling

A beveling method that closely approaches the ultimate in simplicity has been described by Lederer *et al.* (1979). For their research in voltage clamping cardiac Purkinje fibers in sheep, these authors found the jet stream beveler to be effective, but the required beveling time was 'upwards of 30 min'. They then adopted an abrasive formed by mixing Buehler Micropolish (20% by volume) with 3M KCl, which was placed in a flat container such as a petri dish. The

0.05 μm alumina particles quickly precipitated out to form a dense 'settled slurry' beneath the KCl supernatant, as shown in Figure 49. The flat container was then rotated at 10 rpm by a clock motor, micropipettes were lowered until the tips just brushed the surface of the settled slurry, and the progress of beveling was monitored by measuring electrical resistance. Since the abrasive slurry was relatively soft, the tip was unlikely to be damaged by either lowering the tip or rotation of the slurry. Yet the slurry was dense enough for relatively rapid beveling. Within limits, beveling was speeded by thinning the layer of settled slurry. When the slurry was 0.3 mm thick, micropipettes filled with 3 M KCl were beveled from initial resistances of 10–20 MΩ to a final resistance of 3 MΩ in about 10 min, and when the thickness of the slurry was reduced to 0.1 mm, similar results were obtained in only about 1 min. These beveled electrodes were reported to penetrate through the tough connective sheath of cardiac Purkinje fibers, and then into the fibers themselves, as readily as unbeveled electrodes with resistances of 10 MΩ or more. This method seemed promising, but pictures of beveled tips were not provided. Amthor (1984) found the original thick slurry method unsuitable for reliably beveling fine tips and described modifications of the technique that were claimed to work well with fine tips. Though an illustrated tip was well beveled to a tip size of about 0.4 μm, no indication was given of the lower limit of tip size that could be handled. Thus further work is also required to evaluate the capabilities and limitations of slurry beveling.

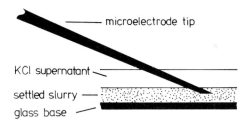

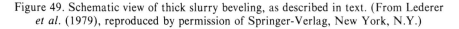

Figure 49. Schematic view of thick slurry beveling, as described in text. (From Lederer *et al.* (1979), reproduced by permission of Springer-Verlag, New York, N.Y.)

V.3   Breaking Tips Preparatory to Beveling or Fire-polishing

If relatively large beveled tips are required, it is helpful to break micropipettes close to the desired tip size prior to beveling. Figure 50 shows a method described by Gardner (1978) and illustrated by McGrath and Solter (1985) as the first step in making beveled Pyrex® tips with outer diameters of about 25 μm. Using a De Fonbrune microforge equipped with a platinum filament of 0.1 mm diameter, a bead of molten Pyrex® is first formed at the tip of the heating filament. The De Fonbrune microforge provides a stream of air over the heating filament, to assure that heat is transferred only by contact, and this air flow should be maximum. As shown in Figure 50(A), the molten glass is brought into contact with the micropipette and allowed to fuse with it where the micropipette has the desired tip size. Upon switching off the heating current, the continuing stream of air rapidly cools the molten glass, which must establish strains in the lower part of the micropipette where it is fused with the glass bead. The heating filament is cooling simultaneously, and as it cools it retracts. It seems unlikely that this retraction would break the micropipette cleanly unless a weak point had been established. But the zone of fusion with the glass bead has been weakened by rapid cooling, and retraction of the heating filament would exert maximum strain where the glass bead loses contact with the micropipette tip. Thus a clean break occurs at that point, as shown in Figure 50(B). This process may be likened to scoring glass tubing and then stressing it, to break the tubing at the desired position. In fact, Brown *et al.* (1984) report that scoring with a diamond knife may also be used to break micropipettes to predetermined diameters. But the microforge method would appear to provide better control and more reliable diameters, particularly in the lower range of tip sizes.

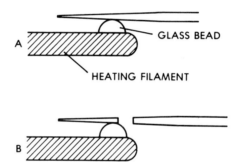

Figure 50. Method of breaking micropipette tips to predetermined size. For details, see text. (Redrawn from McGrath and Solter (1985), reproduced by permission of Plenum Publishing Corporation, N.Y.)

Procedures for controlled breaking of tips may also be used to form suction micropipettes of various sizes, which are then fire-polished by bringing the tip close to an appropriate heat source. Suction micropipettes may be used to hold isolated cells during a variety of procedures. For example, McGrath and Solter (1985) employed the microforge method with a 0.3 mm heating filament to form suction micropipettes with outer diameters of about 75 μm, which were used to hold mouse embryos during microsurgery. Suction micropipettes have also been used to hold isolated cells during penetration by a fine micropipette or during exchange of the cytoplasm by intracellular perfusion (Brown *et al.*, 1984). They may likewise be used for patch clamping (see Chapter 17).

In addition to methods of controlled breaking, recent modifications of our micropipette puller have now made it possible to form tips directly with inner diameters up to at least 19 μm (see Section IV.1 of Chapter 18).

V.4   Forming a Spearpoint on a Beveled Tip

Though beveling sharpens micropipettes, the beveled edge may still encounter considerable resistance to cell penetration when the tip must be large. McGrath and Solter found that their beveled tips of 25 μm outer diameter could not penetrate adequately for transplanting the pronuclei of mouse embryos. Hence they employed a procedure for pointing the tip that had been mentioned by Hoppe and Illmensee (1977). The beveled tip was brought into contact with the 0.1 mm platinum heating filament of a De Fonbrune microforge, and a spearpoint was formed upon the beveled tip when it was withdrawn, as shown in Figure 51. Maximum air flow from the microforge was also used during this procedure. Heat transfer was thus localized to a minimum central portion of the beveled tip, and rapid cooling of the glass prevented the spearpoint from becoming unduly long. This spearpoint sufficiently improved the penetrating abilities of beveled tips to meet their requirements. Hence this technique may be useful in a variety of applications when cell membranes or tissues must be penetrated by unusually large micropipettes.

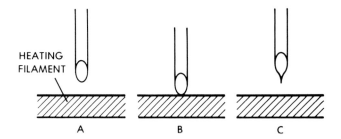

Figure 51. Method of forming a spearpoint on a beveled micropipette tip, as described in text. (Redrawn from McGrath and Solter (1985), reproduced by permission of Plenum Publishing Corporation, New York, N.Y.)

PART VI   COMPARISON OF BEVELING METHODS

The heart of any method of beveling micropipettes is the type of abrasive and how it is applied to the tip during beveling. These factors determine the quality of beveling attainable and also the instrumentation and experience required to attain optimal results.

Abrasives are available that meet all currently envisioned needs for beveling borosilicate glass. In the case of our own beveler, the use of 0.05 μm alumina and various grades of diamond dust has provided tips with extremely sharp cutting edges that closely approach the theoretical limit. The bevel angles can be closely controlled, and tips can be beveled that vary from about 0.06 μm to indefinitely large sizes. In view of these results, the quality of beveling is limited very little, if at all, by the availability of appropriate abrasives. Instead, it is determined by how those abrasives are applied to a micropipette tip, so beveling techniques are best compared on that basis.

Abrasives have thus far been applied by three general methods. (1) The abrasive is suspended in saline that is moved rapidly past an immersed micropipette tip. (2) The abrasive is densely concentrated in a soft medium, such as agar or a slurry of the abrasive itself, that is moved rapidly past an immersed tip. (3) The abrasive is embedded in a surface that is moved rapidly over the tip. Experience has been gained with all three of these methods in the case of 0.05 μm alumina. These methods may also be compared on the basis of some logical consequences, pending the availability of a more complete experimental comparison.

Beveling by Method 1 is much the slowest of the three methods. This limitation was reported by Kripke and Ogden (1974) when 0.05 μm alumina was suspended in saline and rotated upon a glass disc. When a similar suspension of abrasive was applied by the jet stream beveler, Ogden *et al.* (1978) reported more rapid beveling, but Lederer *et al.* (1979) found that the jet stream method was likewise excessively slow, requiring 'upwards of 30 min'. Such slow beveling probably stems from two factors that make this method of applying the abrasive inefficient. First, because the suspended particles are free to move within the saline, they cannot be pressed against the tip. So they only brush lightly over the tip and provide very little abrasive action. Second, with the jet stream method the suspension must be ejected forcefully through a small needle, so its viscosity must be kept low, and the concentration of suspended abrasive cannot be as high as required for efficient abrasion.

Another limitation of jet stream beveling is the considerable difficulty of controlling bevel angles. Ogden *et al.* (1978) state that the stream of abrasive had to be directed at an angle of about 45° from the tip to obtain beveled tips like the one shown in Figure 48, which has a bevel angle of about 30°. This is because the jet stream itself bends the tip to a much smaller bevel angle than the one that is preset. Since the tip is immersed in the stream of abrasive, it cannot straighten as beveling proceeds. Though tip bending may be compensated for, this is inconvenient and can only be approximate because the amount of tip bending will vary greatly with factors such as tip size and tip length. A more surprising difficulty was found in the laboratory of Albert J. Berger at the University of Washington (personal communication), who observed that the jet stream method had a strong tendency to clog fine tips, although that problem was not encountered with Method 3.

With Method 2 the concentration of abrasive may be increased greatly by applying it in a slurry or suspending it in a soft medium such as agar. This method also restricts the movement of abrasive particles, which may be regarded as semi-embedded. With agar, particle movement is restricted by the gelatinous consistency of the medium, while in a slurry the movement of a particle is restricted by the relatively dense packing of the particles themselves. By thus restricting particle movement, each particle is pressed harder against the tip than if it were suspended in saline, and the abrasive action becomes more effective. Hence this method reduces beveling time. But the tip is still immersed in the abrasive, and although this method does not require that the abrasive be moved past the tip at high velocity, the greater density of the abrasive medium must increase drag on the tip. Thus tip bending remains a significant problem in the control of bevel angle. For example, Tauchi and Kikuchi (1977) found that final bevel angles were only 15–20° when micropipettes were held at an angle of 35–40° to the surface of their agar-embedded abrasive.

With Method 3 the abrasive is tightly embedded in a flat surface, so each particle of abrasive may be pressed harder against the tip as the tip passes over it, further improving the efficiency of the abrasive action. Though exact comparisons are not available, beveling time is probably shortened considerably from that of Method 2. In addition, the tip is not immersed in an abrasive medium, but is pressed against a flat abrasive surface, so the tip can straighten to the preset bevel angle as beveling proceeds. Thus the preset bevel angle can accurately and conveniently control the final bevel angle (see Figure 43), despite the many factors influencing how much bending occurs during beveling.

The limited evidence available for Methods 1 and 2 does not permit accurate comparison of the three methods in terms of reliability, sharpness of the cutting edge, or the minimum tip size that may be beveled. Method 3 should produce the sharpest cutting edges, however, for two reasons. First, the abrasive in Method 3 is confined to a single plane and can move over the beveled tip only in that plane. By contrast, in Methods 1 and 2 the tip is immersed in an abrasive medium; as the abrasive material moves past it, the tip must inevitably oscillate in this abrasive medium, which would tend to dull the cutting edge. Second, the termination of beveling by Method 3 need not dull the cutting edge, as indicated in Section III.1 of this chapter. With Methods 1 and 2, however, beveling must be terminated by either withdrawing the tip from the moving abrasive medium or by slowing and stopping the abrasive. In either event the tip would straighten and the cutting edge would tend to be dulled as beveling ceases. It may also be significant that Method 3 has been demonstrated to bevel somewhat finer tips than reported to date for Methods 1 and 2. In the case of Method 2, immersion of the tip in a dense medium is especially likely to break the finest and most delicate tips (Amthor, 1984).

PART VII ADVANTAGES OF BEVELING

VII.1 Some Theoretical Considerations

Of course the difficulty of penetrating a cell membrane, or any other type of tissue, increases with tip size. If the tip is unbeveled, the resistance to its penetration should be roughly proportional to the area of the tip, so the difficulty of penetrating with unbeveled tips probably rises exponentially as the square of the tip diameter. By contrast, beveling forms an almost straight cutting edge, and the resistance to its penetration should increase approximately linearly with tip diameter. Based upon these simplifying assumptions, Figure 52 shows the relative difficulty of penetration as a function of tip size for both beveled and unbeveled tips. The difficulty of penetration with 0.05 μm tips is assigned a value of 1.0, and this same value is used for both beveled and unbeveled tips,

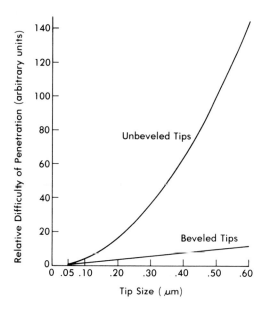

Figure 52. Relative difficulty of penetration, as a function of tip size, for both beveled and unbeveled micropipette tips. Curves are theoretical functions, as described in text.

based upon our results in toad rods (see the following section of this chapter). As tip size increases from 0.05 to 0.50 μm, Figure 52 shows that the difficulty of penetrating with beveled tips rises linearly by a factor of 10, whereas with unbeveled tips it rises exponentially by a factor of 100.

Since it is unlikely that our simplifying assumptions are strictly valid, the numerical values in Figure 52 can only be approximations. But this figure provides a graphic explanation of two important points. (1) It indicates why the size of unbeveled tips is so critical for high quality intracellular work. In toad rods, for example, increasing the size of unbeveled tips from 0.05 to 0.15 μm alters intracellular results from excellent to marginal. In this example the absolute increase of tip diameter is only 0.1 μm, and tip diameter is only tripled, but Figure 52 shows that the difficulty of cell penetration is probably increased by a factor of about nine. (2) The advantages of beveling increase rapidly with tip size, as demonstrated in the following section. Figure 52 also explains this result, since beveling is shown to provide a rapidly increasing reduction in the difficulty of cell penetration as tip size increases.

VII.2   Cell Penetration

When our beveling techniques were developed, they greatly improved the capability of penetrating small cells without significant damage, as indicated by our experience in penetrating photoreceptors and other types of cells in the retina of the snapping turtle. At that time the Industrial Science Associates puller was used to form relatively short tips that were stiff enough to work well in this preparation. But the tip size averaged about 0.15 μm, and unbeveled tips of that size yielded only rare penetrations of cells, which usually deteriorated too rapidly for satisfactory intracellular work. When these tips were minimally beveled, however, stable intracellular recordings were readily obtained (Brown and Flaming, 1974).

During that same period Sheldon S. Miller, working in another laboratory of our department, compared beveled and unbeveled micropipette electrodes for intracellular recording in retinal pigment epithelium cells of the frog. Micropipettes were all formed on the Livingston puller at constant settings. A group of 233 cells was examined with unbeveled electrodes, and another group of 111 cells was studied with electrodes minimally beveled on our instrument. Beveling improved both the frequency of cell penetration and the stability of membrane potentials. In addition, Figure 53 shows that the entire distribution of the number of cells penetrated, as a function of the initial membrane potential, was shifted toward numerically larger membrane potentials. The initial resting membrane potential averaged -82 mV with unbeveled tips and became

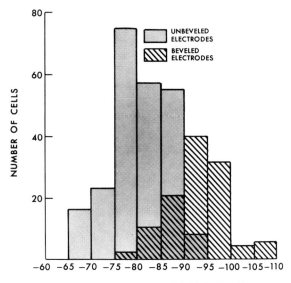

Figure 53. Frequency histogram of number of cells with initial membrane potentials in various ranges, using both unbeveled and beveled micropipette electrodes. Recordings obtained from retinal pigment epithelium cells of the frog. These cells were exposed by removing the retina, and the initial membrane potential was recorded just after penetrating the apical membrane of each cell. The Livingston puller was used at constant settings to form micropipettes, some of which were then beveled on our instrument. (From unpublished work by permission of Sheldon S. Miller, School of Optometry, University of California, Berkeley, CA 94720, USA)

−93 mV when the tips were minimally beveled. Since beveled tips should cut more cleanly through the cell membrane, and thus seal better into the membrane, this probably accounts for both the numerically larger initial membrane potentials and the improved stability of membrane potentials.

Following the development of our micropipette puller, the smaller and shorter tips that it provided gave greatly improved results for intracellular recording in the outer and inner segments of toad rods (see Chapter 13). In that work the tip size averaged only 0.05–0.06 μm, and although beveling seemed to provide a slight improvement of performance, it was no longer required and its effects were minimal in value. Providing that target cells can be reached by ultrafine tips in this size range, it thus appears that beveling is no longer needed or helpful for penetrating small cells to record resting membrane potentials or electrical responses of the cell membrane. But if larger tips must be used, either to reach the target cells or to lower micropipette resistance to the flow of electrical current or experimental substances, then beveling becomes very helpful. Its advantages under these conditions include more frequent penetration of target cells, numerically larger resting membrane potentials, and improved stability of the cell's condition after penetration.

VII.3   Reduction of a Micropipette's Electrical Resistance and Capacitance

In some types of intracellular work, a minimal electrical resistance of the micropipette is either desirable or required. If one starts with a small enough tip to penetrate a given type of cell without damage, an advantage of beveling is that this tip may be enlarged to reduce its electrical resistance, while maintaining a sharp enough cutting edge that the enlarged tip can still penetrate the cell without significant damage.

Reduction of a micropipette's electrical resistance reduces the noise level of all electrical recordings, thus improving the signal/noise ratio, an effect of particular importance in detecting weak signals. In addition to reducing electrical resistance, beveling reduces the micropipette's capacitance, because it removes that portion of the tip where the glass wall is thinnest. The time constant (t) of a micropipette is given by $t = RC$, where R and C are the micropipette's electrical resistance and capacitance. The combined effects of lowering both R and C will thus lower the micropipette's time constant and improve its ability to record accurately the time course of rapid electrical events such as nerve impulses.

VII.4   Injection of Material Into Cells

In many types of intracellular work, it is necessary to inject material from a micropipette into the intracellular medium. This may be done for a variety of reasons. (1) The cell may be marked for later histological identification. (2) The ionic composition of the cytoplasm may be altered experimentally. (3) Substances may be injected to manipulate the cell's genetic makeup or to alter the mechanisms controlling various aspects of the cell's activities. This latter field has already become extremely important in both cell physiology and medicine and it is proliferating rapidly. If the substance to be injected bears a net electrical charge, it may be driven into the cell iontophoretically. If not, pressure may be used, though this 'is generally more difficult. In either event, injections may be greatly facilitated by using beveling to lower the micropipette's resistance to the flow of materials through it.

VII.5 Collection of Fluid Samples

Of course beveling is similarly helpful when micropipettes are used to collect samples from relatively large fluid compartments. In kidney micropuncture work, for example, micropipettes with tip diameters of 4–12 μm may be used to collect fluid from the various segments of a mammalian nephron. Cytoplasm may also be sampled in this way, mainly from relatively large cells.

VII.6 Penetration of Tissues to Reach Target Cells or Target Areas

Beveling can also assist in penetrating tissues that must be traversed to reach a target cell or target area. This advantage is especially great when relatively tough tissues cover a target cell in which intracellular work is to be conducted. In some cases of this type, unbeveled tips small enough for intracellular work in the target cell are broken consistently by the tough overlying tissues. If the micropipette is beveled to a somewhat larger tip with a sharp cutting edge, the tip has greater strength for penetrating tough tissues without being broken, and the sharp cutting edge permits the target cell to be penetrated without damage by the enlarged tip. In other cases the target cell or area is deeply buried in relatively soft tissue such as the brain, and beveling also assists under these conditions, especially if relatively large tips must be used. By smoothing the traverse of overlying tissue, damage to this tissue is reduced. In addition, relatively large unbeveled tips are prone to plugging because tissue can readily enter the orifice, and beveling relieves this problem by permitting the tip to slide through the tissue instead of pressing against it. For example, A.J. Berger (personal communication) finds that beveling with our instrument assists in penetrating the pia mater and in reducing tip plugging en route to target cells in the brain, following which it proved helpful for injecting horseradish peroxidase (HRP) into inspiratory neurons of the tractus solitarius of the cat (Berger *et al.* 1984).

VII.7 Improved Tip Separation with Dual-channel Micropipettes

As shown by Figure 45, beveling may be used to better separate the terminal pores of a dual-channel micropipette. This increases the independence of the two channels, as indicated by the decreased coupling resistance, thus improving the performance of dual-channel micropipettes for a variety of applications, such as voltage clamping.

VII.8 Microsurgery

By improving the penetration of cell membranes, beveling improves the performance of micropipettes in certain types of microsurgery, such as the transplantation of intracellular organelles. An excellent example is the work of McGrath and Solter (1985), who used beveled and spear-pointed micropipettes to extract the pronuclei from one mouse embryo and insert them into another mouse embryo from which the original pronuclei had been removed. This operation was performed with a high success rate, as judged by subsequent viability of the embryo with the transplanted pronuclei.

CHAPTER 10

Filling Micropipettes: Techniques and Solutions

PART I   FILLING TECHNIQUES

I.1   Why Micropipettes Are Difficult to Fill

As stated by Purves (1981), 'Water would rather be in contact with glass than with air, as illustrated by the well-known phenomenon of capillary rise.' Hence the surface energies assist in filling the tip of a micropipette with an aqueous solution. The difficulty results from viscous resistance to flow, which according to Purves (1981) is inversely proportional to at least the third power of tip radius in the case of a long conical tube. Since viscous resistance to flow rises rapidly as tip size decreases, the filling of fine and ultrafine tips can be particularly difficult.

I.2   Early Methods of Filling Micropipettes

Following the work of Graham and Gerard (1946), many methods were devised for filling micropipettes, each of which had distinct limitations and

149

disadvantages. Purves (1981) describes 12 such methods and discusses the advantages and disadvantages of each. Since these early methods have been well described elsewhere and have all become either obsolete or little used, they will not be treated here.

I.3   The Fiber Filling Method

I.3a   The original technique

A highly satisfactory method of filling fine micropipette tips was first developed by Kyoji Tasaki and his co-workers (Tasaki *et al.*, 1968). This method was quickly adopted by almost all investigators using micropipettes, and its advantages proved so compelling that it has remained the method of choice.

As originally described, a small bundle of glass fibers was inserted through a piece of capillary tubing before mounting the tubing in a micropipette puller. The glass fibers were about 20 μm in diameter, and 5–10 of them were used with capillary tubing of about 1.0 mm outer diameter. A pair of micropipettes was then formed in the usual manner. Later examination by both light and electron microscopy revealed no traces of glass fibers in the orifice of the tip, but light microscopy showed that the individual glass fibers tapered toward the micropipette tip. Though Tasaki *et al.* (1968) did not describe the fate of these fiber terminals, we have also used this filling method and have noted that the fiber terminals fuse to the inner wall of the micropipette. This occurs far enough behind the tip itself that the fiber terminals may be observed by light microscopy. To fill the tip, a long 30-gauge hypodermic needle was inserted until it was stopped by the tip taper, and electrolyte was injected by a syringe while the needle was withdrawn. Filling of the tip was usually completed during this process, so microelectrodes could be used immediately.

Dye solutions were used to observe directly the filling of a tip under the microscope. Fluid was noted to flow rapidly along the glass fibers by capillary action and to reach the tip 'almost instantaneously', while air in the fiber-free portion of the shank moved backward and formed a bubble in the shaft that could be removed readily by reinjection. In a gradually tapering shank 20–30 mm in length, several bubbles usually formed that were not removed. But they did not appear to affect the quality of the microelectrodes, since electrical continuity was maintained through the fine channels that were filled with electrolyte by capillary action.

Since this method introduces glass fibers that fuse with the wall just behind the tip, these fibers must thicken the wall at the tip. As in the case of a single large Omega Dot (see Sections I.1 and II.4 of Chapter 7), these multiple fibers must thus increase OD_t/ID_t and decrease tip size. We were originally surprised that it was possible to obtain an occasional ultrafine tip from the Industrial Science Associates puller, as reported in Section III.2 of Chapter 9. But at that time we were inserting a rather large bundle of glass fibers, for purposes of filling the tip, and these fibers must have decreased tip size according to the principles revealed in Part III of Chapter 6. We have also noted that with this filling method the electrical resistance of micropipettes increases when more glass fibers are inserted. This may be similarly explained, since more fibers should further decrease tip size and thus increase electrical resistance.

I.3b   The 'Omega Dot' method

Though the original fiber filling method worked well, it was quickly simplified and improved. This resulted from the observation that a single glass fiber, fused to the inner surface of a glass capillary over its entire length, could replace the original bundle of glass fibers. For reasons given in the first paragraph of Chapter 7, we refer to such a fiber as an Omega Dot. Its diameter is not crucial, but in the case of Standard Tubing its diameter is 100 μm. Figure 29 shows that both sides of an Omega Dot form acute angles with the inner surface of the capillary tubing, and these acute angles provide strong capillary action. Figure 29 also shows that during tip formation the Omega Dot fuses more completely with the wall of the tubing, a progressive effect that becomes maximum at the tip itself. As this occurs, angles between the Omega Dot and tubing become less acute and thus less favorable for capillary action. A significant capillary action undoubtedly remains at the tip itself in cases like the one shown in Figure 29, but capillary action would be greatly reduced and perhaps negligible at the tip shown in Figure 31.

The mechanism of filling the tip by an Omega Dot is shown in Figure 54. When solution is injected at the shoulder of a micropipette, it flows toward the tip by capillary action in the hydraulic channels on both sides of the Omega Dot, as shown in Figure 54 (A and B). Though rapid, this capillary flow may be observed under a microscope if the tapering tip is watched closely. The tip itself then suddenly fills with a rush. This very sudden filling of the fine tip makes it unlikely that fluid is carried all the way to the tip by the Omega Dot channels. Instead, when the Omega Dot has carried the solution close to the tip, a critical point is probably reached in the narrowing lumen where the solution suddenly fills the lumen and then rushes toward the tip by capillary action of the lumen itself. Of course this would only be possible by ejecting air from the tip; apparently this occurs readily because very little air must be ejected from the short and very small final section of the tip. If the terminal section of the tip fills by capillary action of the lumen, a greatly reduced capillary action of the Omega Dot at the tip itself (in certain cases like the tip shown in Figure 31) would have no adverse effect upon filling of the tip. The situation just after filling the tip itself is shown in Figure 54(C). The shaft has also been filled by continuing to inject while withdrawing the needle, and these two volumes of solution are connected by the hydraulic channels beside the Omega Dot. This leaves in the shank at least one bubble, which sometimes separates into several bubbles. These have little or no significance in many cases because of the electrical continuity provided by the Omega Dot channels. As shown in Figure 54(C), however, a bubble in a tapered channel with tip downward will have a smaller radius of curvature in its lower meniscus than in its upper meniscus. Thus surface tension will be stronger in the lower meniscus, producing a tendency for the bubble to rise. But this could not occur unless fluid could move from the upper compartment into the lower one. The Omega Dot also solves this problem by providing the requisite channels for the upper compartment to fill the lower one as the bubble rises. So any bubbles originally trapped in the shank will rise up to the shoulder of the micropipette, where they may be removed by reinjection. In our laboratory we usually fill the tips late one afternoon, store them tip downward in a closed moist chamber, then reinject them the next morning just before use.

Of course bubbles are most readily removed from tips that taper rapidly, and their removal can become difficult in the case of long tips with little taper. When bubbles must be removed from such tips, it is helpful to apply mild heat, especially in combination with mechanical agitation.

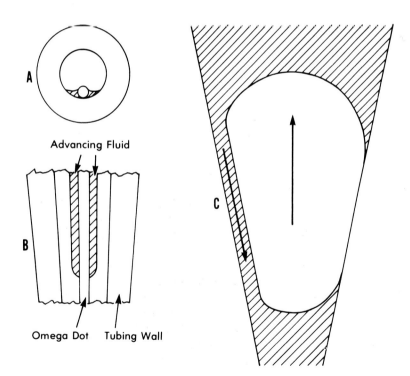

Figure 54. The mechanism of tip filling by an Omega Dot. (A) Cross section of the shank showing the fluid channels that form on either side of the Omega Dot. (B) Longitudinal section of a segment of the shank showing fluid advancing toward the tip on either side of the Omega Dot. (C) Schematic illustration of the shank after injection of fluid at the shoulder. As described in text, the bubble moves upward while fluid continues to flow toward the tip through the Omega Dot channels. (Part (C) of this illustration redrawn from Purves (1981), reproduced by permission of Academic Press, Orlando, Florida)

I.3c   Injection of solution

Commercial hypodermic needles are not long enough to inject solution at the shoulders of micropipettes with relatively long shafts. This problem may be handled by obtaining stainless steel tubing, cutting and dressing it to the requisite length, and then sealing it into a larger hypodermic needle. For glass capillary tubings that have minimal clearance for injection, such as our Tubings 1 or 9 for fine tips (see Sections I.2 and I.4 of Chapter 8), stainless steel tubing can be obtained with values of OD and ID as small as about 0.2 and 0.1 mm, respectively. Such tubing is available from Tube Sales (2211 Tubeway, Los Angeles, CA 90040, USA).

I.3d   Advantages of the fiber filling method

Compared with the 12 earlier filling methods described by Purves (1981), the fiber filling method has important advantages. There is no need for special equipment to provide a partial vacuum or heating of the filling solution, and the method is relatively insensitive to particulate contamination because the filling solution need not pass through the tip. Tips are filled with minimal effort and sufficiently rapidly that an entire batch of micropipettes may be filled within a few minutes. If the initial bubbles are not a problem, filling may thus be done just before an experiment, and additional micropipettes may even be filled during an experiment. If micropipettes are filled with a strong K^+ solution, which is well known to attack either soft or borosilicate glass, rapid filling also reduces the time during which K^+ can attack and enlarge the tip and reduce its efficiency in penetrating cells. Tips are also filled reliably and well. When Tasaki *et al.* (1968) compared fiber filling with the 'boiling' or 'alcohol' methods described by Purves (1981), the fiber method was reported to reduce electrode resistance by about half. Finally, in the case of multi-barrel micropipettes, the various barrels may readily be filled with different solutions.

I.3e   Advantages of Omega Dot over the original fiber filling method

In this comparison the Omega Dot offers at least four improvements. (1) Considerable time is saved by not having to insert a bundle of fibers into each section of capillary tubing before mounting it in the puller. (2) Unless special precautions are taken, inserted glass fibers fall out of a capillary tube mounted in a vertical puller, so the Omega Dot is more convenient for vertical pullers. (3) Inserted glass fibers are often broken by the needle when solution is injected at the shoulder, andthe resulting loose fibers can be a nuisance, a problem eliminated by the Omega Dot. (4) The electrical resistance of a micropipette increases with the number of fibers inserted, which is difficult to control. Thus the electrical resistance of micropipettes is more reliable with the Omega Dot.

PART II   FILLING SOLUTIONS

II.1   High Molarity Potassium Solutions

II.1a   Composition of solutions

In the early work of Graham and Gerard (1946) and Ling and Gerard (1949), micropipettes were filled with 'isotonic KCl'. Soon thereafter, it became common practice to use 3 M KCl as the filling solution. This higher molarity is close to the saturation point of KCl, and it was adopted to reduce the resistance of micropipette tips. According to Purves (1981), this strategy is not very successful because of mixing between solutions inside and outside the tip. As a consequence, he states, raising the molarity of KCl in the micropipette from 0.15 to 3.0 (a factor of 20) only decreases the tip resistance by a factor of about 7. Still later, many workers adopted K-acetate to further reduce tip resistance, since it could be used in a concentration as high as 5 M without becoming saturated. We thus used 5 M K-acetate as the filling solution in much of our early work, and it is probably the solution of choice for minimizing micropipette resistance.

II.1b   Micropipette electrical resistance

Using 5 M K-acetate as the filling solution, and with the tips in a bath of 0.15 M KCl, we measured the electrical resistance of a batch of 18 micropipettes. These were formed from Standard Tubing by our model P-77B puller, using puller settings that produced consistent ultrafine tips averaging about 9.0 mm in length. Though the Omega Dot filling method is not very sensitive to contaminants in the solution, we routinely distill and de-ionize the water and then filter the filling solution through a 0.1 μm Nuclepore filter. When first tested about 40 min after filling, the average micropipette resistance was 172 MΩ; after another 4 hr the average value was 140 MΩ, and when first tested the next morning it was 93 MΩ. Micropipettes were then reinjected to remove bubbles at the shoulder, after which the average resistance was 84 MΩ and the range was from 70–130 MΩ. These are the values that would have pertained if we had used these micropipettes for an experiment. On the next two successive mornings, the average resistance dropped further to 65 and then 51 MΩ.

These results illustrate three points. First, these resistances are quite low compared with ultrafine tips formed on a Livingston puller (and resistance may be lowered still further by reducing tip length from 9.0 to about 6.0 mm). Second, micropipette resistances fell consistently when measured on successive days, almost certainly because of strong K$^+$ solution attacking and enlarging the tips. Third, the measured variability of electrical resistance among a batch of ultrafine tips seems satisfactory for most purposes. Though it may be higher than desired for some special cases, it can undoubtedly be reduced significantly by making all ultrafine tips from a single section of tubing only a few feet long (see Section IV.2c of Chapter 15). In addition, the variability of both tip size and electrical resistance drop markedly at tip sizes larger than the ultrafine range (see Section IV.2b of Chapter 15 and Section IV.2 of Chapter 5).

II.2   Isotonic KCl

It is generally assumed that minimizing tip resistance will minimize the noise level of a micropipette electrode. Some years ago, however, we accidentally learned that this is not always the case. For injections of Procion yellow into toad rods, we mixed the Procion yellow into 0.15 M KCl and filled micropipettes with this solution. Since Procion yellow has low conductivity, the KCl was added to improve intracellular recordings of light-evoked responses from photoreceptors. But the molarity of KCl was kept low, so that passage of current would be effective in driving Procion yellow into cells. The noise levels of these micropipettes proved surprisingly low. Compared with 5 M K-acetate, we then found that micropipettes filled only with 0.15 M KCl had higher resistances by a factor of about 10, but the noise level of intracellular recordings was consistently decreased. At this point we had come full circle and were back to the isotonic KCl of Graham and Gerard (1946). Since this solution closely matches the concentration of KCl in the cytoplasm, it should minimize any tendency for the *net* movement of K^+ between micropipette and cytoplasm to vary from moment to moment, and this is probably why the noise level is reduced. The actual extent of noise reduction is difficult to document, since the same micropipettes cannot be used to compare different filling solutions during intracellular recordings. As a rule, however, the reduction of noise level when using 0.15 M KCl instead of 5 M K-acetate was at least 50%. The typically low noise levels thus obtained during intracellular recordings from toad photoreceptors are illustrated in Figures. 74, 76 and 77. Mainly because of its low noise level, which is particularly helpful when recording small signals, 0.15 M KCl has now been adopted as a filling solution by a number of investigators.

This filling solution offers several other advantages. Compared with more concentrated K^+ solutions, the problem of K^+ attack upon fine tips is doubtless reduced, while the contribution of a K^+ diffusion potential to the tip potential should be eliminated entirely. In addition, Stoner *et al.* (1984) demonstrated by direct measurement that K^+ leaks from tips of micropipettes filled with 3 M KCl, and this effect increases with lowered micropipette resistance (presumably associated with the larger tips in a given batch). With relatively low resistance micropipettes, impaled red blood cells of *Amphiuma* were also shown to swell and depolarize, presumably due to K^+ leaking into the cells. Fromm and Schultz (1981) have shown by direct measurement that K^+ leakage decreases about five-fold when the molarity of KCl in micropipettes is decreased from 3.0 to 0.5. Tips filled with 0.15 M KCl should either eliminate K^+ leakage entirely or reduce it to an insignificant level, even in the case of relatively large tips.

A final point concerns pH of the filling solution, which has been little studied. Purves (1981) suggests that a pH below 7 is desirable to prevent 'alkaline attack of the glass' and recommends a pH of about 4 to reduce the tip potential of micropipettes filled with KCl. In our case we buffer 0.15 M KCl to a pH of 7. Empirically this appears close to the optimal pH for the minimal noise level of intracellular recordings, but this subject requires further investigation.

CHAPTER 11

Advancing Micropipettes through Tissues
and into Cells

PART I   MICROMANIPULATORS

Many types of research require the positioning of micropipettes in three-dimensional space, and various micromanipulators have become available for this purpose. Pneumatic, hydraulic, and piezoelectric instruments have been designed, many of which have been discussed by Ellis (1962). See also Corey and Hudspeth (1980). These devices offer remote control of all three axes, which is helpful in special cases but rarely needed for research with micropipettes. Hence most commercially available micromanipulators use only mechanical movements. Other features being equal, mechanical micromanipulators of rather large size and weight offer the advantage that strong construction can prevent many types of vibrations or inadvertent movements from disturbing the microelectrode. For example, the hand movements required to turn a micrometer in a direct drive can be well tolerated in a sturdy instrument but can be a severe problem with miniature direct drives. Some sturdy micromanipulators provide mechanical motions sufficiently fine and well controlled to position a micropipette against a cell under visual control, as in patch clamping (see Chapter 17). Though our experience with such instruments is not extensive, ones that we have found satisfactory are available from Leitz and the Sutter Instrument Co. For advancing a micropipette through tissue or into cells, however, it is usually necessary or advisable to mount a special micropipette advancer upon the micromanipulator. For our intracellular work in toad rods, for example, we assembled a sturdy micromanipulator from high quality components (see Part VIII of Chapter 12) and mounted upon it a micropipette advancer of our own design (see Section III.6 of this chapter).

Unfortunately, many types of research require micromanipulators that are quite small and light. Various designs have become available for these special cases and they are usually to be found in the literature of specific research areas. Though a fine control is always required for advancing the micropipette along its own axis, only coarse controls are usually required along the other two axes. Thus miniature micromanipulators frequently use a remotely operated hydraulic advance of the micropipette, supplemented by mechanical coarse controls for the other two axes. The micropipette may be aimed by the coarse controls before it enters the preparation, and it may then be advanced by the remote hydraulic control. Inadvertent motions of the micropipette by hand movements are thereby avoided.

An example of an especially small micromanipulator of this type is a device for intraretinal recording with micropipettes in the closed mammalian eye (Brown, 1964). A ball joint is placed directly against the sclera, and the ball is drilled for a needle that is inserted into the eye. A micropipette is then introduced through the needle. The ball joint may be used to aim the micropipette at any desired retinal area, and the micropipette may then be advanced along its own axis by a remotely operated hydraulic control. The hydraulic system can be constructed quite simply by connecting two small glass syringes with a polyethylene tube and filling the system with mineral oil. A micrometer then drives the remote syringe, which is spring-loaded to provide the return movement. This simple hydraulic advancer can be adequate for many types of extracellular research (see Brown *et al.*, 1965; Brown, 1968).

PART II   ADVANCING A MICROPIPETTE THROUGH TISSUES

Even for extracellular work, however, special devices are often required to control the advance of a micropipette through tissue. A micropipette advancer for this purpose should permit accurate positioning of the micropipette tip to an accuracy of about 1.0 μm, and the range of motion should be adequate for the research conducted. If it is desirable to compare micropipette positions during advance and withdrawal, it is also necessary that backlash be either absent or well-specified.

An instrument that has been much used as a micropipette advancer is the Kopf stepping hydraulic microdrive (David Kopf Instruments, 7324 Elmo St., Tujunga, CA 91042, USA). This device provides 1.0 μm steps over a total range of 25 mm, and micropipette position is displayed on a digital counter. In our experience the backlash of this instrument varies from about 3–8 μm. This device is adequate for most extracellular work, and other instruments suitable for that purpose are described in Sections III.6, III.7, and III.8f of this chapter. Additional provisions are required, however, to penetrate cells efficiently for intracellular work.

PART III   PENETRATION OF CELL MEMBRANES

III.1   Nature of the Problem

If cells are penetrated under visual control, during *smooth* advancement of the micropipette, severe dimpling of the cell membrane is seen before penetration occurs. When finally penetrated the membrane is usually damaged, as indicated by rapid decline of both the resting membrane potential and the cell's electrical responses to stimulation. Of course dimpling stretches the membrane, and when penetration occurs the membrane must snap back over the micropipette tip in much the manner of a released rubber band. Penetrating a cell membrane by advancing slowly will thus build up and suddenly release a relatively large amount of energy, which tends to damage the membrane at the site of entry.

III.2   Crudely 'Tapping Into' Cells

Dimpling should be avoided or minimized by a high velocity advancing step that takes advantage of the inertia of the cell membrane and the fluids surrounding it. In theory the membrane may thus be penetrated too quickly for significant dimpling to develop. This has long been recognized, and rapid steps have often been provided crudely by tapping or scratching the recording table or micromanipulator and learning from experience a type of movement that gives occasional cell penetrations. While this method can be helpful, it leaves much to be desired. The distance and velocity of the penetrating motion are poorly controlled, and penetration is followed by relatively large continuing vibrations that only die out slowly (Fromm *et al.*, 1980). Hence this method also causes frequent damage to the membrane, as indicated by rapid deterioration of the cell's electrical activity. As a result, much attention has been given to improved methods of providing the requisite high velocity steps.

III.3   Penetrating Cells by 'Buzzing' the Micropipette

As described in Section I.1 of Chapter 3, cells may sometimes be penetrated by imposing a high frequency current across the micropipette. This procedure is presumably effective by reversing the mechanoelectric transducer properties of micropipettes discussed in Section IX.1a of Chapter 12, thus setting up very fine vibrations of the tip that facilitate cell penetration. When we directly compared the penetration of toad rods by our high speed hydraulic stepper (see Section III.6 of this chapter) and by 'buzzing', both methods proved quite effective. But after 'buzzing' the cells more often showed significant deterioration of the resting membrane potential and could not be maintained in stable condition. Hence 'buzzing' seems to carry a higher risk of damage at the site of penetration, probably because of continuing tip vibrations, so it is preferable to penetrate the membrane by a single high speed advancing step.

III.4   Characteristics of an Ideal Step Advance for Cell Penetration

For optimal cell penetration the advancing step must be short, to minimize cell damage, and to avoid passing all the way through small cells, nerve fibers, or organelles such as mitochondria. Since the step must be short, rapid acceleration is required to reach the requisite velocity for efficient cell penetration, and deceleration at the end of the step must be similarly rapid. Of course high acceleration and deceleration tend to set up tip vibrations, which can damage the membrane if they persist after cell penetration, so after-vibrations must also be eliminated or minimized. Though the requirement of high acceleration and deceleration conflicts with the need to minimize after-vibrations, both requirements must be met to penetrate cells efficiently without significant damage.

III.5   Early Electromagnetic and Piezoelectric Steppers

Early devices for generating rapid steps were either electromagnetic or piezoelectric, stepping motors having been introduced more recently. Electromagnetic devices were described by Tomita (1965), Fish *et al.* (1971), and Van der Pers (1980). Though all of these authors reported improved cell penetration, none of these devices has been widely adopted, perhaps because of after-vibrations. These were severe in the rapid steps recorded by Tomita (1965) and less severe but noteworthy in the records of Fish *et al.* (1971).

Piezoelectric devices for rapid steps subdivide into two main categories. In one case the piezoelectric effect is used directly by employing the sudden change in thickness of a piezoelectric material when the voltage across it is altered. Such piezoelectric elements are often called monomorphs. The other case employs bimorph 'bender elements' that are described in detail by Corey and Hudspeth (1980). Briefly, a bimorph consists of two piezoelectric elements bonded together and so oriented that application of an electric field across them causes one element to expand while the other contracts. This provides a bender element in much the manner of a bimetallic strip that bends in response to temperature changes. While a monomorph is strong and can be quite compact, displacements can only be a few microns unless very high driving voltages are employed. On the other hand, if a bimorph is fixed at one end, the other end can provide movements of considerable extent; but this arrangement is flimsy, and less force can be obtained. Methods of handling these problems have been devised, and we shall return to this subject later in the present chapter. Devices providing rapid steps with monomorphs have been described by Chen (1978), Fromm *et al.* (1980), and Hengstenberg (1981), while bimorph bender elements have been incorporated into a greater variety of designs (Corey and Hudspeth, 1980; Lassen and Sten-Knudsen, 1968; Pascoe, 1955; Peters and Tetzel, 1980; Prazma, 1978; Rikmenspoel and Lindemann, 1971; Tupper and Rikmenspoel, 1969).

To our knowledge a piezoelectric element was first used for intracellular work by Pascoe (1955), who employed a 'bender crystal' to provide a rapid 20 μm step for penetrating cells in the rat's superior cervical ganglion. These cells were reported to have diameters up to 39 μm, and the technique of penetrating them was described as promising. But all resting potentials decayed rapidly, so even these large cells must have been damaged markedly during penetration. Lassen and Sten-Knudsen (1968) mounted four bender elements in a radial configuration within a tube, one end of each element being attached to the inside of the tube, while the central ends of all the bender elements were attached to a lightweight electrode holder. This configuration brought all four bender elements into play at the same time, thus improving the force of the piezoelectric step. In response to a step voltage of 50–250 V, the microelectrode was reported to advance 10–50 μm in 2 msec, and this device was used for early measurements of membrane potentials and membrane resistance in human red blood cells. It is impressive that results could be obtained at all at that time in such a difficult preparation. On the other hand, the authors were clearly unsatisfied with the performance of the device and the quality of results that it provided. Tupper and Rikmenspoel (1969) made minor improvements on this design, using eight bender elements to provide a much shorter step of 1 μm, which was said to be completed within 1 msec. Though insufficient data were provided to evaluate its experimental performance, this device was used to impale human red blood cells, isolated rat liver nuclei, and large mitochondria (3–4 μm in diameter) from *Drosophila*. Rikmenspoel and Lindemann (1971) made further refinements and reported an 80 V step to give an advance of 3 μm within 4 msec, while

150 V provided 10 μm within 5 msec, their device having been used to impale the heads of bull spermatozoa.

Unfortunately, none of these early reports of piezoelectric devices provided records of the step movements, as required to assess step velocity and after-vibrations. In addition, there was no evidence that the potential importance of after-vibrations was considered or that the designs contained features to minimize them. Hence after-vibrations were probably also the main limitation in the usefulness of these early piezoelectric devices.

In seeking improved methods of cell penetration, we first tested an early version of the 'Inchworm' (Burleigh Instruments, Inc., Burleigh Park, Fishers, NY 14453, USA). This uses a piezoelectric clutching system to provide an advancing series of piezoelectric steps without the usual requirement to retract each step before making another advance. Though toad rods seemed to be penetrated, resting membrane potentials declined to zero almost instantly and no light-evoked responses could be obtained. Thus all cells seemed badly damaged. When advancing steps were observed under a microscope, each step caused such severe lateral vibrations of the micropipette tip that it disappeared entirely and then gradually reappeared. So this experience dramatically demonstrated the importance of minimizing vibrations. At that time the Inchworm was being used mainly for delicate positioning of devices such as laser beams. Recently, however, it has been modified to be more suitable for cell penetration, as described in Section III.8f of this chapter.

III.6   Our High Speed Stepping Hydraulic Advancer

III.6a   Description of the instrument

Since no device that was optimal for cell penetration could be found, we developed our own instrument for this purpose. A remotely controlled hydraulic drive seemed desirable, because this is one of the surest ways to prevent vibrations of the drive unit from reaching the slave unit upon which the micropipette is mounted. For this purpose we used a modified hydraulic unit from a Kopf stepping microdrive. All hydraulic units seem to lose fluid slowly, and in the Kopf unit this is minimized by sealing both ends with rolling diaphragms, as described by Lutz and Wagman (1965). Though the complete Kopf microdrive employs a stepping motor, each step is relatively slow; in addition, the angular step is sufficiently large that gears are employed between the motor and a micrometer to provide step advances of 1.0 μm. These gears introduce backlash and their inertia further slows the velocity of a step. When the complete Kopf microdrive was tested for intracellular work in toad rods, very few cells were penetrated by its step advances, and most of these deteriorated rapidly. We thus developed an improved drive unit, and our micropipette advancer is shown in Figure 55. This device has previously been described in detail (Brown and Flaming, 1977a) and will thus be covered only briefly here.

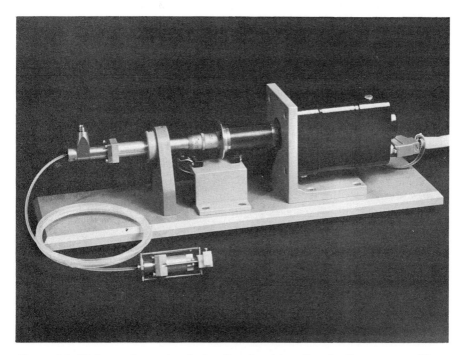

Figure 55. High speed stepping hydraulic microdrive. For details, see text. (From Brown and Flaming (1977a), reproduced by permission of Pergamon Press, Oxford, England)

Fortunately, the design of stepping motors had considerably improved by that time. The one we used was a Model HDM-150-500-4-HS (made by Responsyn Products, USM Corp. Bldg. 3G, Sixth Road, Woburn Industrial Park, Woburn, MA 08101, USA). The angular step is sufficiently small to provide advancing steps of 1.0 μm when directly coupled to a fine-thread micrometer. In addition, this motor may be driven at stepping rates up to 1500/sec, so each step requires only about 2/3 msec. Though this motor is no longer available, it has been replaced by a heavier and quieter Model HDM-185-2000-8. A special power supply must be provided for these motors, but they may otherwise be controlled by the electronic control unit of the Kopf microdrive. A critical feature is the method of coupling the motor to the micrometer, since this coupling must take up the axial motion of the micrometer. This was accomplished by a metal bellows designed to transfer torque without any rotary twisting of the bellows itself, though the bellows can change in length to take up the axial motion of the micrometer (custom design No. SK-7160, Servometer Corp., 501 Little Falls Road, Cedar Grove, NJ 07009, USA). This coupling introduced no detectable backlash, and when attached with light magnesium adaptors it added a minimum of rotary inertia. The hydraulic unit was also modified in an important respect. The tube provided was too small to transfer a fluid pulse with the desired speed. The length of this tube is also important, since added length decreases the transfer of axial vibrations but also decreases the velocity of each advancing step. An adequate compromise was obtained by using a Teflon® tube 8 ft long with an ID of 0.06 in. and an OD of 0.12 in.

III.6b   Recording of high speed steps

By the time our micropipette advancer was developed, a very useful device had become available for recording small high speed movements. The Unimeasure/80 utilizes the Hall effect and may be obtained from Unimeasure Incorporated (909 Williamson Loop, Grants Pass, OR 97526, USA). In our application, movements of 0.1 μm could be resolved and the response time was 0.25 msec or less, so this instrument proved quite satisfactory. It is also reasonable in cost and may conveniently be read out with an oscilloscope. In our work it was invaluable for evaluating specific design factors, such as the size and length of the Teflon® tube, and for evaluating the overall design. It should also be helpful in any case where it is occasionally necessary to check the movement of a high speed stepping device.

Figure 56 shows recorded movements of the slave end of the hydraulic device, to which a micropipette may be attached. The control record is a 1.0 μm step by an unmodified Kopf microdrive, which may be compared with a 1.0 μm step after the same hydraulic unit had been modified and provided with a high speed drive as shown in Figure 55. The control record shows a long latency, and the step required about 7.0 msec from onset to completion, during which the maximum velocity attained was about 0.27 μm/msec. By comparison, a 1.0 μm step with our instrument begins with much shorter latency and is always completed in two phases. Both phases are about 0.5 μm in amplitude and they are separated by a notch that seems to result from the inertial and resonant characteristics of the system. As required to attain high velocity during a small step, the initial movement rises from the baseline almost instantaneously, so acceleration is very high. Records with higher gain and expanded time scales were used to measure velocities of these rapid steps, and the respective velocities of the first and second phases of a 1.0 μm step proved to be 0.94 and 0.69 μm/msec. Owing to inertia, our stepping motor does not reach full velocity during a single 1.0 μm step, and higher velocities were achieved by preset bursts of steps at about 1500/sec. As shown in Figure 56, these bursts essentially fuse into a single large step, but the total motion is always separated into two phases. For a 2.0 μm advance the first and second phases had respective velocities of 1.56 and 0.85 μm/msec, while a 3.0 μm advance yielded respective velocities of 2.0 and 1.4 μm/msec. The velocity of 2.0 μm/msec during a 3.0 μm step is close to the maximum attainable with this instrument, since bursts of 4 or 5 steps yielded little further increase of movement velocity. Figure 56 shows that after 1–3 μm advances the deceleration was likewise extremely rapid, but after-vibrations were very small on both an absolute and relative basis, being effectively damped by the hydraulic system.

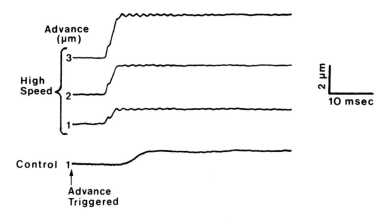

Figure 56. Records of a 1.0 μm advancing step by a standard Kopf hydraulic micro-drive (labeled 'control') and 1.0–3.0 μm steps by the same hydraulic unit after the high speed modifications shown in Figure 55. The recording instrument for all records was a Unimeasure/80 using a bandpass of 0–10,000 Hz. For further details, see text. (From Brown and Flaming (1977a), reproduced by permission of Pergamon Press, Oxford, England)

Though only axial vibrations were recorded, these should be dominant because of the axial direction of the hydraulic pulse. In addition, lateral vibrations should always be damped to some extent by the tissue within which the highly flexible micropipette tip is located. Hence very small lateral vibrations of the slave unit holding the micropipette should not be serious.

III.6c   Automatic stopping upon cell penetration

Electromagnetic or piezoelectric devices (aside from the Inchworm) require that the advancing step be taken back and the micropipette advanced by other means before another rapid advancing step can be utilized. This limitation does not apply to stepping motors, which permit a long train of successive advancing steps, each of which has a good chance of penetrating any cell that has been closely approached by the micropipette. This feature is particularly advantageous for deep penetrations through tissues, in which all cells must be approached blind. To obtain intracellular recordings quickly and efficiently under these conditions, it would also be useful if the stepping rate could be relatively high and if the micropipette could be stopped automatically following the step that penetrates a cell.

As previously described (Brown and Flaming, 1977a), these features have also been incorporated into our high speed stepping device. This was done by programming its operation from a Nova 2/10 minicomputer, with specification of the stepping rate and the total distance the micropipette was to be advanced. When the stepping rate was too high, interactions between long trains of steps led to undesirable vibrations. So we used 10/sec, which was somewhat lower than necessary. The DC potential recorded by the advancing micropipette was monitored continuously by an A-D converter, and the advance was stopped automatically whenever there was a negative DC shift exceeding a preset trigger level. In brief, electrode advancement at 10 μm/sec was initiated by pressing a button, and this advance stopped immediately when a cell was penetrated. After recording from a given cell, an override signal was provided to restart the advance. Upon reaching the total preset distance, the advance stopped automatically, and the micropipette was withdrawn at high speed (1000 μm/sec). Since the retina is relatively thin, we relied mainly upon 3.0 μm steps without automatic control. But automatic advance by 1.0 μm steps quickly provided many intracellular recordings, and programming for automatic advance by 3.0 μm steps should be even better. In any event, automatic control is feasible with this device and should be especially worthwhile for penetrating deep tissues such as those of the central nervous system. With present computer technology, this could be achieved with relatively low cost and effort.

III.6d   *Evaluation in preparations*

While physical measurements are useful in designing a device for improved cell penetration, its performance can only be evaluated accurately during intracellular work. As described in detail in Chapter 13, our high speed stepping hydraulic drive proved highly satisfactory for intracellular work in toad rods. In this preparation 3.0 μm steps proved superior to 1.0 μm, probably because penetration was aided by moving at a higher velocity. In any event, 3.0 μm steps yielded frequent cell penetrations. Equally important, many of these intracellular recordings showed no significant deterioration of either the resting membrane potential or light-evoked responses over periods of several hours. Our high speed stepping device has also been used by a number of other laboratories at our institution, and it has provided satisfactory results during intracellular work in a variety of preparations.

III.6e   *Limitations of this instrument*

Though the performance of this instrument for intracellular work is close to ideal, it has not been made available commercially, mainly because further improvements were desired in convenience of use, and a simpler type of instrument could greatly reduce the cost. Most notably, hydraulic systems are subject to slow leakage, which is undoubtedly exacerbated in the Kopf unit by maintaining spring pressure upon the fluid to assure smooth movement during withdrawal. Leakage may occur partly through the rolling diaphragms, but probably occurs mainly through minute pores of the Teflon $^{\circledR}$ tube. In fact, a slight porosity for water is characteristic of many plastics, so this problem is difficult to avoid in high speed hydraulic systems, since more viscous fluids would be less suitable for transferring a rapid fluid pulse. In both the unmodified Kopf unit and in our instrument this slow leakage causes a withdrawal of the micropipette at about 1.0 μm/hr. In our experience this does not disturb intracellular recordings, even those held as long as 4 hr. And this steady withdrawal could be compensated, if required, by small periodic advances. Slow leakage requires an occasional replacement of water, however, which is inconvenient and must be done carefully to avoid introducing air bubbles. It should also be noted that rapid steps, such as those recorded in Figure 56, require the rolling diaphragms to be well exercised to avoid undue stiffness. This must be done when the high speed advancer is new or when it has remained unused for a long period. In our case this was done by a computer program that drove the advancer back and forth over its full range for about 250 cycles. In summary, though a hydraulic system can be incorporated into a high speed stepping device that performs very well for intracellular work in small cells, the hydraulic system requires special care for adequate maintenance.

III.7　A High Speed Stepping Direct Drive

III.7a　Description of the device

In recent years stepping motors have been further developed in the direction of smaller stepping angles, smaller inertial mass of the rotor, and improved circuitry for generating single steps. These developments should permit smaller steps and higher step velocities, and we hoped that manipulation of the stepping circuit could reduce after-vibrations to an acceptable level. We thus experimented with these improved miniature stepping motors, for driving a micropipette without an interposed hydraulic unit, and were unsatisfied with the vibrations. But an instrument of this type has now been described (Sonnhof *et al.*, 1982). Of course a micropipette cannot be attached directly to the shaft of a stepping motor, so it was attached to a 'high precision microdrive' driven by the stepping motor, and the driving circuitry was modified to reduce vibrations. In this instrument a microstep was 0.125 μm, and the total range of motion was about 25 mm. A single microstep proved too small to assist materially in cell penetration, but 2–5 microsteps were sometimes helpful for repositioning a micropipette after penetrating a cell. The velocity during a microstep at maximum energizing voltage was only about 0.625 μm/msec. Thus high frequency trains of steps were used in this instrument, as in ours, to generate larger steps at higher velocity.

III.7b　Simultaneous recording of step advance and membrane potential

An important contribution of Sonnhof *et al.* was recording the axial advance of the micropipette holder while intracellular work was conducted under visual control, as shown in Figure 57. In this case a 2.0 μm step was used to penetrate a glial cell (about 20 μm in diameter) in tissue culture from a mouse spinal cord. During the high velocity advancing step, the resting membrane potential appeared very suddenly, and this finding was obtained consistently. Though this result has commonly been assumed, confirmation is valuable because it has sometimes been argued that vibrations associated with a step advance are useful or even necessary for cell penetration. Of course vibrations may be useful if advancing velocities are insufficiently high. But Figure 57 shows that when the velocity during an advancing step is above some critical level, only the rapid step is required for cell penetration. In such a case the vibrations occur after penetration and can play no useful role, but they may damage the cell membrane and should thus be eliminated as completely as possible.

In Figure 57 the step advance accelerates rapidly to a high velocity and is followed by vibrations of notable amplitude. Though the final amplitude of the step was only 2.0 μm, the initial penetrating advance measures about 3.0 μm and is followed by an initial oscillation with a peak-to-peak amplitude of almost 2.0 μm, after which the remaining oscillations rapidly become smaller. In the illustrated case these vibrations caused no discernible damage, at least during the first 18 msec after cell penetration, during which the membrane potential remained stable. But these vibrations may cause damage that appears later, and they are probably more significant in small cells.

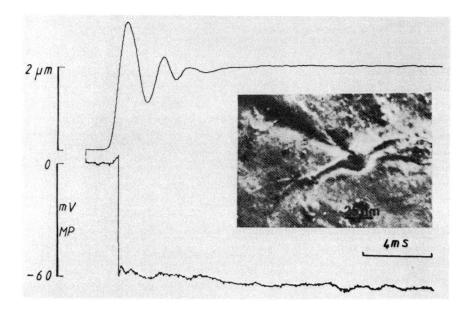

Figure 57. Simultaneous recording of a 2.0 μm advancing step by a direct drive stepping motor device (upper trace) and the membrane potential of a glial cell at the time of penetration and shortly thereafter (lower trace). Axial motion of the stepping device measured at the micropipette holder by an inertia-free differential magneto resistor. The glial cell was in tissue culture from a mouse spinal cord and was observed through a microscope, as shown by the inset photograph. (From Sonnhof *et al.* (1982), reproduced by permission of Springer-Verlag, New York, N.Y.)

III.7c   Determination of minimal and optimal penetrating velocities

It may be expected that some minimal velocity is required to penetrate cells without dimpling or significant damage. There should also be an optimal velocity, above which further increases of velocity become ineffective. Another contribution of Sonnhof *et al.* was determination of these velocities under specified conditions. Their electrodes were either single-barrel tips of diameter less than 1.0 μm or dual-channel theta tubing (see Chapter 16) with tip diameters of 1.5–2.0 μm (used as ion-specific electrodes). Their main preparation was frog spinal motoneurons, but some other rather large cells were also used. While the relatively large tips should penetrate only with considerable difficulty, the relatively large cells should resist damage from penetration. When a step advance was composed of a number of microsteps, the velocity developed could be controlled by either the voltage energizing each microstep or the microstep frequency. Below about 2 μm/msec the number of successful impalements dropped markedly, while optimal penetration with insignificant damage occurred at about 4 μm/msec, and higher velocities offered no clear advantage. Thus 4 μm/msec was the approximate optimal velocity under these conditions. With maximum energizing voltage and microstep frequency, a step size of 1.5 μm was necessary to reach the minimal velocity of 2 μm/msec, so step sizes for suitable cell penetration ranged from 1.5–4.0 μm. The authors state that 'In the isolated frog spinal cord a great number of motoneurons and glial cells were penetrated with ion-sensitive microelectrodes and stable recording for many hours allowed detailed analysis of ionic movements across the neuronal membrane.' Thus many cells were penetrated without significant damage, in spite of the relatively large tips and the relatively large after-vibrations shown in Figure 57. Considerably smaller cells such as vertebrate photoreceptors cannot tolerate such large tips, and the effect of the after-vibrations in small cells needs to be determined.

III.7d   Summary and comments

In summary, this stepping device appears useful for large cells, but its performance in small cells was not evaluated. In addition, the advancing head that carries the micropipette appears rather large, which might limit its application in some cases. According to Fromm *et al.* (1980), this direct drive stepper is now available from B. Marcinowski (Biotechnische Geräte, 6900 Heidelberg, FRG).

The obtained values for minimal and optimal velocities seem especially helpful in designing micropipette advancers for intracellular work. Using tips 1–2 μm in diameter, the respective minimal and optimal velocities were 2 and 4 μm/sec. By comparison, our stepping hydraulic advancer attains a velocity of 2 μm/msec, which has now been shown adequate though not optimal for some of the largest tips used in intracellular work. More important, the minimal and optimal penetrating velocities must decrease with tip size. Hence 2 μm/msec is probably at or above the optimal velocity for ultrafine tips, as strongly indicated by the ease with which we obtained and held stable recordings in toad rods (see Part III of Chapter 13). Thus hydraulic advancers, which can provide remote control and freedom from after-vibrations, can also attain the requisite step velocity for excellent or adequate performance in many types of intracellular work. If the value of 4 μm/msec can be taken as at or near the highest velocity required for optimal cell penetration under all but the most extreme conditions, this is also helpful for the design of piezoelectric advancers. Some recent devices of that type are reported to attain considerably higher velocities, but for many applications the extra velocity may not serve any useful purpose, while generating undesirable vibrations.

III.8   Recent Piezoelectric Stepping Devices

III.8a   A three-dimensional micromanipulator

A number of recent developments have been reported with piezoelectric advancers. Corey and Hudspeth (1980) describe a three-dimensional micromanipulator in which each motion is accomplished by two bimorphs that form parallel sides of a hinged parallelogram, thus providing movements with a range of about 100 μm at a sensitivity of 0.56 μm/V. The rise-time for a movement along the slowest of the three axes was 2.9 msec, and after-vibrations were reduced by rounding both the onset and termination of the driving pulse. Though this device was described as a remotely controlled and sensitive manipulator, which could also be adapted as a mechanical stimulator, A.J. Hudspeth (personal communication) has also found it helpful for penetrating hair cells in the bullfrog sacculus.

III.8b   Amplification of the maximum step amplitude with a single monomorph

Though bimorph bender elements can provide relatively large steps, as desired in some cases, their application for this purpose presents difficulties. When mounted radially in a tube, as described in Section III.5 of this chapter, the arrangement is rather flimsy. More important, alignment of the bender elements to obtain an axial movement of the micropipette has proved difficult (Rikmenspoel and Lindemann, 1971), and this problem is exacerbated if there are slight differences between the response amplitudes of the various bender elements. Chen (1978) alleviated these problems by bonding a circular monomorph to one side of a thin brass disc, which was mounted around its rim. When the monomorph expanded in diameter, the brass disc became 'dished' in one direction, while contraction caused a similar effect in the other direction. When a microelectrode holder was then bonded to the center of the brass disc, rapid axial movements were produced that varied in amplitude from 0.25–100 μm. An activating step of 136 V elicited an advance of 50 μm in 2 msec, this being the maximum movement on either side of the neutral position. Starting from full withdrawal and then suddenly reversing the activating polarity, both the distance and velocity of the movement were doubled. Though such large advances are seldom required for cell penetration, Chen found them useful for the exceptionally large cells represented by the free-swimming protozoan *Stentor*. The after-vibrations of this device were not evaluated, and means of suppressing them were not reported.

III.8c   A sturdy step advancer using bimorphs

Peters and Tetzel (1980) describe a similar design based upon circular bimorph bender elements that were originally developed for loudspeaker applications. Two of these are held together only around their rims and are so oriented that an activating voltage pulse will cause them to become 'dished' in opposite directions, thus doubling the range of movement. In this case the micropipette holder is axially mounted on one side while the other side is axially bonded to a rod that is firmly attached to a micromanipulator. Though small, this device is reported to be 'robust', and only 40 V are required for a full excursion of about 140 μm. Records of sample movements show high velocities but without sufficient resolution to provide accurate values, and after-vibrations appear to be small. The device was reported to greatly facilitate penetration in preparations used by the authors, as illustrated for muscle cells of the snail, which are probably quite large though the cell size was not stated.

III.8d   Increase of step amplitude with stacked monomorphs

Fromm *et al.* (1980) increased the range of motion by the different expedient of using a stack of ceramic monomorph discs bonded together. With 60 discs an advance of up to 40 μm could be elicited by a 1000 V exciting pulse, but their device normally contained 36 discs and gave a maximum advance of 20 μm. The stacked discs were mounted upon a 1.0 kg block of lead to dampen after-vibrations, and the lead block (of dimensions 40 $\times$ 40 $\times$ 80 mm) was mounted in turn upon a Leitz micromanipulator. This sturdy piezoelectric device could accelerate relatively large masses and it was used by the authors to support and advance an entire electrometer input stage. When this instrument was compared with the direct stepping drive of Sonnhof *et al.*, as shown in Figure 58, steps of 25 μm were generated at higher velocity and with much reduced after-vibrations. For cell penetration the step advance was usually 10–15 μm, and this device was reported to aid penetration and decrease cell damage in a variety of preparations.

III.8e   An extremely high speed step with a monomorph

Hengstenberg (1981) employed a piezoceramic tube and used the fast relaxation from electrostriction to greatly speed the velocity during an advancing

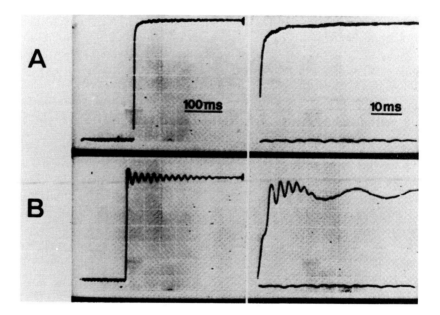

Figure 58. Records of 25 μm advancing steps by two instruments. (A) The piezoelectric device of Fromm *et al.* (1980) consisting of stacked monomorphs. (B) The direct drive stepping motor design of Sonnhof *et al.* (1982). Records obtained by mounting upon a micropipette an opaque 'flag', which was advanced over a scanning slit, while light through the slit was detected by a photomultiplier and displayed upon an oscilloscope. The time constant of the piezoelectric device was adjusted to 0.5 msec and the stepping motor was run at maximum speed. (From Fromm *et al.* (1980), reproduced by permission of Springer-Verlag, New York, N.Y.)

step. The tube was first contracted in length by an applied voltage and then released to provide the high speed advancing step. As shown in Figure 59(a), the movement during release was much faster than that during contraction, and Figure 59(b) shows the advance during release at faster time scale. The step amplitude for penetrating cells was usually 0.2–0.5 μm, but it could be as large as 2.0 μm. For a step of about 0.5 μm the recorded time constant was 5 μsec, from which the calculated velocity attained was at least 60 μm/msec. But the recorded time constant was limited by the recording bandwidth, so the velocity attained was presumably even higher. In addition, Figure 59 shows that the after-vibrations were quite small. Since no special provisions were described for suppressing vibrations, they were probably small because of the light piezoceramic tube mounted upon the much larger mass of a micromanipulator. Though such high accelerations and step velocities might be suspected to break micropipette tips, ultrafine tips in saline showed no change of electrical resistance or steady-state noise after these high speed step advances. This device was used to penetrate and stain fibers as small as 1.0 μm diameter and cell

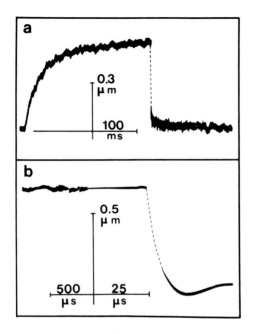

Figure 59. Movements during contraction and relaxation of a piezoceramic tube, recorded by mounting a razor blade in a narrow light beam and using a phototransistor to record the transmitted light flux. (a) slow retraction (upward) and much more rapid expansion (downward) of the piezoceramic tube in response to the application and release of a 120 V step. (b) the rapid advancing step, recorded at a fast time scale, upon release from a 140 V step. For further details, see text. (From Hengstenberg (1981), reproduced by permission of Elsevier Biomedical Press B.V., Amsterdam)

somata as large as 20 μm diameter. Membrane potentials were demonstrated to be quite stable after penetration, and in excitable cells there was no 'injury burst' of impulses associated with cell penetration. Hence this device appears able to penetrate cell membranes without significant damage.

III.8f   The recently modified 'Inchworm'

Finally, the Inchworm has now been modified to reduce vibrations. As mentioned in Section III.5 of this chapter, this instrument contains a unique piezoelectric clutching system that permits a high frequency series of steps in a given direction. Current models generate single steps of 10 nm. For positioning a micropipette these microsteps may be delivered in high frequency runs, and the total range of travel may be either 25 or 50 mm, depending upon the model. For cell penetration the microsteps may be delivered in short bursts for advances of 1.0 μm, or for greater advances by increments of 1.0 μm. During a high frequency burst the average velocity of movement is specified to be at least 2 μm/msec; but the instrument comes to a complete stop at the end of each microstep, so the velocity during each microstep must be greater than this average velocity. Vibrations associated with the stepping action are now reduced by an optional attachment bringing spring-loaded wires to bear against the advancing spindle. These wires dampen lateral vibrations with minimal friction against the spindle. We are informed by Burleigh Instruments that each Inchworm intended for cell penetration is now tested to assure that advancing steps do not set up tip vibrations sufficiently large to be detected under a microscope.

Thus far this modified Inchworm does not appear to have been used extensively for cell penetration, but it has been tested rather thoroughly by Burks Oakley II at the University of Illinois (personal communication). Since Oakley had previously used our high speed hydraulic stepper (Oakley *et al.*, 1979), his comparative experience with the Inchworm should be especially useful. In both cases ultrafine micropipettes were formed by our puller and used for intracellular recording in toad rods within an isolated and inverted retinal preparation. Under these conditions he finds that the Inchworm performs similarly to our advancer. Toad rods have been readily penetrated, and stable recording conditions have been maintained for at least 30 min.

We have also found three investigators at different institutions who are using the Inchworm for cell penetration in hippocampal or hypothalamic brain slices. Of these, the best results have been reported from Dr. Robert W. Snow at Tulane University (personal communication). In one of his setups a recent model of the Inchworm (No. IW 601-2L) is being used for cells of about 20 μm diameter in hypothalamic slices, which are penetrated with tips formed by our puller. About half the penetrations result from advancing the Inchworm, while the other half result from 'buzzing', but cells penetrated by the Inchworm tend to remain more stable than those penetrated by 'buzzing'. These results are very similar to ours when the high speed hydraulic stepper was compared with 'buzzing' for penetrating toad rods (see Section III.3 of this chapter). The other two investigators contacted, however, report less satisfactory results in brain slices. So it appears that the Inchworm can now be useful for cell penetration, at least under some conditions, which may need to become better defined.

PART IV   SUMMARY AND PROSPECTS

In summary, it appears that much progress has been made in recent years in the design of devices for advancing micropipettes through tissues and into cells. But this field is in a state of flux, and no instrument has emerged that provides ideal performance over a wide range of conditions, while offering simplicity of design, moderate initial cost, and freedom from maintenance problems. Recent developments with stepping motors and piezoelectric devices, however, are particularly promising. Good results can be obtained by coupling a stepping motor to an appropriate hydraulic unit, if one can tolerate the nuisance of slow leakage. Promising results have also been obtained by using a stepping motor without a hydraulic unit, but in this case after-vibrations have thus far been notable and may cause significant damage in small cells. The Inchworm is also promising now, for cell penetration as well as positioning of micropipettes.

While bimorphs have been used to provide single piezoelectric steps of 100 μm or somewhat larger, this range of movement appears useful for cell penetration only in the case of exceptionally large cells. Though it remains to be demonstrated, it seems likely that a much smaller step could also suffice for these large cells if the step velocity could be made sufficiently high. As shown by Hengstenberg, a monomorph can provide a step velocity of at least 60 μm/msec over a distance of 0.5 μm, providing that the step is generated by release from an applied voltage, and this unit can generate steps as large as 2.0 μm. Such short steps at such a high speed may well be adequate for penetrating even the largest cells, and this needs to be tested. Advantages of this type of unit are its small size and the simplicity of its required circuitry. After-vibrations appear suitably small and, if necessary, could be reduced further by mounting the piezoelectric unit upon a small block of lead, which could be advanced directly by a miniature stepping motor to position the micropipette over a long range. Hence this type of device might prove close to ideal both for positioning a micropipette and for penetrating cells of virtually all sizes without significant damage, while the simplicity of the design should permit a moderate initial cost and high reliability with minimal maintenance. In view of these possibilities, a micropipette advancer is now being developed along the described lines.

CHAPTER 12

Ancillary Techniques for Conducting Intracellular Research

PART I INTRODUCTION

Previous chapters have covered the fabrication and filling of micropipettes and methods of advancing micropipettes through tissues and into cells. This chapter will describe ancillary techniques that are commonly required or helpful for conducting intracellular research. Though these techniques are adapted most specifically to our work in photoreceptors of the toad retina, where they have proved very useful, they should be similarly helpful in a wide variety of preparations. Our retinal preparation will also be described, since it has been used to test various aspects of our microelectrode techniques, as reported in Chapters 13 and 14.

PART II TOAD PHOTORECEPTORS

In any given retina the types of photoreceptors and their main anatomical features may be determined most readily by SEM. Thus Figure 60 shows a retina of the toad (*Bufo marinus*) that has been fixed and cracked to expose the photoreceptors, which are then viewed perpendicularly to their long axis. Details of this procedure have been described by Steinberg (1973). The various types of photoreceptors may thus be revealed with considerable three-dimensional detail and in their normal anatomical relationships and relative densities. The toad retina contains predominantly rods, which are of two types. They are conventionally called red and green rods, because of their colors when a fresh retina is transilluminated by white light and the tips of the outer segments are observed under a light microscope. Intracellular recordings are most readily made from the outer and inner segments of red rods. As shown in Figure 60, the red rods are numerically predominant and may readily be identified by their long columnar outer segments. The diameter of these outer segments ranges from 5.0–7.5 μm and averages about 5.9 μm (Brown and Flaming, 1977a), while their length averages about 42 μm. The outer and inner segments are separated only by a narrow gap crossed by many fine calycal processes, which are shown at higher magnification in Figure 61(B). By comparison with the outer segments, the inner segments are much shorter and taper slightly toward their bases at the level of the external limiting membrane of the retina. This is not a true membrane, but a dense collection of microvilli which may be seen in Figures 60 and 61. These microvilli arise from the outer terminals of Müller cells, the glial cells that extend through the retina to its inner margin, where their inner terminals expand and fuse together to form the internal limiting membrane. By comparison with red rods, the green rods are much less numerous, only two being clearly visible in Figure 60. One of these is slightly left of center, and another is farther left and partially obscured by overlying cells. The green rods have outer segments that are likewise columnar, and their diameters are similar to those of red rods. But the outer segments of green rods are considerably shorter and their tips extend beyond the tips of most of the outer segments of red rods. In addition, the inner segments of green rods taper rapidly to a thin process. Figure 60 also shows a few single cones, the short and quite slender photoreceptors interspersed among the bases of the rods.

In addition to single cones, the toad retina contains double cones, the least common of the four types of photoreceptors in the toad retina. A double cone, along with several well preserved single cones, may be seen in Figure 61(A). Double cones typically consist of a chief cone similar to a single cone, and a

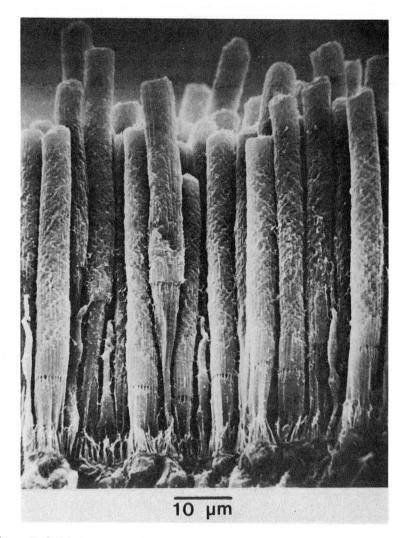

10 µm

Figure 60. SEM photograph of the receptor layer of a retina from the toad, *Bufo marinus*. The retina was fixed and then cracked to expose the long axis of the receptors. Types of photoreceptors present include red rods, green rods, and single cones, all of which are readily identified by distinctive features described in the text. (From Brown and Flaming (1977a), reproduced by permission of Pergamon Press, Oxford, England)

considerably smaller accessory cone, fused together at their inner segments (Walls, 1963, p. 60). These features are evident in the double cone near the center of Figure 61(A).

The basic structural features common to all vertebrate photoreceptors have been summarized by Brown (1980). For all photoreceptors the connection between the outer segment (which contains the photopigments leading to excitation) and the inner segment is exceptionally fragile. The entire outer segment is

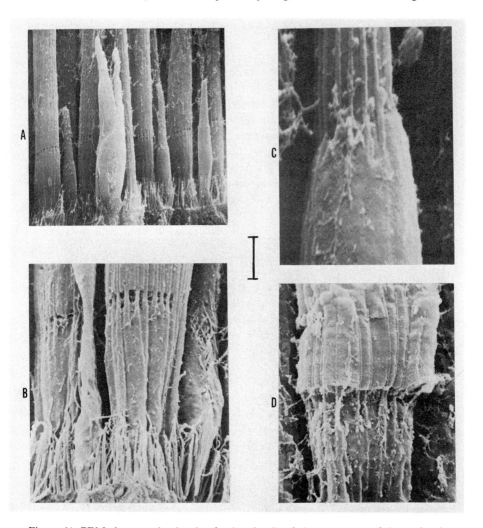

Figure 61. SEM photographs showing further details of photoreceptors of the toad retina. Retina prepared in the same manner as for Figure 60. (A) View similar to that of Figure 60; in this case a double cone may be seen, as well as three well-preserved single cones. (B–D) Details of the connecting zone between outer and inner segments; (B) a red rod, (C) a single cone, (D) a green rod. The calibration mark indicated for (A) 10.0 μm, (B) 3.09 μm, (C) 1.06 μm, and (D) 2.0 μm.

a modified cilium, and the typical ciliary structure is maintained at the connection between outer and inner segments. In other words, the only true connection between outer and inner segments is a single cilium. In response to mechanical stress, the outer segment readily separates from the inner segment. This must be taken into account in preparing an isolated retina for experimental work and in conducting intracellular work in photoreceptors. Though the connecting cilium cannot be seen in SEM photographs like those of Figures 60 and 61, the calycal processes that cross the connecting zone between inner and outer segments are clearly visible. These processes, which are consistent features of vertebrate photoreceptors, arise from the inner segment and extend outward for some distance in longitudinal grooves of the outer segment. Though the calycal processes are not connected to membranes of the outer segment, their intimate apposition in grooves of the outer segment, combined with their relatively dense representation around the base of the outer segment, may supplement the cilium in strengthening the connection between outer and inner segments. Figure 61 shows details of the connecting zone between outer and inner segments of toad photoreceptors in the respective cases of a red rod (B), green rod (D) and a single cone (C). When retinas are fixed and cracked for SEM observations, as in Figures 60 and 61, some receptors are damaged. The green rods are especially fragile, the outer segment often being broken off at the connecting zone.

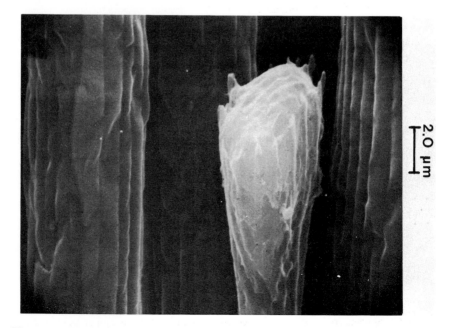

Figure 62. SEM photograph of a green rod that was damaged when the retina was prepared as in Figures 60 and 61. The outer segment was torn off at the connecting zone with the inner segment, leaving only the inner segment and stumps of some of the calycal processes.

As shown in Figure 62, this leaves only the inner segment and short projecting stumps of some of the calycal processes, but little or no sign of the connecting cilium. Similar effects occur, though less often, in the case of red rods. These results illustrate the special fragility of the connection between outer and inner segments.

PART III   RECORDING CHAMBER FOR ISOLATED AND SUPERFUSED RETINA

III.1   Description of Recording Chamber

Toad retinas were isolated and mounted, receptor side up, in a recording chamber illustrated by Figure 63. This chamber provided a stable mounting of the retina in its normal shape. It also provided the continuous superfusion of a bathing medium to maintain the retina in physiologically normal condition, and the composition of this medium could be changed during intracellular recordings to investigate the effects of specific ions upon the resting membrane potentials and light-evoked responses of impaled cells. The chamber itself was mounted on the stage of a special microscope (see Figure 65). This permitted

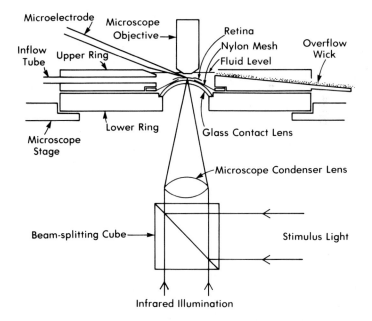

Figure 63. Schematic drawing of the recording chamber for mounting and superfusing isolated toad retinas, with the recording chamber itself mounted on the stage of a modular microscope (see Figure 65). View is from the front of the microscope, as seen by the experimenter, with the stimulus beam entering from the experimenter's right. For details, see text.

the retina to be viewed continuously by infrared light, which was supplied by an illuminator in the base of the microscope. It also permitted the introduction of stimulus flashes, which could be accurately focused upon the retina, for eliciting light-evoked responses of photoreceptors. As shown in Figure 63, the infrared illumination and stimulus flashes were combined by a beam-splitting cube and then focused upon the retina by the microscope's condenser lens. The retina was viewed by a 40× water immersion lens, modified to provide increased working space (see Figure 64), so that micropipette electrodes could be introduced at appropriate angles for retinal penetrations. Our micropipettes usually approached the retina at 16–17° from the horizontal, and they were advanced by our high speed stepping hydraulic microdrive described in Section III.6 of Chapter 11. Micropipettes were mounted upon the slave portion of the hydraulic microdrive, which was mounted in turn upon a 3-dimensional micromanipulator (see Figure 69), for positioning the micropipette tip prior to penetrating the retina.

Figure 63 shows that the recording chamber consists of two main components, the upper and lower rings, both of which are made from Plexiglas®. The lower ring is attached to the microscope stage by a waterproof seal, and into this ring is sealed a glass contact lens that serves as a mounting surface for the isolated retina. The lens for this work was previously used as a contact lens during intraretinal microelectrode work in the intact cat eye (Brown and Wiesel, 1959, 1961a, b). Though glass contact lenses are no longer readily obtainable, they are well suited for mounting isolated retinas. A plano contact lens has no focusing action, and glass surfaces may be maintained indefinitely, whereas plastic surfaces are readily scratched during cleaning. The spherical surface of the contact lens supports the retina in its normal shape. The radius of curvature of our lens is slightly greater than that of the toad eye, so that the rod outer segments are slightly squeezed together (see Figure 67). This facilitates penetrating rod outer segments by assuring that each one is held in position by its neighbors. In brief, the glass contact lens supports the isolated retina in its normal shape and with its normal tight packing of rod outer segments, thus providing a relatively large receptor area to work with, and facilitating intracellular work in rod outer segments. By contrast, a retina mounted on a flat surface becomes severely folded, with very limited areas that are suitable for intracellular work in either receptors or higher-order cells of the retina, since the rod outer segments in most areas are disarranged from their normal orientation.

As shown in Figure 63, a piece of retina is mounted over a small hole cut in a circular piece of nylon mesh (readily obtained from a ladies' stocking), which is cemented to a small Plexiglas® ring fitted into a recess in the upper ring of the recording chamber. This upper ring contains an inflow tube for the superfusate, and on the other side is a flat-bottomed overflow channel, which contains a cotton wick about 10 mm wide. The overflow channel is open at the top and angled slightly downward, so that outflow will be maintained by gravity after the wick has become saturated. The overflow is then collected in a large container. If the superfusate drips from the end of the wick into the overflow vessel, flow through the recording chamber will be pulsatile and each drip will give an artifact in the electrical recording. Thus the wick should extend into the fluid in the overflow vessel. The reference electrode for all electrical recordings (not shown) is an Ag–AgCl plate permanently mounted under the overflow wick near its exit from the chamber; this reference electrode leads to a pin for making contact with the recording system.

III.2   Mounting of Retina in Recording Chamber

Toads were dark adapted for 2–4 hr in a chamber that was well ventilated but insulated from sound and placed in a quiet location. Experience suggests that if toads are subjected to stress, the release of adrenalin or some other circulating substance may make the retina more difficult to detach from the pigment epithelium without damaging rod outer segments. Thus stress was avoided as far as possible during dark adaptation. When the animal was sacrificed by guillotine, this was done as rapidly as possible to minimize the chance that adrenalin could reach the head by the time it was severed. The head was then pithed immediately, through the open spinal cord, to assure that the severed head was free from pain. An eye was enucleated, the front of the eye was carefully removed, and the eyecup was cut into three pieces. One of these contained the optic disc and could not be used, since the retina cannot be detached in the region of the optic disc. The other two pieces were placed immediately into a dissecting chamber containing superfusate, into which the nylon mesh was also placed. The pieces of eyecup were soaked in the superfusate for about 5 min, since this seemed to facilitate retinal detachment. At a cut edge of one of the pieces of eyecup, the sclera was then grasped with a forcep; the retina was grasped with another forcep, gently peeled away from the pigment epithelium, and floated receptor-side-up over the hole in the nylon mesh. At this stage the entire upper ring of the recording chamber had been removed from the microscope. The nylon mesh was quickly lifted from the dissecting chamber and sealed into the upper ring with silicone vacuum grease. The upper ring was then similarly sealed to the lower ring of the recording chamber, to which it was firmly clamped by two screws (not shown), and superfusion of the retina was initiated. When the upper ring was mounted to the lower ring of the recording chamber, the nylon mesh was stretched upward by the contact lens, and this tension helped bring the retina into close contact with the surface of the lens. In addition, two fine stainless steel wires on top of the chamber (not shown) were used as delicate hold-downs at opposite sides of the piece of retina.

All procedures for isolating and mounting a piece of retina were conducted under dim red light. This was partly to avoid damage to rod outer segments, since dark adapted retinas separate more readily from the pigment epithelium, and partly to avoid the bleaching of photopigments that might not regenerate fully in isolated retinas. For the latter reason, all experimental work was likewise conducted with only dim red illumination in the recording room.

PART IV   SUPERFUSION OF THE RETINA

IV.1   Composition of Control Superfusate

Our control superfusate for maintaining the isolated toad retina in good condition during long experiments contained NaCl (94 mM), KCl (2 mM), MgCl (1 mM), $NaHCO_3$ (15 mM), glucose (10 mM), and $CaCl_2$ (1.8 mM). The pH was adjusted by bubbling this solution with 98.5% O_2 and 1.5% CO_2, which provided a pH of 7.7–7.8, and the temperature of the solution was usually held constant at 22 °C. The concentration of bicarbonate in this solution, and the pH at the maintained temperature, were based upon an analysis of blood plasma from *Bufo marinus* (Howell *et al.*, 1970).

IV.2   Superfusion Technique

The control superfusate, and the experimental solutions for a given experiment, were mounted on a shelf high enough to provide a gravity feed. Source chambers were made of either Pyrex ® or Plexiglas ®, and at the outlet of each source chamber was a precision flow valve that allowed only glass and Teflon ® to contact the solution (Roger Gilmont Instruments, Inc., 161 Great Neck Road, Great Neck, NY 11021, USA). The outflows of the source chambers all fed into a switching valve that allowed only Teflon ® to contact the solution (Rheodyne, Inc., P.O. Box 996, Cotati, CA 94928, USA). This device permitted any one of six source chambers to be connected to a common outflow channel, and this was controlled from outside the shielded recording cage. The outflow channel from the switching valve passed through a stainless steel loop, the temperature of which was controlled by a Peltier device (Cambridge Thermionic Corp., 445 Concord Ave., Cambridge, MA 02138, USA), and the solution then passed to the recording chamber. The temperature of the solution near the retina was monitored by a miniature thermistor probe (Yellow Springs Instrument Co., Box 279-T, Yellow Springs, OH 45387, USA). By varying the current through the Peltier device in either direction, the solution could be either warmed or cooled, and the temperature of the solution in the recording chamber could be set and maintained at any value between 10–30 °C. Though the temperature was normally maintained at 22 °C, it has also been deliberately varied in experiments upon rod receptor potentials (Oakley *et al.*, 1979).

At the beginning of each experiment, prior to mounting a retina in the recording chamber, the outflow from the switching valve was disconnected from the recording chamber and connected to either a vacuum line or a glass flowmeter (Roger Gilmont Instruments). The outflow from the flowmeter was at the same height as the fluid level in the recording chamber, to duplicate the pressure head in the gravity flow. Each source chamber was connected first to the vacuum line to initiate flow and remove bubbles, following which it was connected to the flowmeter for adjustment of the flow rate at 5.0 ml/min. After completing these adjustments, which required only a few minutes, outflow from the switching valve was closed off. The wick was then primed by flushing with distilled water to remove precipitated salts and to saturate the wick. Immediately after mounting the retina in the recording chamber, the upper ring of this chamber was connected to the outflow of the switching valve, and superfusion was initiated from the appropriate source chamber.

The described superfusion technique has proved quite satisfactory. Retinas have been maintained in good condition for up to 4 hr, as indicated by very little decline in either resting membrane potentials or light-evoked responses during intracellular recordings from photoreceptors (see Chapter 13). The wick could handle an outflow greater than the inflow, so the chamber did not overflow. Yet the flow rate of 5.0 ml/min was high enough to avoid any significant effects of oxidation at the surface of the superfusing solution in the recording chamber. It also provided a rapid change of superfusate upon switching solutions, since the volume of the recording chamber was only about 1.5 ml, and the retina was located directly between the inflow and outflow ports of the recording chamber. It might be expected that the turbulence from such a high flow rate would disturb intracellular recordings. Electrical recordings during continuous flow, however, contained no artifacts that were eliminated by temporarily stopping the flow. We likewise experienced no loss of intracellular recordings, or deterioration of resting membrane potentials, associated with changing the superfusate by switching between source chambers.

PART V　MODIFICATION OF THE ZEISS 40× WATER IMMERSION OBJECTIVE FOR INCREASED WORKING SPACE

As described in Part VII of this chapter, many aspects of our intracellular work have been conducted under direct visual control, with the aid of infrared illumination and a high resolution image converter. This required a water immersion microscope objective with relatively high magnification and resolution, yet enough working space under the objective to permit a micropipette electrode to approach the photoreceptor surface at a relatively high angle. An objective often used for such purposes is the Zeiss 40× water immersion lens with a numerical aperture of 0.75 and a working distance of 1.6 mm. Though this objective provided adequate resolution of toad rods, as shown in Figures 67 and 68, the working space proved inadequate for our short and rapidly tapering micropipette tips. As shown in Figure 64, this lens may readily be modified to improve its working space. The outer lens of the objective is mounted as shown, with the metal casing extending slightly beyond the lens. More important, this metal casing extends laterally to form a shoulder, which causes the main limitation of working space. With reasonable care this shoulder may be filed away, all the way around the lens, to the dotted line in Figure 64. If a straight line is passed through the focal point of the objective, this line will contact the shoulder of the unmodified lens when it is tilted up to about 27° from the horizontal, but it will not contact the modified lens until it is tilted up to about 38°. Though the angular difference is not great, the increased working space permits micropipettes with short and rapidly tapering tips to approach the photoreceptor surface at adequate angles for retinal penetrations.

For electrical recording under microscopic control, it is usually necessary or helpful to isolate the microscope from the recording circuit and then ground the microscope. Since the metal casing of the Zeiss water immersion lens extended into the solution bathing the preparation, it was necessary to insulate this metal from the solution. This was done by painting a thin layer of silicone rubber (Dow Corning 734 RTV) over the lower end of the metal casing, and this coating was extended slightly over the margin of the outer lens of the objective. This insulating layer has proved satisfactory and durable.

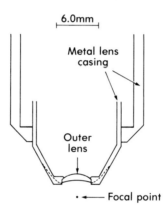

Figure 64. Scale drawing of outer end of Zeiss 40× water immersion lens. The working space under and beside this lens may be increased by filing off the outer end of the metal casing to the dotted line.

Many types of research require micropipettes or other elements to be manipulated under visual control at relatively high magnification. Hence our described modification of the Zeiss 40× water immersion objective may be helpful in many other preparations. If the metal casing of this lens were slightly redesigned by its manufacturer, it appears that micropipettes or other elements could approach the focal point of this lens at even higher angles. A. J. Hudspeth of our department has found the modified lens helpful for electrical recordings from hair cells in the sacculus of the bullfrog. In this application he coated the lens casing with Sylgard® 184, a silicone elastomer that is also made by Dow Corning. The Sylgard® was mixed as instructed by the manufacturer, applied as a thin coating with a small brush, and cured for about 30 sec by hot air from a hair dryer. This material can be applied in a thinner coat than the Dow Corning 734 RTV, and it has proved satisfactory for both electrical and thermal insulation of the microscope from the preparation. Either of these insulating materials, if damaged, can readily be stripped off and replaced.

For cases that require approaching the preparation at even higher angles, such as intracellular recording in hair cells of the bullfrog sacculus, Hudspeth and Corey (1978) have described a simple and effective method for controlled bending of micropipettes very close to the tips.

PART VI   A MODULAR RESEARCH MICROSCOPE

Most microscopes are compactly constructed and offer very limited possibilities for inserting additional optical elements. This was an acute problem in our work, mainly because the condenser systems of conventional microscopes could not be readily modified to meet our needs. This problem was solved by assembling a modular microscope based upon the Nikon 'Measurescope', a microscope originally designed for metallurgical work, with other microscope elements being used as required. Though the Measurescope has been discontinued, similar results may be obtained by using modular components based upon the Nikon 'Optiphot', as demonstrated by J. Sherwood Charlton (Department of Electrical Engineering, Univ. of Arkansas, Fayetteville, AR 72701, USA). In assembling our instrument we received helpful advice from the Technical Instrument Co. (348 Sixth St., San Francisco, CA 94103, USA), which handles the necessary modular components.

As shown in Figure 65, the Measurescope features a heavy vertical support column upon which focusing blocks may be positioned as required. In our case the vertical column is mounted to a heavy metal base attached directly to a large steel baseplate. The main elements of the microscope are then attached to upper and lower focusing blocks, which provide coarse and fine focusing controls. The lower focusing block supports an EPOI microscope stage, upon which the preparation chamber is mounted. This stage features X–Y micrometer controls for selecting the retinal area to be studied. The condenser lens is also mounted on the lower focusing block but has its own focusing control.

Intense white light, plus abundant infrared illumination, is provided from a tungsten source by a Tiyoda microscope base illuminator. This light is usually passed through a high-pass infrared filter (Schott, RG-850) to supply infrared illumination of the retina. With the infrared filter removed, white light is supplied for making optical alignments prior to mounting the preparation. Since this light source illuminates a large area of the preparation, it may also be used to provide a white background illumination of the retina during experiments on light adaptation. The background illumination is turned on and off by an electromagnetic shutter, and its intensity is controlled by neutral density filters (not shown). A beam-splitting cube, which has its own mount, is used to combine light from the microscope base illuminator and from the stimulus beam; as shown in Figure 63, the stimulus beam enters from the right as the microscope is viewed by the experimenter. Stimuli are delivered by a special optical device (not illustrated), which forms stimuli controllable in shape, size, position, color, intensity, and flash duration.

The upper focusing block supports a turret for up to three microscope

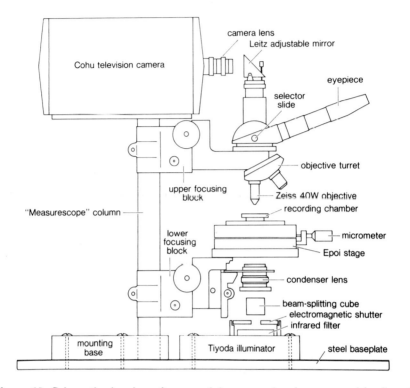

Figure 65. Schematic drawing of our modular research microscope, with all major components labeled. For details, see text.

objectives. In addition to the Zeiss 40× water immersion lens for experimental work, objectives with lower magnification are useful for making optical adjustments. The upper focusing block also supports a Leitz adjustable mirror for directing infrared light into the lens of a closed circuit television camera mounted directly upon the heavy column of the Measurescope. Alternatively, a selector slide may be used to direct light to an eyepiece, which is used mainly for making initial alignments by direct viewing with white light.

PART VII   A HIGH RESOLUTION INFRARED IMAGE CONVERTER

VII.1   Description of Image Converter

The television camera (Cohu 5000 series) is provided with a Vidicon image tube with a silicon target (Model SVC-A), which has high sensitivity in the infrared, and the camera's output is fed to a high resolution monitor (Conrac Model SNA 9/C). Thus equipped, the camera functions as an efficient infrared image converter. When light from our tungsten source is passed through the Schott RG-850 high-pass filter, this camera is sufficiently sensitive to the supplied infrared illumination that there is no significant light adaptation of photoreceptors. This has been demonstrated by the high stability of photoreceptor response amplitudes over a period of several hours, during which the retina was monitored continuously with infrared illumination, as documented in Chapter 13. This camera also permits the tips of toad photoreceptors to be viewed with high resolution, as shown by Figures 67 and 68. Hence this image conversion system seems ideal for the described purpose, and it is quite reasonable in cost. The camera, image tube, and monitor are available from Cohu, Inc. (5725 Kearny Villa Rd., San Diego, CA 92138, USA).

VII.2   Infrared Monitoring of Photoreceptor Surface

As a reference point for infrared views of the photoreceptor surface, Figure 66 is an SEM photograph of the tips of photoreceptors in an isolated toad retina. The outer segments of scattered photoreceptors project well beyond the majority of outer segments. These projecting outer segments are mainly green rods, as shown by Figure 60. This may also be confirmed by examining a fresh retina with white light; if one focuses the tips of the red rods, the objective must be raised slightly to focus sharply upon tips of the green rods.

In Figure 67 the receptor surface was photographed directly from our television monitor, while illuminating the retina with only infrared light. Though the

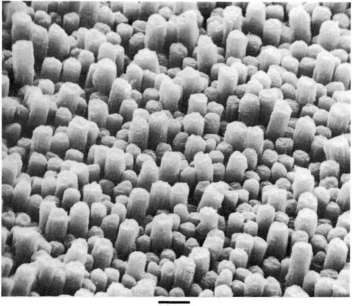

10 µm

Figure 66. Scanning electron micrograph of the tips of outer segments at the photoreceptor surface of an isolated toad retina.

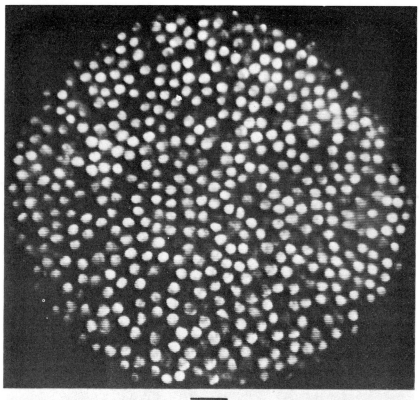

20 μm

Figure 67. The photoreceptor surface of a toad retina that was mounted in the recording chamber of our modular microscope, illuminated only with infrared light, and then photographed directly from the monitor screen of our infrared image conversion system.

outer segments average only about 6.0 μm in diameter, individual outer segments are well resolved, and the pattern of their distribution may be seen at a glance. This permitted the photoreceptor surface to be scanned quickly to find areas in which the outer segments were tightly packed in their normal hexagonal array, as shown in Figure 68. Only areas of this appearance, which showed little or no distortion from detaching and mounting the retina, were used for intracellular work.

In Figure 67 the microscope was focused upon the majority of photoreceptor tips, the red rods, each of which is sharply outlined and quite bright. Scattered among these red rods are green rods, which are less well focused and dimmer. These could be focused better by slightly raising the microscope objective. Since the inner segments of red rods are almost columnar, they function well as light pipes in passing light to the outer segments, which likewise act as light pipes;

thus light is conducted rather efficiently to the tips of outer segments of red rods, and they photograph quite well in Figure 67. By contrast, Figure 60 shows that the inner segments of green rods change rapidly from a thin fiber to a much larger one as light passes through them. This form of the inner segment is inefficient for transferring light to the outer segment, so the outer segments of green rods photograph much less brightly. From these criteria of focusing depth and relative brightness, the red and green rods could be readily identified in infrared views like the one illustrated.

Our infrared viewing system also permitted precise determination of when a micropipette contacted the tips of photoreceptors. The advance of a micropipette tip beyond the photoreceptor surface could thus be measured accurately. Combined with the measured angle of approach to the photoreceptor surface, depths of recordings from the photoreceptor surface could be determined with satisfactory accuracy.

In Figure 68 an initial contact is illustrated by photographs of the television monitor printed at higher magnification than in Figure 67. At this higher magnification the scan lines of the monitor become apparent but do not impair the resolution required for these purposes. In View 1 the arrow points to a red rod centrally located in a hexagonal array of other red rods. A micropipette tip has just made contact with this central rod, along an axis of approach indicated by the arrow, and the position of the contacted rod has not yet been disturbed relative to the surrounding rods. In View 2 the micropipette was advanced an

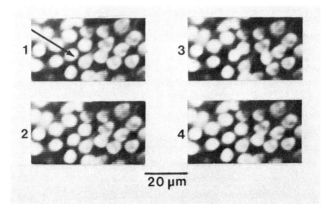

20 µm

Figure 68. Photographs of the photoreceptor surface of a toad retina, taken as described for Figure 67, to illustrate our method of determining when a micropipette initially contacted the tip of an outer segment. In View 1 the arrow indicates the orientation of the micropipette and it points to the red rod that has not yet been moved from its normal position in the surrounding hexagonal array of red rods. In View 2 the micropipette has been advanced 3.0 µm, with a resulting displacement of the contacted outer segment, and in View 3 a further advance of 3.0 µm has increased the displacement. In View 4 the micropipette has been withdrawn 6.0 µm to its original contact point, and the outer segment has also returned to its original position among the surrounding red rods.

additional 3.0 μm, which is indicated by a displacement of the central rod within the surrounding hexagonal array, and in View 3 a further advance of 3.0 μm displaced the central rod even further. In View 4 the micropipette was withdrawn 6.0 μm to the contact point, and the position of the central rod was restored. This result was not an isolated case but was used routinely to determine when the micropipette tip had reached the photoreceptor surface. The depth counter of our micropipette advancer was then set to zero, so that further advances along the electrode track could be measured from the photoreceptor surface.

PART VIII   MICROMANIPULATOR

A three-dimensional micromanipulator was required to position the micropipette tip near photoreceptor outer segments in the retinal area selected for study, prior to using our micropipette advancer to penetrate the photoreceptor layer. For this purpose we needed a micromanipulator sturdy enough to resist being moved by inadvertent hand contacts or by vibrations of the supporting table top when other elements of the experimental equipment were manipulated. Though relative compactness was also desired, we considered sturdiness as being much more important.

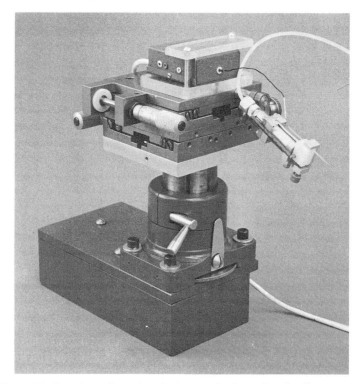

Figure 69. Our three-dimensional micromanipulator. For details, see text.

A micromanipulator with these features was assembled and is shown in Figure 69. The vertical movement was taken from an Emerson micromanipulator. It features a 2-in steel column driven by an axial screw with a smooth round head bearing against the surface upon which the device is mounted. The screw has fine threads (24/in.) and is moved by a knurled wheel of 3–5/8 in. diameter, so the vertical movement is sufficiently fine for most purposes. Rotation of the steel column is prevented by a spring-loaded key that travels in a V-groove, and when desired the movement may be locked firmly. In our experience this device is particularly helpful in supplying a fine vertical control that can also act as a sturdy base for elements providing movements along the other axes. Two micrometer-driven translation devices for X–Y movements, obtained from the Lansing Research Corporation (P.O. Box 730, Ithaca, NY 15851, USA), were mounted directly upon the vertical column. The headstage of our preamplifier, and the slave end of our hydraulic microdrive that carried the micropipette electrode, were then mounted upon the upper translation device. The entire micromanipulator was mounted upon a steel plate, which was mounted in turn upon a lead brick. This mass of lead (about 26 lbs) conferred additional resistance to vibration and eliminated the necessity of attaching the micromanipulator to the table top.

This micromanipulator has proved highly satisfactory and should be similarly useful in other applications where a sturdy micromanipulator is required for either the preparation or the micropipette advancer. For some applications a useful modification would be an adjustable tilt of the upper translation device, and the fineness of the X–Y motions may be adjusted by choosing appropriate micrometers.

PART IX ISOLATION OF PREPARATION FROM VIBRATION AND ELECTRICAL INTERFERENCE

IX.1 Vibration Isolation

IX.1a The mechanoelectric transducer action of micropipette tips

As shown by Brown and Wiesel (1959), in experiments where micropipette tips were advanced against a glass surface at an acute angle, the tip of a micropipette electrode is an extraordinarily sensitive mechanoelectric transducer. This property, which resides in the extreme tip, causes any deformation of the tip to be converted into a voltage signal.

IX.1b Isolation of preparation from floor vibrations

When using micropipette electrodes, inadvertent movements of either the micropipette or preparation can thus be troublesome. Though intracellular recordings may even be lost in extreme cases, the more usual problem is introduction of artifacts into electrical recordings. A common source of such movements is building vibrations, which will occur at a characteristic frequency for any given building, and of course the vibration amplitude increases at higher levels of the building. Our building vibrates at about 4 Hz, which identifies this type of artifact, and in our 7th floor laboratory the vibrations from wind and traffic cause almost continual recording artifacts unless appropriate precautions are taken. In some laboratories the floor vibrations resulting from walking in the experimental room or adjacent rooms can also be a problem.

Investigators have long handled such problems by mounting the preparation and micropipette holder on some type of heavy recording table that is shock-mounted to the floor. Figure 70 shows a relatively simple and inexpensive type of recording table that has long been used successfully in our laboratory. The base is cast of concrete in an H-form, as shown in the top view. Then a 2-in. slab of stone (the type used in chemical table tops) is set in mastic upon the

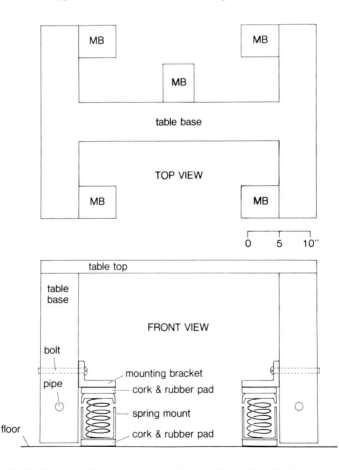

Figure 70. Scale drawing of our heavy recording table and its shock mounting to the floor, to isolate the preparation from floor vibrations. (MB) mounting bracket. For details, see text.

concrete base. Such a table in the indicated dimensions weighs about 1600 lbs. Pipes are cast into the base, as shown in the front view, for the insertion of rods to facilitate moving the table into position. It was originally placed on heavy rubber pads, but these proved inadequate for vibration-isolation. Following the advice of Alfred Strickholm, five vibration-isolators of the type shown in the front view were positioned as shown in the top view. Vibration-isolation pads containing layers of rubber and cork were placed both above and below an industrial vibration-isolating machinery mount containing a heavy coil spring. The internal damping provided especially by the cork significantly improves the vibration-isolation provided by the spring mount. Recording artifacts from building vibrations were then eliminated entirely. Such a table also provides an excellent base for mounting the preparation and equipment directly associated with it. This is mainly because the thick stone top transmits vibrations very poorly, particularly when mounted as described to the concrete base. During an experiment the recording table will sometimes be touched, either by necessity or inadvertently. If the resulting vibrations were readily transmitted through the table top, they would cause the micropipette to move relative to the preparation, but no significant problem of that type has been experienced with the illustrated design.

In recent years relatively heavy tables supported by a cushion of compressed air have become commercially available from a number of companies, and these tables have become rather popular. We have not tried any of them, but they have proven to be satisfactory in several laboratories in our department where the requirements are similar to ours. An improvised inexpensive version of this type of table is a heavy table top supported by inner tubes from small tires, such as those used on motor scooters. We understand this method is also being used by a number of investigators.

IX.1c   *Taking advantage of the mechanoelectric transducer action of micropipette tips*

Though this property of micropipette electrodes is usually a disadvantage, because of movement artifacts, there are also cases where it can be used to advantage. For example, it was used by Brown and Wiesel (1959) to detect contact of the micropipette with the retinal surface in an intact and circulated cat eye, as shown in Figure 71. Since the retina was moving slightly in response to both respiration and the pulse beat, these movements were first recorded upon contacting the retinal surface. With minimal contact the pulse beat was recorded only during late inspiration and early expiration of each respiratory cycle (Figure 71A). After advancing another 6 μm, the pulse beat was recorded continuously and was superimposed upon the full respiratory cycle, with the pulse beats becoming maximal in amplitude during late inspiration and early expiration (Figure 71B). Since the circulatory supply of the mammalian retina is layered, similar methods provided identification of certain deep levels of the retina. So these techniques also assisted in determining the depths of cells

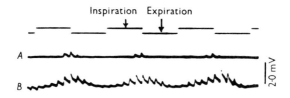

Figure 71. Recording of pulse and respiratory movements at the retinal surface in an intact and normally circulated cat eye. In Record A the tip of a micropipette electrode contacted the retina only during late inspiration and early expiration, as indicated by brief recordings of pulse movements. In Record B the micropipette tip was advanced a further 6 μm, which was just sufficient to establish continuous retinal contact. Pulse movements were then superimposed continuously upon the full respiratory cycle, with the amplitude of pulse movements becoming maximal during late inspiration and early expiration. Artificial respiration at 2.7 sec per cycle; negative deflections shown upward. (From Brown and Wiesel (1959), reproduced by permission of The Physiological Society, Cambridge, England)

yielding various types of electrical responses to light, thus aiding the identification of those cells (Brown and Wiesel, 1959). In addition, these methods permitted determination of the depth at which each major component of the local ERG becomes maximum in amplitude, thus establishing the retinal level at which each major ERG component is generated (Brown and Wiesel, 1961b).

As previously mentioned (Chapter 3, Section I.1), it is also quite possible that reversal of the mechanoelectric transducer action provides the mechanism whereby an oscillating current across the micropipette can improve cell penetration, presumably by causing the very tip of the micropipette to vibrate.

In short, though opportunities to take advantage of the mechanoelectric property of micropipettes are rather rare, this property can be quite helpful under certain conditions.

IX.2   Isolation from Electrical Interference

When recording small electrical signals at high gain with micropipette electrodes, interference from unwanted electrical signals generated within or outside the recording room is a problem for all investigators. The usual solution is to place the preparation (and the headstage of the preamplifier) in a grounded metal cage that shields the preparation from electrical interference. The main difficulty is isolating the preparation electrically while keeping it accessible to adjustments that must be made within the shielded cage either during or between experiments.

Figure 72 shows the design of a shielded cage that has long solved this problem in our laboratory. As shown in front view, the cage contains an access door in front of the modular microscope. This door is small enough to operate easily without disturbing an intracellular recording, yet it is large enough to permit almost all manipulations that are required within the cage during experiments.

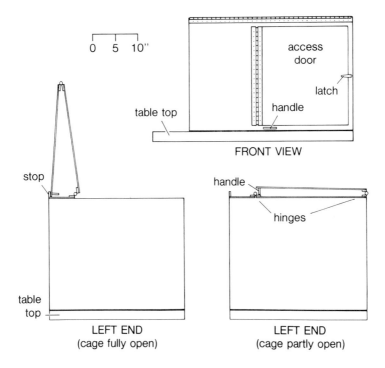

FRONT VIEW

LEFT END
(cage fully open)

LEFT END
(cage partly open)

Figure 72. Scale drawing of our shielded cage to isolate the preparation from electrical interference. During experiments a front door provides access to the preparation. For greater access the entire front of the cage may be opened, and the top of the cage may be opened as well, as shown in the two end views. Such complete access is seldom required during experiments but is very helpful between experiments.

For greater access the cage may be opened further in two stages. The entire front of the cage is supported by a piano hinge along its upper edge, as illustrated in the front view. This allows the entire front of the cage to be opened and folded onto the top of the cage, as shown in one of the end views. For further access the top of the cage is also attached by a piano hinge permitting the front and top to be lifted together to stand upright, as shown in the other end view. The contents of the shielded cage thus become fully accessible. Though we have never needed to open the cage completely during an intracellular recording, this capability has proved very helpful at other times during or between experiments.

In our work the preparation must be protected not only from electrical interference, but from light in the recording room. We thus construct the cage from sheet aluminum about 1.5 mm thick, which provides adequate electrical shielding for our needs, and its light weight facilitates opening the front and top of the cage.

PART X   RECORDING, ANALYSIS AND STORAGE OF ELECTRICAL RESPONSES

X.1   Introduction

Experiments involving electrical responses of excitable cells often present difficulties in recording and analyzing the responses efficiently and in storing them with easy access for further analysis. The traditional method of photographing each response from the face of an oscilloscope has many shortcomings. Most of these may be alleviated by computer techniques, as a number of investigators have discovered. Our own applications of computer techniques to these problems have proved very useful and should be adaptable to a large range of experimental problems; hence these applications will now be described.

X.2   Equipment

Our recording system is illustrated by the block diagram of Figure 73. A chlorided silver wire contacts the solution in the shaft of the micropipette, and a chlorided silver reference electrode contacts the solution in the recording chamber. The signal between these electrodes first enters a Model 1090 Micro-Electrode Pre-Amplifier (Winston Electronics, 1090 Ahwahnee Dr., Millbrae, CA 94030, USA). This unit has an input impedance of 10^{12} Ω, an adjustable negative capacitance, and output terminals with gains of either $1\times$ or $10\times$. The headstage of this unit is in the shielded cage; this permits a short lead to the micropipette for the further reduction of noise pickup. A shielded lead then carries the signal outside the cage to the preamplifier. The $1\times$ output is used to record light-evoked responses, while the $10\times$ output is used without further amplification for the recording of resting membrane potentials. Since the light-evoked responses require relatively high gain, they are passed first into a recentering unit to compensate for drift and to maintain all signals within the operating range of our recording equipment. This recentering unit also amplifies the responses by $100\times$, and they are then passed through a low-pass filter with a bandwidth of 0–30 Hz. This filter is of the 'active' type, by comparison with the 'passive' type of filter provided by an RC network. Above 30 Hz this active filter provides an attenuation of 12 db/octave, compared to only 3 db/octave obtainable with a passive filter. This sharp cutoff eliminates the 60 Hz line frequency from our recordings, but a 60 Hz notch filter may also be needed in some other applications. For intracellular work in toad rods, the filtering of frequencies above 30 Hz does not distort light-evoked responses, and the reduction of high-frequency noise reduces the noise level of all records.

During an experiment, light-evoked responses are displayed upon a storage oscilloscope and also recorded upon a 4-channel FM tape recorder for permanent records that may be analyzed later as desired. An S-100 computer triggers light stimuli at the desired frequency, which is set at the beginning of each experiment. These timing pulses trigger the shutter control and the sweep of the

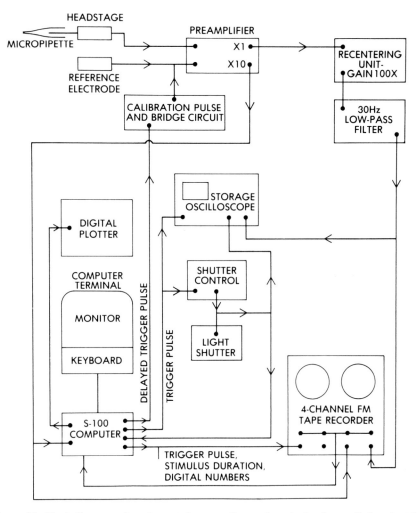

Figure 73. Block diagram of equipment for recording and analyzing intracellular electrical responses of vertebrate photoreceptors.

storage oscilloscope. After a slight delay the computer also triggers a calibration pulse, which is delivered through a bridge circuit to the reference lead of the preamplifier. Upon receiving its trigger pulse, the shutter control provides a variable delay and then opens an electromagnetic shutter for a variable duration of the light stimulus. The signals for opening and closing the shutter are fed to the storage oscilloscope, and also into the computer, from which they are fed to the tape recorder. The computer thus acts as the master timer initiating each stimulus, and it assigns a number to each stimulus that codes the elicited response. This number appears upon the computer terminal and is also fed to the tape recorder. The resting membrane potential is fed from the preamplifier to the computer, where it is read by analog-to-digital converter and signal-averaged. The digital resting membrane potential then appears on the computer terminal just after the number of the response with which it is associated. The tape recorder receives the resting membrane potential directly and it also receives the digital value from the computer in coded form.

Following an experiment the tape recording is played back through the computer, which is also programmed to measure the amplitude of each light-evoked response, and permanent records are made by a digital plotter as illustrated in the following section. When used in this way, an important function of the computer is to store signals that were originally recorded with a relatively fast time base and then feed them more slowly into a digital plotter which lacks the response speed of an oscilloscope but provides more convenient permanent records.

X.3   Results

Figure 74 shows sample records reproduced directly from our digital plotter. Three light-evoked responses are shown that were recorded intracellularly from a red rod of the toad retina, the micropipette tip having probably been located in the inner segment. These responses are from a series in which a well dark adapted retina was stimulated by light flashes of increasing intensity from threshold to the maximum response amplitude that could be elicited. The illustrated responses are from the central portion of this series, and the light intensity was increased 1.0 log unit for each record, reading from top to bottom.

Just after the beginning of each record, a square calibrating pulse provides voltage and time calibrations. This is followed shortly by the light flash, which is displayed as a bar just above the onset of the response. The illustrated changes in latency, amplitude and time course of light-evoked responses, as a function of stimulus intensity, are typical of vertebrate photoreceptors. Just before the onset of each record there are three numbers, which the computer was programmed to provide. The upper one is the coded number of the response, the middle one is the resting membrane potential in mV, and the bottom number is the amplitude of the light-evoked response in mV. The resting membrane potential was determined by signal-averaging a sample of 1000 points during the 1.0 sec interval just prior to each calibration signal. Response amplitudes were determined as the difference between the signal-averaged baseline (just before onset of the light stimulus) and the maximum negativity attained during the light response.

The records of Figure 74 illustrate a number of points. The insertion of a calibration signal for voltage and time at the beginning of each record is a useful convenience. During an experiment the gain and time base must often be changed, and these changes are registered automatically by the calibration signal. This eliminates the need to record every change of this type in the protocol, and errors resulting from failure to record such changes are abolished. By inserting the calibration signal well ahead of the response, this signal may readily be cut from published records if that is desired.

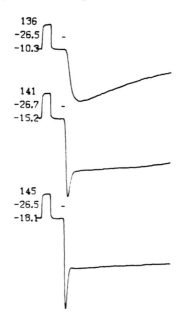

Figure 74. Sample experimental responses that have been stored on tape, computer-processed, and recorded by a digital chart recorder. Responses obtained intracellularly from a red rod in the isolated and inverted toad retina. Micropipette electrodes formed by our puller and filled with 0.15 M KCL adjusted to a pH of 7.0. Ancillary recording techniques were as described in this chapter. Stimulus was a focused spot of 500 nm light that was 10 mm in diameter, centered upon the micropipette tip, 100 msec in duration, and delivered once every 30 sec to the well dark adapted retina. Reading from top to bottom, the stimulus intensity was increased 1.0 log unit for each record. At the left of each record the number of the response is given at the top, followed by the computer-averaged resting membrane potential in mV, and the third number is the computer-measured baseline-to-peak amplitude of the light-evoked response in mV. Just after the beginning of each record is a calibration signal 5.0 mV in amplitude and 250 msec in duration. Duration of the light stimulus is indicated by a bar over each record. For further details, see text.

The computer-generated numbers are helpful in a variety of ways. The number of each response appears on the computer terminal during the experiment, as well as in the permanent records. This makes it easy to keep an accurate protocol, which only needs to record the relevant conditions under which each numbered response was obtained, since the responses are similarly numbered in the permanent record.

In Figure 74 the resting membrane potential of about 26.5 mV might be thought quite low, but for vertebrate photoreceptors this is in the normal range of values. Unlike most excitable cells, vertebrate rods and cones respond to light only by hyperpolarization, as Figure 74 illustrates. The relatively low resting membrane potential seems a necessary feature of this photoreceptor activity, since it permits a relatively long range for the hyperpolarizing responses to light. The digital recording of signal-averaged resting membrane potentials is more accurate than hand measurement of records. Note in Figure 74 that values are given to the first decimal place, and that the membrane potential is quite stable from one recording to the next, even when it is expressed with this accuracy. This is not a misleading result of careful record selection but was typical of many of our intracellular recordings. In short, our intracellular techniques permit sufficiently stable resting membrane potentials to take advantage of the improved accuracy of this method of measuring them. The provision of resting membrane potentials associated with each response is helpful both during and after experiments. By following these values on the computer terminal, one may decide when the resting membrane potential has become sufficiently stable to carry out any given type of experiment with intracellular recording, while the permanent records reveal the stability actually obtained for the resting membrane potential during the experiment. In some cases the experimental procedure will alter the resting membrane potential, which is one of the dependent variables, and in such cases the desired data are accurately provided. In all cases where resting membrane potentials must be measured, of course the illustrated method saves the labor of measuring records by hand. In our work, response amplitude is almost always a significant dependent variable. Thus the provision of digital values of response amplitude for each recording is also useful because of the improved accuracy and saving of labor, compared with measuring records by hand.

X.4   Storage of Records

Our records are read out by the digital chart recorder in vertical columns, as shown in Figure 74, and the columns progress from left to right upon a continuous strip of paper that is accordion-folded into 8 1/2×11 in. sheets. This format is convenient for storage and all records are readily accessible, since the accordion-folded records may be read like a book. For each experiment we attach the protocol to the records and file them together. Information from the protocol is sometimes transcribed so that the relevant experimental facts are also indicated beside each response. This takes little time, and thereafter the entire experiment may be read quickly without referring to the protocol.

X.5   Comparison with Conventional Methods

In addition to points already covered, there are other comparisons to be made between conventional methods of record handling and those just described. Conventional photography of the oscilloscope face requires a camera that interferes to some extent with visibility of the oscilloscope, unless a separate slave oscilloscope is used for photography. More important, the experimenter must give thought to taking appropriate photographs during the experiment, and this extra burden can distract from the main purpose of performing the experiment as well as possible. In addition, if the photographs do not come out well for any reason, the results of an entire crucial experiment may be lost. After the experiment the film must be developed, an inconvenient and time-consuming step, and we do not know of any fully satisfactory method of storing the negative film (usually 35 mm) so that all records are readily available. Finally, when illustrations are made for publication, each record must usually be printed as a positive enlargement, which requires further darkroom work before the individual records may be assembled into an illustration.

Of course all of these disadvantages of oscilloscope photography are avoided by the methods just described. In addition, when responses are tape-recorded and transcribed later, they may be recorded in various ways. For example, the gain and time scale may be altered as desired, and records are readily superimposed when this is required. Though computers and digital plotters were expensive when they first became available, comparative cost of photographic and computer-based recording equipment is no longer a significant factor. In deciding whether to use computer-based methods, of course the saving in labor and the flexible capabilities of the equipment should also be considered. In our experience the only significant limitation of the described methods is the need for a person who can program the computer to do the experimenter's bidding. But even this limitation is now becoming less critical as improved package programs are becoming available for laboratory research.

CHAPTER 13

Evaluation of Improved Intracellular Recording Techniques in Vertebrate Photoreceptors

PART I METHODS

Much can be learned about micropipettes, and methods of advancing them through tissues, from physical measurements. Performance in an experiment, however, must always be the critical test. We thus tested micropipettes in a series of intracellular recording experiments. Some preparations are more suitable than others for this type of work. We used the isolated and inverted toad retina for intracellular recording from the exposed rod photoreceptors, as described in Part II of Chapter 12. As a preparation for testing microelectrodes, toad rods offer two major advantages. First, they provide a dense population of cells of quite uniform size, so the size of each cell penetrated is known within narrow limits. Second, these cells are small enough to provide a rigorous test of how well microelectrodes can penetrate small cells without significant damage.

For all intracellular work in this preparation, micropipettes were formed by our Model P-77 puller with the round loop filament, since this work was conducted before the rectangular trough and square loop filaments were adopted.

All micropipettes were filled with 5 M K-acetate by the Omega Dot method, as described in Section I.3b of Chapter 10. Microelectrodes were advanced through the photoreceptor layer by our high speed stepping hydraulic advancer, as described previously (Brown and Flaming, 1977a) and in Section III.6 of Chapter 11. The step size was 3.0 μm, during which a velocity of 2.0 μm/msec was attained without any significant vibrations after termination of the step (see Figure 56). All ancillary techniques for this work have been described in Chapter 12.

PART II   RECORDING SITES

The outer and inner segments of red rods are both cylindrical in form, with diameters varying from 5.0–7.5 μm and averaging about 5.9 μm, as may be noted in Figure 60. In the case of green rods, the outer segments are similar in form and diameter, but the inner segment tapers rapidly to a thin fiber that is very unfavorable for intracellular recording. Almost all recordings were from red rods, because of their strong numerical predominance and because their inner segments are favorable for intracellular work. Occasional recordings were also obtained, however, from the outer segments of green rods (Brown and Flaming, 1977b). Green and red rods have respective absorption maxima of their photopigments at 432 and 502 nm (Gordon and Hood, 1976). Thus green and red rods were readily distinguished by observing relative response amplitudes to stimuli of equal quantum content at wavelengths of 429 and 509 nm. Whereas the green rod gives a larger response to the shorter wavelength, the red rod responds more strongly to the longer one. Initial contact of a micropipette with the exposed tip of an outer segment could be directly visualized with infrared light (see Figure 68). Intracellular recordings were sometimes obtained at that point. Additional intracellular recordings could be positively identified with outer segments when they were obtained at distances beyond the contact point that were too short to be from inner segments. Though recordings from inner segments could not be so surely identified, inner segments of red rods are favorable for intracellular recording because they are held to some extent by the terminals of Müller fibers that form the internal limiting membrane (see Figure 60), and intracellular recordings were most frequently obtained from red rods at depths appropriate to their inner segments. Red rod responses that appeared to be from inner segments showed no distinct difference in form or amplitude from the outer segment responses.

PART III   IMPROVEMENT OF INTRACELLULAR RECORDINGS BY OUR TECHNIQUES

III.1   Overall Improvement by Comparison with Previous Techniques

Though we have not tested the separate effects of each of our techniques upon intracellular recording, the combined effect of some of our main improvements of technique has been assessed. In this comparison the baseline results were those obtainable during intracellular recordings from photoreceptors of cold blooded vertebrates (such as toad rods) prior to developing our improved techniques. The methods and results obtained at that time have been given in some detail in Section I.1 of Chapter 3. Briefly, micropipettes were usually formed by the Livingston puller (which then gave the best results for this type of work), and micropipettes were advanced through the preparation by an advancer providing relatively slow steps, such as the unmodified Kopf hydraulic microdrive (see Figure 56). Cell penetration was often assisted by tapping the recording table, moving the preparation rapidly with a 'jolting' device (Tomita, 1965), or passing brief pulses of alternating current through the microelectrode (see Section I.1 of Chapter 3). These techniques yielded useful results but had many disadvantages, as reflected by experience in our own laboratory and many others. Intracellular recordings were difficult to obtain, and those obtained usually deteriorated rapidly. Typically, a week of daily experimentation would yield only one or two recordings of publishable quality, and even the best recordings were rarely held for more than 15 min, during which the resting membrane potential and light-evoked responses were almost always declining in amplitude. Thus results were costly in time, effort, support funds, and experimental animals. In addition, the quality of data that could be obtained, and even the types of experiments that could be performed, were severely limited.

Shortly after our improved techniques were developed, we performed many intracellular experiments in toad rods (Brown and Flaming, 1977b, 1978, 1979b; Flaming and Brown, 1979a; Oakley *et al.*, 1979). This work was done with Standard Tubing, since the advantages of special tubings using a thick wall or large Omega Dot had not yet been demonstrated. Nevertheless, the improvement of results was astonishing. Impalements of outer and inner segments of toad rods became so easy that several were commonly obtained during a single traverse through the photoreceptor layer. With impalements this common, there was no longer any temptation to waste time on a recording that was not promising. So we immediately left any recording in which the resting membrane potential and light-evoked responses were undesirably small or showed any sign of significant deterioration. In a typical experiment only 10–20 min was required to obtain a high quality impalement. By that time 20–30 other recordings had usually been obtained and rejected. Impalements accepted for study had resting membrane potentials of at least 25 mV (up to 46 mV) and maximum (saturated) light-evoked responses of at least 15 mV (up to 25 mV). In recordings of this initial quality, both the resting membrane potential and light-evoked responses frequently remained stable in amplitude within 1–2 mV for 3–4 hr. Thus all the data of a given experiment were often obtained from the same photoreceptor. In short, intracellular recordings were much more easily obtained, with little or no indication of damage to the cells penetrated, and stable recording conditions could thereafter be maintained for exceptionally long periods.

III.2 Specific Capabilities of Our Techniques

III.2a *Increased efficiency of intracellular work*

Improved cell penetration yields major advantages in the efficiency with which experiments may be conducted. Before developing our improved techniques, almost all of our time during experiments was spent searching for adequate intracellular recordings. By contrast, the improved techniques permitted experiments to be devoted almost entirely to the collection of high quality data. This provided major savings of experimental time and effort, while reducing requirements for animals and research funding. Of course reducing the animals needed for a given project is always desirable from a humane standpoint. When scarce animal populations are involved, it also becomes both ecologically important and a helpful strategy for accomplishing research with the limited animals available. In recent years improved research efficiency has likewise become increasingly desirable to help maintain the pace of scientific work in the face of budgetary restrictions.

III.2b *Improved results in experiments requiring prolonged intracellular recording*

A major advantage of the improved stability of intracellular recordings is that observations may be made under control conditions, followed by an experimental condition, followed again by control observations. This permits an accurate comparison of experimental and control observations in the same cell. In addition, the before-and-after control observations permit determination of whether experimental effects, such as an altered ion concentration in the perfusate, are fully reversible. In some cases this has permitted experiments to be performed in a more critical manner than previously possible.

For example, in an experiment requiring at least 2 hr of stable recording, we examined effects of altering external Ca^{2+} concentration upon the sensitivity of toad rods (Flaming and Brown, 1979a). As shown in Figure 75, an entire curve was first obtained showing the response amplitude of a red rod as a function of stimulus intensity in a normal external Ca^{2+} concentration. A curve was then obtained in elevated Ca^{2+}, followed by another control curve in normal Ca^{2+}, then Ca^{2+} was lowered, followed by a final control curve. The five curves in Figure 75 are numbered in the order in which they were obtained, and $[Ca^{2+}]_0$ indicates the Ca^{2+} concentrations in mM. The resting membrane potential in control solution was -38 mV throughout the experiment, but it hyperpolarized about 1.0 mV in elevated Ca^{2+} and depolarized about 6.0 mV in lowered Ca^{2+}. The effects of raised Ca^{2+} mimicked light adaptation by hyperpolarizing the resting membrane potential, reducing the maximum light-evoked response, and shifting the entire response curve toward higher stimulus intensities, while lowered Ca^{2+} produced the opposite effects. Shifts of the curves along the stimulus intensity axis were indicated by altered values of σ,

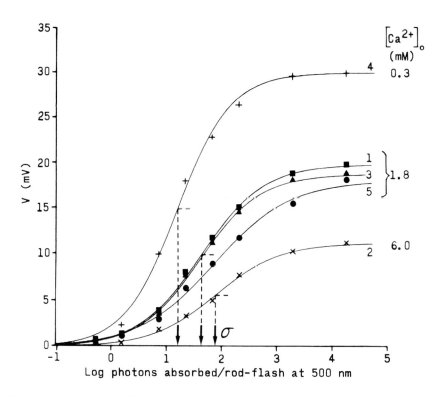

Figure 75. Effects of $[Ca^{2+}]_o$, the external Ca^{2+} concentration, upon the V-log I curve of a well dark adapted red rod in the toad retina. V is the peak response amplitude in mV, while the stimulus intensity (log I) is given in log photons absorbed/rod flash at 500 nm. Each curve is numbered at the right in the order in which curves were obtained. For further details, see text. (From Flaming and Brown (1979a), reprinted by permission from *Nature*, Copyright 1979 by Macmillan Journals Ltd., London.)

the stimulus intensity evoking a response of one-half the maximum (saturated) response amplitude. In earlier work Lipton *et al.* (1977) had failed to find any shifts of σ and had thus concluded that Ca^{2+} cannot exert the major control of adaptive changes in light sensitivity. The different findings and conclusions of our work were strongly dependent upon our greatly improved conditions for intracellular recording (Flaming and Brown, 1979a, 1979b).

III.2c   The extension of systematic intracellular work to new cell types

Among the various types of cells in a given preparation, there are typically large differences in the difficulty of obtaining intracellular recordings. Toad rods provide an example of this, green rods being much more difficult to impale than red rods. This is partly because of the considerably lower density of green rods and partly because the inner segments of green rods are too small

for intracellular work. Previous intracellular techniques yielded only very rare
penetrations of green rod outer segments, combined with rapid deterioration of
the recordings, so only fragmentary observations could be made. By improving
both the frequency of impalement and the stability of our recordings, our techniques made it possible to perform systematic experiments with green rods. Of
course impalements of green rods remained rare compared with red rods, but
by immediately rejecting red rods and searching diligently, enough green rods
were impaled that stable recordings were obtained. Figures 76 to 78 were all
taken from the same green rod during an afternoon that yielded experiments on
three different green rods. Though this work has been reported in abstract form
(Brown and Flaming, 1977b), the figures have not been published previously.
They are presented here as an example of how our improved techniques have
brought a new type of cell within the scope of systematic intracellular work.
In addition, some of the findings are of interest in the physiology of vertebrate
photoreceptors.

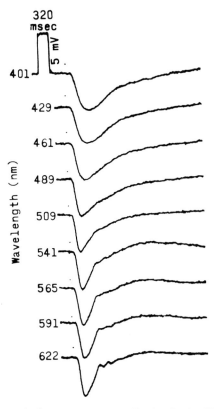

Figure 76. Responses evoked at a constant amplitude of 5.0 mV by light stimuli of varying wavelength, recorded intracellularly from the outer segment of a green rod in the toad
retina. Resting membrane potential was stable at 28 mV. Light stimuli were centered and
focused upon the recording area, 10 mm in diameter, and delivered in 100 msec flashes
at 10 sec intervals. Onset of light flash indicated by a dot over each recording.

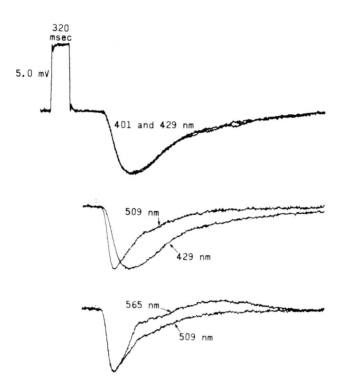

Figure 77. Selected pairs of superimposed responses from the experiment of Figure 76, to better illustrate changes in the time course of responses as a function of stimulus wavelength.

Figure 76 shows light-evoked intracellular responses of a green rod to stimuli of varying wavelength, with stimulus intensity adjusted at each wavelength to evoke responses of 5.0 mV peak amplitude. If the responses were generated entirely by light absorption in the impaled photoreceptor, constant amplitude responses to stimuli of varying wavelength should all be identical in form (univariant). Though red rods have thus far proved univariant, Figure 76 shows that green rods are not. At short wavelengths the response is a hyperpolarization of relatively slow time course. At longer wavelengths the response is more rapid, showing a faster rise to an earlier and sharper peak, from which decay is also faster. Finally, at the longest wavelengths, there is also a delayed slow wave of after-depolarization.

In Figure 77 these results are examined further by superimposing selected pairs of responses. The responses to 401 and 429 nm have identical time courses and are thus generated by a single type of photoreceptor. When responses to 429 and 509 nm are compared, the 509 response shows a distinctly more rapid time course, so this response must be generated largely by light absorption

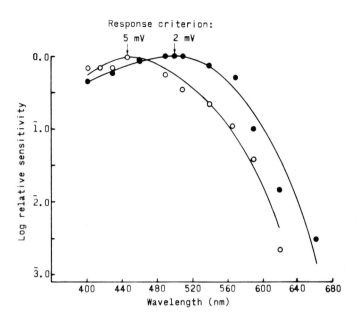

Figure 78. Log relative sensitivity as a function of stimulus wavelength for criterion response amplitudes of 2.0 and 5.0 mV. Data obtained from the green rod of Figure 76. Log relative sensitivity plotted from stimulus intensities required to elicit responses of constant amplitude.

in another type of photoreceptor. Finally, when responses to 509 and 565 nm are superimposed, their time courses remain identical until shortly after the response peak. Thereafter, the 565 response exhibits a slow depolarizing wave that is not seen in the 509 response.

Since each type of photoreceptor contains a distinctive photopigment, curves that exhibit sensitivity as a function of stimulus wavelength are especially helpful for identifying the type of photoreceptor generating a given response. For the experiment of Figure 76 with a criterion response amplitude of 5.0 mV, data were replotted in Figure 78 to show sensitivity as a function of stimulus wavelength. This was readily done from the relative stimulus intensities required to elicit responses of constant amplitude. Just before the experiment of Figure 76, data had been obtained from the same green rod at a criterion response amplitude of 2.0 mV. These results are also plotted in Figure 78 and are strikingly different. The sensitivity function for 2.0 mV responses corresponds closely to the absorption spectrum of red rods, which peaks at 502 nm, while the sensitivity function for 5.0 mV responses fits well to the absorption spectrum of the green rod photopigment, which peaks at about 432 nm (Gordon and Hood, 1976). Thus Figure 78 shows that red rods, as well as green rods, contribute to hyperpolarizing light-evoked responses recorded intracellularly from the outer segments of green rods.

As pointed out in Section VII.2 of Chapter 12, the inner segments of red rods convey light to the outer segments by internal reflection, and this process is much less efficient in the case of green rods. This appears to account for red rods having a higher brightness than green rods when the outer segments are viewed end-on by transmitted light (see Figure 67). This must also provide red rods with a higher sensitivity than green rods and thus account, at least in part, for red rods dominating the 2.0 mV responses of a green rod in Figure 78. Since the effects of light absorption in red rods could be recorded in a green rod, of course this also implies that red rods are synaptically connected to green rods. At the higher response amplitude of 5.0 mV, Figure 78 shows that the green rod photopigment dominates the sensitivity function. Thus, when the stimulus is sufficiently strong to activate the green rod directly, light absorption in the green rod photopigment becomes more effective than that absorbed by the red rods.

At the shortest wavelengths of Figure 78, the green rod photopigment would have the greatest advantage for light absorption compared with the red rod photopigment. Hence the green rods probably contribute the slow hyperpolarizing responses to short wavelengths that are shown in Figure 76. At longer wavelengths the excitation of red rods would increase relative to green rods, so in Figure 76 the red rods probably contribute the more rapid hyperpolarization to long wavelengths, especially since Figure 78 clearly demonstrates that red rods can generate hyperpolarizing responses in green rods. The slow wave of after-depolarization in Figure 76 is probably contributed by cones, since it is only seen at wavelengths above 509 nm and becomes maximum in the range of 541–565 nm.

As summarized by Brown (1980), it is well known that summative hyperpolarizing interactions can occur between vertebrate photoreceptors of the same class, and that delayed inhibitory interactions can occur between cones of different classes. Our findings in green rods of the toad indicate a notable exception to these rules, since green rods appear to be influenced by summative interaction from a different class of receptor (the red rod). It has also been shown in Macaque monkeys that photopic stimulus intensities which activate cones strongly suppress the rod receptor potential (Whitten and Brown, 1973). The rod receptor potential decays much more slowly than that of cones, especially when pure rod responses are evoked at photopic stimulus intensities. Hence the photopic suppression of rods by cones appears to be an important mechanism permitting cones to take advantage of their superior ability to resolve stimuli that are separated in time. Since this mechanism has not been observed by previous intracellular work in cold blooded vertebrates, it may have been a rather late development in the evolution of mammals. But it is also noteworthy that green rods of the toad retina appear to be influenced by a delayed inhibitory interaction from cones, as indicated by the after-depolarization evoked by light stimuli of relatively long wavelength. These findings suggest that more detailed studies of green rods, which are now feasible, might well be of special interest.

III.2d   Instructional intracellular demonstrations

As a further consequence of the new-found ease of intracellular work in this preparation, we began using it for live demonstrations of intracellular recording in vertebrate photoreceptors. To our knowledge this had never before been attempted, but these demonstrations were conducted for a number of years as part of a course in Visual Physiology. During a designated afternoon, students came into the laboratory in several successive small groups. Each group was shown the satisfactory impalement of a toad rod and the effect of stimulus variables such as intensity, duration, and color upon the amplitude and time course of light-evoked responses. Though the quality of recordings and the amount that could be illustrated in such a short time inevitably varied between groups, these demonstrations were always successful.

PART IV   INTERPRETATION OF IMPROVED CAPABILITIES FOR INTRACELLULAR WORK

In the absence of detailed analysis, of course we cannot be certain which of our techniques contributed the most to the described improvement of intracellular recording in this preparation. But we believe the most important factor to be the ultrafine short tips provided by our airjet micropipette puller. Undoubtedly the high speed stepping hydraulic microdrive also contributed, because its short high speed steps frequently impaled cells. Many impalements, however, were still obtained by passing a burst of 60 Hz current through the micropipette. Some other aspects of our technique may also have assisted. For example, our methods of mounting and superfusing the toad retina may have significantly improved the mechanical stability of the preparation and its maintenance in good physiological condition for several hours.

It should be emphasized that the much improved intracellular recording capabilities, as described in Part III of this chapter, were obtained with Standard Tubing and the original round loop heating filament. Our Tubing 9 can provide a further major improvement in the ease of penetrating small cells, as reported in Section II.2 of Chapter 14, and Tubing 1 probably has similar advantages since it provides smaller tips than Standard Tubing (see Section III.2e of Chapter 6). In addition, our square loop filament can markedly reduce tip size in the case of Tubing 9, and a similar effect may be expected with Tubing 1 (see Section III.1 of Chapter 14). Finally, the use of aluminosilicate tubing can provide still smaller tips, as shown in Section VII.1 of Chapter 18.

In summary, though this chapter has demonstrated major improvements of intracellular recording, the use of a square loop filament in conjunction with borosilicate Tubings 1 or 9, or aluminosilicate tubing, should provide significant further improvements in the ease of obtaining and maintaining high quality intracellular recordings in small cells.

CHAPTER 14

Evaluation of Tubing Designs for Intracellular Work

PART I   METHODS

The basic methods for this work were as described in the preceding chapter. Micropipettes were formed on our Model P-77 puller with the round loop filament, filled with 5 M K-acetate by the Omega Dot method, and advanced by our stepping hydraulic advancer, using a step size of 3.0 μm. The preparation remained the isolated and inverted toad retina, with intracellular recordings being obtained from the outer and inner segments of red rods and the outer segments of green rods.

When comparing capillary tubings that may be used for micropipettes, a number of precautions were necessary. In each experiment of this type, micropipettes were formed from Standard Tubing and a comparison tubing at constant puller settings. The difficulty of obtaining intracellular recordings can vary greatly from one toad retina to another, and it can even change markedly during an experiment on a given retina. These factors were rendered negligible by alternating, throughout each experiment, electrodes made from Standard Tubing and from the comparison tubing. Each electrode was used for only one retinal penetration, to minimize breakage of tips in the retina. At the angle of penetration in this work, a distance of about 200 μm was required along the electrode track to pass the inner segments of the red rods; hence each penetration consisted of a 200 μm advance beyond initial contact with the tip of a photoreceptor. During each penetration the retina was stimulated repetitively with light delivered through the condenser system of our microscope (see Figure 63). This stimulus was a 100 msec flash of 500 nm light centered upon the recording electrode and covering a circular retinal area 1.0 mm in diameter. The flash was delivered every 10 sec and had an intensity at which about 26 photons were absorbed/red rod/flash. Details of this calculation have already been given, and at this stimulus intensity fully dark adapted responses are only about 38% of the maximum response amplitude to a saturating stimulus intensity (Brown and Flaming, 1979b). The repetitive low-intensity flash also maintained the retina at a constant low level of light adaptation.

During each retinal penetration we counted all intracellular recordings yielding initial light-evoked responses of 1.0 mV or larger. The amplitudes of light responses just after cell penetration were also recorded. While the number of intracellular recordings per retinal penetration indicates the ease with which cells were impaled, the relative response amplitude indicates the condition of the cell and the quality of recording conditions just after impaling the cell.

PART II   COMPARISON OF CAPILLARY TUBING DESIGNS

For intracellular work in any given type of cell, one may ask two main questions relative to micropipette design. One concerns how much the tip can be enlarged by lowering OD/ID while still obtaining satisfactory cell penetration. This is particularly important if it is necessary to increase the internal tip diameter as much as possible for injecting a solution or material into the cell. The second question concerns how much cell penetration may be improved, relative to results with Standard Tubing, by manipulating the factors of tubing design examined in this work.

II.1   Tubing Design for Microinjections into Cells

Table 5 shows the results when electrodes formed from Standard Tubing were compared with those formed from the thin-walled Tubing 3. The OD_t averaged 0.08 μm for Standard Tubing and increased to 0.17 μm for Tubing 3 (see Table 2). Table 5 shows that the mean number of rods impaled per retinal penetration dropped from 3.19 with Standard Tubing to only 1.05 for Tubing 3. This difference was statistically highly significant ($p = 0.00001$). Also, with Tubing 3 the responses after impalement deteriorated much more rapidly in most cases.

By contrast, the average response amplitude just after penetration dropped only from 4.01 mV with Standard Tubing to 3.67 mV with Tubing 3. This 8.5% reduction is in the expected direction and is probably meaningful but did not prove statistically significant ($p = 0.26$). In measuring the effectiveness of micropipette electrodes for intracellular work, the frequency of impalements is thus a much more sensitive index than average response amplitude just after impaling cells. We have noted this principle consistently, and it also holds when frequency of impalements is compared with maximum response amplitudes.

Table 5. Intracellular recording performance of two experimental tubings compared with Standard Tubing. For details, see text

Designation of tubing	OD (mm)	ID (mm)	Omega Dot diameter (mm)	Wall thickness (mm)	OD/ID	Predicted F_o	No. of electrodes tested	Mean No. of rods impaled/retinal penetration ± S.E.M.	Mean amplitude of light-evoked rod response (mV) ± S.E.M.
Standard	0.98	0.49	0.10	0.24	2.00	1.00	21	3.19 ± 0.38	4.01 ± 0.27 (N=67)
No. 3	1.02	0.74	0.10	0.14	1.38	1.82	22	1.05 ± 0.28	3.67 ± 0.49 (N=23)
Standard	0.98	0.49	0.10	0.24	2.00	1.00	23	1.91 ± 0.18	3.78 ± 0.31 (N=44)
No. 9	1.85	0.81	0.56	0.52	2.28	0.89	23	3.39 ± 0.47	4.02 ± 0.17 (N=78)

It should be recalled that Tubing 3 is the thin-walled tubing advertised by Frederick Haer & Co. as giving 'ultra-small tips' (see Section IV.1 of Chapter 6). Compared with Standard Tubing, the OD_t approximately doubled for Tubing 3, while the frequency of penetrating toad rods decreased by a factor of about three, and cells were usually much less well maintained after penetration.

In spite of the disadvantages of Tubing 3, it provided a few light-evoked responses of 9.0 mV, similar to the largest obtained with Standard Tubing. Unlike the relatively small responses obtained with Tubing 3, these initially large responses were usually well maintained. Thus high quality intracellular recordings could still be obtained, though they were much fewer in number. In summary, tips provided by Tubing 3 proved at or very near the practical upper limit of OD_t that permitted rare high quality intracellular recordings in this preparation. But Tubing 3 provides a marked increase of ID_t that can be a decisive advantage in any experiment requiring injection of material into cells.

II.2   Tubing Design for Improved Cell Penetration

We tested all experimental tubings that gave any theoretical promise of improved cell impalement relative to Standard Tubing. Among these, the greatest improvement was obtained with Tubing 9, which is described in Table 5. This tubing was designed to give an OD/ID slightly greater than 2.0 in conjunction with an Omega Dot as large as possible in relation to wall thickness. This was done by using an OD of 1.85 mm and an ID of 0.81 mm to achieve an OD/ID of 2.28, while also providing room for an Omega Dot with a diameter of 0.56 mm, which was somewhat greater than the wall thickness of 0.52 mm. It should be noted that the full advantages of a large Omega Dot and of increasing OD/ID cannot be obtained in combination, because these two strategies for reducing tip size require that the space in the capillary lumen be used in different ways. In one case the lumen must accommodate a large Omega Dot, while in the other case it must be reduced as much as possible.

When compared with Standard Tubing, Table 5 shows that Tubing 9 improved the number of impalements per retinal penetration from 1.9 to 3.4, which was statistically significant ($p = 0.003$). Here also the average response amplitude was affected only slightly, increasing from 3.78 to 4.02 mV. Though this 6.3% increase is in the expected direction, it proved too small to be statistically significant ($p = 0.17$). In short, Tubing 9 improved the frequency of impalements by a factor of 1.8 but gave little indication of improving response amplitude.

By reference to Figure 23, an increase of OD/ID from 2.0 (Standard Tubing) to 2.28 (Tubing 9) would only reduce OD_t from about 0.081 to 0.074 μm. As shown in Chapter 7, enlargement of the Omega Dot can significantly reduce tip size, and this is the probable reason for much of the improved cell penetration by Tubing 9. The heavier Omega Dot should further aid cell penetration by stiffening the tip. Finally, the large Omega Dot may have led to formation of an occasional spade-like spear at the tip (see Sections I.2 and II.3 of Chapter 7).

This possibility is supported by an unusually high variability in the performance of electrodes formed from Tubing 9. The number of cells impaled per retinal penetration varied only from 0–4 for Standard Tubing but from 0–8 for Tubing 9. This high variability would be explicable if the performance of Tubing 9 was based partly upon chance factors governing the formation of an occasional spear.

PART III   THE OPTIMAL DESIGN OF CAPILLARY TUBING FOR INTRACELLULAR WORK

III.1   Optimal Penetration of Small Cells

In much intracellular work the main requirement is to penetrate cells as readily as possible with minimal damage. This is typically the case when the main goal is intracellular electrical recording without any need to inject material into the cell.

In evaluating the more frequent penetration of cells by Tubing 9, it should be remembered that this work was conducted with our original round loop filament, prior to the improved filament designs described in Sections III.7 and III.9 of Chapter 3. The square loop filament provides an increased heat delivery, which can be particularly important when forming fine tips on tubing containing a heavy Omega Dot or having thick walls associated with a high OD/ID. It is thus unlikely that the full advantage of Tubing 9 for improved cell penetration was demonstrated in this early experiment. This is strongly suggested by the fact that SEM measurements, at the time of the Table 5 experiment, showed little reduction of tip size when Tubing 9 was compared with Standard Tubing. But when this same comparison was made with the $2 \times 2 \times 2$ mm square loop heating filament, and improved SEM mounting methods, Tubing 9 reduced the average OD_t from 0.091 to 0.051 μm (see Section I.4 of Chapter 8). If the experiment of Table 5 were repeated with the square loop filament, therefore, it seems almost certain that Tubing 9 would exhibit a considerably greater advantage over Standard Tubing in the frequency of cell penetration.

At the time of the work in Table 5, the thick-walled Tubing 1 showed no significant reduction of tip size and no improved cell penetration, when compared with Standard Tubing. Later comparisons of tip size reported in Chapter 6, still using the round loop filament but with improved SEM mounting methods and more rigorous precautions for maintaining a constant tip temperature, showed that Tubing 1 can provide significantly smaller tip sizes than Standard Tubing. Furthermore, when the square loop filament was used, the difference in tip size was increased (see Section III.2e of Chapter 6). This may be expected because the thick-walled Tubing 1 also requires considerable heat to form ultrafine tips. Compared with Standard Tubing, Tubing 1 should have advantages for cell penetration similar to those of Tubing 9, since it can provide smaller tips which should also be stiffer because the walls thicken more rapidly behind the tip itself.

In summary, the data of Table 5 for improved penetration by Tubing 9 should be considered preliminary. It would be desirable to repeat this type of experiment for both Tubing 9 and Tubing 1, using the $2 \times 2 \times 2$ mm square loop filament, but this has not been done. Under these conditions we would expect both tubings to greatly improve the frequency of cell penetration by comparison with Standard Tubing, but we cannot predict which would give the better result. Furthermore, aluminosilicate tubing has recently been found to provide even finer tips than our special designs of borosilicate tubing, as documented in Section VII.1 of Chapter 18. Though these extremely fine aluminosilicate tips have not been tested systematically in preparations, they should improve still further the penetration of small cells and fibers.

It is also of special interest that we found the quality of cell penetration by various tubing designs to be much better indicated by the frequency of cell penetration than by the maximum response amplitude that could be obtained. For example, when Tubing 3 was compared with Standard Tubing, the frequency of cell penetration decreased by a factor of about 3.0, but the largest light-evoked responses obtainable remained unchanged. This clearly indicates why so much work with larger-than-ideal micropipettes has produced useful intracellular results based upon strong experimental efforts. Ironically, however, the fact that marginal micropipette techniques can produce valuable results has probably had the unfortunate consequence of retarding the development of more effective techniques.

III.2 Maximizing the Inner Tip Diameter for Injecting Materials into Cells

The other main requirement of intracellular work is to facilitate the injection of material from a micropipette into a cell. In forming micropipettes, this will be assisted by either increasing ID_t or decreasing tip length. When strategies for increasing ID_t are considered, it is clear that one efficient method is to decrease OD/ID. For example, Equations 1 and 2 in Chapter 6 show that when OD/ID drops from 2.0 (the value for Standard Tubing) to 1.33 (the value for a much-used thin-walled tubing), F_o doubles but F_i triples. Since electrode resistance is inversely proportional to ID_t (Chowdhury, 1969), electrodes formed from this thin-walled tubing should have electrical resistances only about 1/3 that of electrodes formed from Standard Tubing at similar puller settings and then similarly filled. This has been confirmed as an approximation of the relative electrode resistances (D.H. Feldman, personal communication). The special advantage of this strategy is that decreasing the OD/ID causes the ID_t to become a larger fraction of the OD_t. In applying this strategy, OD/ID should be decreased until OD_t has become as large as feasible for penetrating the target cells without significant damage. In our test preparation of toad rods, the minimal value of OD/ID proved to be about 1.33. In larger cells this minimal value of OD/ID could obviously be less, while in smaller cells it would have to be greater.

Of course the other main strategy for increasing ID_t is precision beveling of the micropipette tip. Compared with decreasing the OD/ID, this strategy is less efficient because ID_t and OD_t increase proportionately. On the other hand, beveling permits a greater increase of OD_t without damaging the cell by penetration. The limitation of increasing ID_t by beveling is when OD_t has become as large as permitted by the sharpening effects of beveling, a limitation that will also be more severe with small cells than with large ones.

These two strategies for increasing ID_t may be combined, and tip length may be minimized by the airjet effects provided by our puller (see Part III of Chapter 5). Hence all three of these strategies are advisable when serious difficulties are encountered with injecting materials into cells, providing that the target cells are large enough to increase OD_t significantly above the smallest tips that may be formed.

CHAPTER 15

The Structure and Properties of Glasses for Fabricating Micropipettes

PART I   INTRODUCTION

In fabricating micropipettes for applications in cell physiology, borosilicate glass has long been used and found satisfactory for most purposes. Hence composition of the glass used in making micropipettes has not been discussed earlier in this book. But this subject has recently gained renewed interest, especially in connection with ion-specific and patch clamping electrodes. For example, Corey and Stevens (1983) have treated this subject in relation to patch clamping. So we shall now discuss some of its main aspects that apply to the fabrication of micropipettes for biological work. More detailed information may be obtained from specialized treatises on glass, such as those by Warren (1940), Morey (1954) and Volf (1961).

PART II   TYPES OF GLASS

II.1   Quartz

All glasses in common use are silicate glasses composed largely of silicon dioxide, and among these the simplest is quartz, which is composed of pure SiO_2. In crystalline quartz each silicon atom is surrounded by a tetrahedron of four oxygen atoms, each of which forms a bridge between two silicon atoms. The interatomic distance between silicon and oxygen is about 1.6 Å. As shown

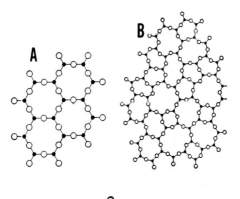

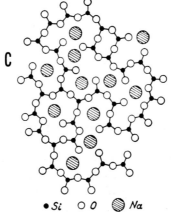

Figure 79. Two-dimensional representation of the molecular structure of crystalline quartz (A), quartz glass (B), and a soft glass composed only of silicon dioxide and sodium oxide (C). Though Zachariasen (1932) used illustrations (A) and (B) to show the generalized alteration of structure between the crystalline and glassy states of a glass-forming oxide, Warren (1940) showed by X-ray diffraction that these illustrations apply to the relation between crystalline quartz and quartz glass. (Parts (A) and (B) from Zachariasen (1932), reproduced by permission of the American Chemical Society; Part (C) from Warren and Biscoe (1938), reproduced by permission of The American Ceramic Society)

in the two-dimensional representation of Figure 79(A), this provides a strong and orderly molecular structure. When crystalline quartz is softened the interatomic distances are unchanged, but the tetrahedra become deformed and are not restored during normally rapid cooling. In this state it is a quartz glass often called fused quartz or fused silica. Since the basic molecular structure is retained in spite of the deformations, as illustrated in Figure 79(B), this accounts for the great strength of quartz glass. In fact, quartz is the ultimate silicate glass with respect to mechanical strength, electrical resistivity, and chemical durability. For these reasons it has long been attractive for making micropipettes, but this has been prevented by its high working point. The Corning Glass Works gives the softening point of quartz as 1580 °C, but does not give a working point, perhaps because the working point of quartz is less clearly defined than for most other glasses. In any event, platinum–iridium melts at 1815 °C, and we have noted that a platinum–iridium filament always burns out before supplying enough heat to pull quartz tubing. Tungsten filaments, on the other hand, oxidize too severely to be useful at the temperatures required by quartz (see Section III.10 of Chapter 3). Flame heaters are used to work quartz industrially, but these are too difficult to control to be useful in micropipette pullers, where heat delivery must be well specified and highly reliable.

II.2   Soft Glass

Because of the high temperatures required by quartz glass, all commonly used glasses contain additives that lower the working point. In so-called soft glasses the main additive is Na_2O, so they are often called soda glasses. These are commonly used for making items such as windows, largely because they are easy to work.

For the case of a glass formed only from SiO_2 and Na_2O, its structure is represented in two dimensions in Figure 79(C). Compared with quartz, the addition of Na_2O provides an excess of oxygen atoms, each of which carries a negative charge and is bonded to a single silicon atom. An oxygen bound to only one silicon causes a break in the Si–O framework, as shown in Figure 79(C), and of course these breaks become more numerous as more Na_2O is added. Thus the overall network becomes less rigidly braced in three- dimensional space, accounting for both its lowered mechanical strength and its lowered softening point. Sodium does not become part of the Si–O network but is incorporated as Na^+ ions within the holes of the network. Under the influence of an electric field, Na^+ ions may move readily from one hole of the network to another, which accounts for the increased electrical conductivity of soda–silica glass compared with quartz.

Though Na_2O is the main additive in soft glasses, other additives are typically used in small amounts. In fact, there are many types of soft glass with greatly varying properties, depending upon the exact amounts of the various additives. According to Volf (1961), a typical example of soft glass contains 72.2% SiO_2, 15% Na_2O, 5.1% CaO, 3.5% MgO, 1.7% B_2O_3, 1.5% Al_2O_3, and 1.0% K_2O.

The effects of an additive upon the properties of a silica glass depend largely upon whether it functions as a network-former, which joins with oxygen to form networks such as that of SiO_2, or whether it is a network-modifier, which fills the interstices of a network. Like Na^+, Ca^{2+} is a network-modifier, and glass containing significant amounts of both Na_2O and CaO is often referred to as soda–lime glass. Aside from silicon, the most useful network-former for our purposes is boron, which is introduced as B_2O_3. It may be added either as a minor component of soft glass or as a more major component of borosilicate glass. Many other types of atoms play more complex roles, acting partly as network-formers and partly as network-modifiers. Of special interest here is aluminum, which is introduced as Al_2O_3, either as a minor component of soft glass or as a more significant component of aluminosilicate glass.

Though soft glass is readily worked, it has disadvantages for many applications of micropipettes. Because of its relatively weak structure, micropipettes readily bend or break. Since the electrical conductivity of a glass depends mainly upon its Na^+ content (Morey, 1954), the electrical conductivity of soft glass is undesirably high. In addition, soft glass is of low chemical durability, so it is strongly attacked by certain filling solutions such as KCl.

II.3   Borosilicate Glass

The limitations of soft glass are much alleviated by borosilicate glasses, sometimes called hard glasses, in which the additive is predominantly B_2O_3 instead of Na_2O. This type of glass was first patented by the Corning Glass Works in 1919. Though a variety of such glasses were originally described, they differed little in composition, and only one of them (Corning No. 7740) continues to be available under the trade name of Pyrex®. According to Volf (1961) its composition is 80.9% SiO_2, 12.9% B_2O_3, 4.4% Na_2O, and 1.8% Al_2O_3. X-ray studies of glass formed from pure B_2O_3 indicate that '... each boron is triangularly bonded to three oxygens, and each oxygen is bonded to two borons' (Morey, 1954). In a glass formed only from silica and boric oxide, the structure is a random pattern of silica and boric oxide networks joined by oxygen atoms. In borosilicate glass, however, this structure is modified by small amounts of Na_2O and Al_2O_3. Compared with soft glass, the improved properties appear to result from the decreased sodium content and fewer oxygen atoms with single bonds. On the other hand, the structural network is less regular than that of quartz. Thus the properties of borosilicate glass are intermediate between those of soft glass and quartz with respect to mechanical strength, chemical durability, electrical resistivity, ability to withstand thermal stress, and ease of working. The working point of a typical soft glass (Corning No. 0080) is 1005 °C, while that of Pyrex® is 1252 °C. So Pyrex® can also be handled by a platinum–iridium heating filament, but it requires more heat. As a result, the types of micropipettes that may be formed are more limited unless appropriate precautions are taken.

II.4   Aluminosilicate Glass

In recent years there has been a developing interest in making micropipettes from aluminosilicate glass, especially for ion-specific and patch clamp electrodes (see Chapters 16 and 17). But it has thus far been little used for these purposes. The main additive in this type of glass is Al_2O_3. According to Volf (1961) the hardest aluminosilicate glass contains 35.5% SiO_2, 29.1% Al_2O_3, 13.8% ZrO_2, 9.5% B_2O_3, 6.9% BeO, and 5.3% CaO. Like silicon, aluminum combines with oxygen to form tetrahedral networks, and the Al–O bonds are very strong. When compared with borosilicate glass, aluminosilicate glass provides increased hardness, improved chemical durability, reduced electrical conductivity, and a lower coefficient of thermal expansion. Yet Corning aluminosilicate glasses (Nos. 1720 and 1723) have respective working points of only 1202 and 1168 °C. These working points are somewhat lower than that of Pyrex ®, so a filament system adequate for Pyrex ® can likewise handle aluminosilicate tubing. It should be noted, however, that glasses also differ in their 'working range'. While this term lacks precise definition, it has great practical significance and is widely used by glass workers. It refers roughly to the temperature range over which a glass is soft enough to be worked without becoming so fluid that it falls apart from its own weight. In forming micropipettes the lower limit of this range is the working point, while the upper limit is the temperature at which the micropipette tip becomes too long and slender to be useful. Though exact measures of working ranges are not available, we have noted the working range of aluminosilicate glass to be much narrower than those of either soft glass or Pyrex ®. As a result, aluminosilicate glass requires the factors controlling its temperature to be adjusted with special care. To that end the recent P-80 models of our micropipette puller contain a new design feature to initiate the fast pull when the slow pull has reached a criterion velocity. Of course attainment of any given velocity will be at a given viscosity, thus a given temperature, of the glass. Hence this design feature has proved especially helpful in handling aluminosilicate glass (see Parts V and VII of Chapter 18).

PART III   THE ELECTRICAL CONDUCTIVITY OF GLASSES

For our purposes the electrical conductivity of glasses is particularly important. This is usually expressed as electrical resistivity in ohm-cm (the electrical resistance in ohms of a one centimeter cube of material to a current perpendicular to one of its faces). This type of data is seldom available for room temperatures, and the electrical resistivity of glass drops markedly at higher temperatures. But the Corning Glass Works provides resistivities, expressed as log_{10} ohm-cm at 25 °C, for most of its glasses. The value given for their No. 0080 soft glass is 12.4, while Pyrex ® (No. 7740) is rated as 15, and their aluminosilicate glasses and fused quartz are all rated at 17+. The lack of discrimination between these latter glasses probably reflects the great difficulty of measuring such high resistivities. Though Corey and Stevens (1983) do not indicate the source of their values, they indicate that the resistivity of quartz is about 4 log units higher than that of borosilicate glass. Based upon discussions with industrial glass specialists, the resistivity of quartz likewise exceeds that of aluminosilicate glass. Since resistivity is strongly dependent upon contained impurities, most notably sodium, it is also noteworthy that the resistivity of quartz can vary considerably with the purity of its composition.

PART IV   NONHOMOGENEITIES OF COMPLEX GLASSES

IV.1   Chemical and Structural Nonhomogeneities

Aside from quartz glass and a few other glasses formed from pure substances, glasses appear to contain significant departures from homogeneity. Though these are not apparent in most applications, they are probably important for micropipettes, especially those with ultrafine tips in which the tip itself is formed from a very small sample of glass.

It appears that nonhomogeneity can come about in at least two ways. First, glasses formed by mixing additives to SiO_2 cannot be homogeneous when examined on a fine scale. Since glasses are relatively viscous, even when melted, perfect mixing is not possible. So the exact proportions of the additives must vary somewhat from point to point, which we shall refer to as a chemical nonhomogeneity. Since the properties of glass depend critically upon the proportions of the additives, the properties of a complex glass will thus vary from point to point, and this factor must contribute to the variability of tip size among micropipettes pulled under well controlled conditions.

The second factor is illustrated by Figure 79(C). Though the molecular structure of a soda–silica glass exhibits a definite pattern, the 'cells' of this pattern vary considerably in size and shape, which we shall refer to as a structural nonhomogeneity. The strength of the structure, and hence the softening point as well, thus vary from one locus to another. These local variations of the softening point explain why glass does not soften completely at a specific temperature but instead softens gradually over a considerable temperature range. They probably contribute also to the variability of tip size. This is because even if the tip temperature could be held entirely constant, its effects would vary with the softening points in the extremely small samples of glass at the forming tips of ultrafine micropipettes. Since the structural nonhomogeneities of glass occur on an especially fine scale, they may influence only the very smallest micropipette tips, whereas chemical nonhomogeneities probably exert an influence over a greater range of tip size.

IV.2   Effects of Nonhomogeneities upon Tip Size

IV.2a   *Different tip sizes with slightly separated double-barreled tips*

Using borosilicate glass (Corning No. 7740), we have obtained three separate types of evidence for effects of nonhomogeneities within this complex glass upon

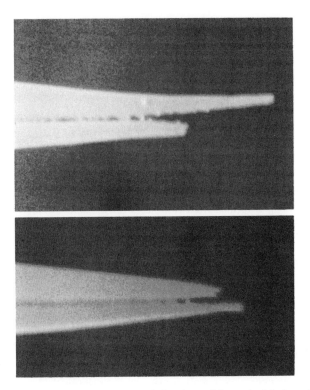

Figure 80. Examples of slightly separated tips formed from double-barreled tubing that consists of two fused lengths of Standard Tubing. Note the marked difference in tip size between a given pair of tips, though the pulling conditions for both tips may be assumed to be identical (see text). Calibration mark is 1.0 μm.

tip size. Effects of this type would be clearly confirmed if significant variability of tip size could be demonstrated with pulling conditions constant. This cannot be assumed for micropipettes formed on successive pulls, especially since small variations of tip temperature may produce significant changes of tip size, but a chance observation offered a much more critical test. While pulling double-barreled micropipettes consisting of a pair of fused capillary tubes, attempts to form particularly short tips often resulted in a splitting apart of the two tips. This occurred over such a short distance that it could be observed only by SEM. In such cases the two tips are formed from separate samples of glass but at tip temperatures that may be assumed identical. As shown in the examples of Figure 80, the two tips of a given pair sometimes differ in both tip size and tip length. The difference in tip size seems to vary randomly between successive pulls, ranging from undetectable to the examples of Figure 80, where the size differences are marked and near the maximum that we have observed. The difference in tip length also seems to vary randomly between pulls. In the two cases illustrated the longer tip is the smaller one, but the opposite relationship has also been observed. Sometimes the two barrels also differ in size at some

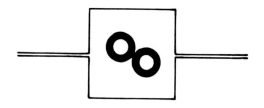

Figure 81. Scale drawing of double-barreled tubing positioned within the square loop filament of our micropipette puller. The square loop filament measures 3.0 mm in both the horizontal and vertical dimensions. Though the two halves of this filament are actually in contact, they are shown slightly separate for purposes of illustration. The double-barreled tubing is formed from two pieces of Standard Tubing fused together (the contained Omega Dots are not shown). In clamping this tubing, we place one tube in the V-grooves of the pipette carriers, and the other tube lies slightly lower on the flat surfaces of the pipette carriers. As illustrated, this results in the two tubes being tilted at an angle of about 30° from the horizontal axis of the heating filament.

distance behind the tip itself, as in the examples of Figure 80. But in one case the larger barrel provided the smaller tip size, while in the other case the opposite occurred. Thus relative tip size varies considerably and is not clearly associated with other relationships between the tips of a given pair. This strongly indicates that tip size is determined partly by structural or chemical aspects of glass that can differ significantly between the very small samples of glass contributing to a given pair of tips.

Though one cannot be certain that double-barreled tips are formed at identical tip temperatures, both theory and evidence support this assumption. Precautions were taken to assure that the two capillary tubes were not heated unequally during the early stages of pulling. A square loop filament was used, and the double-barreled tubing was carefully centered within the filament, as shown in Figure 81. The heat delivery by a square loop filament should be rigorously symmetrical about a vertical axis through the center of the filament, and symmetry should also pertain about the horizontal axis, aside from possible effects of convection currents. Although the double-barreled tubing was mounted at a slant within the heating filament, as shown in Figure 81, heat delivery to the two capillary tubes should thus be the same within a small margin of error. Even if slight differences do occur in the initial heating of the two tubes, these are probably eliminated as pulling proceeds. This is expected in part because the fused tubes quickly become so small that they occupy essentially the same position within the heating filament. Also, as this occurs the capillary walls become so greatly thinned that their temperature becomes readily changed toward the ambient temperature at the center of the heating filament. In any event, we tested the final result by SEM, and the smaller tip of a pair proved to be formed at either position within the heating filament. So unequal initial heating of the two tubes is not a critical factor, unless the direction of the inequality varies significantly between pulls, which seems quite unlikely.

It is a good rule of thumb that in a group of 10 ultrafine tips formed on our puller from borosilicate tubing, the ratio between the largest and smallest tips is about 3/2 (see Section IV.3 of Chapter 5). When two tips are formed simultaneously on double-barreled tubing, the chance of observing similarly large and small tips in a single pair becomes only 1 in 100 pulls. Nevertheless, cases were found where the two tips had a size ratio of about 3/2, as shown in Figure 80. So the variability of tip size remains about the same when all pulling conditions, including tip temperature, may safely be assumed to be identical for two tips of any given pair.

IV.2b   The reduced variability of tip size with enlarged tips

The importance of nonhomogeneities in glass has also been shown by examining the effect of enlarging tips upon the variability of tip size. If there are significant differences between the very small samples of glass that contribute to ultrafine tips, of course these differences should decrease and disappear when tip size becomes sufficiently large that the samples of glass forming the tips are no longer significantly different.

For this test the puller was our Model P-80C, as described in Chapter 18, this being a recent revision of our P-77 series to fulfill also the requirements of patch clamping, and to permit the convenient handling of aluminosilicate glass. The heating filament was a rectangular trough measuring 3 mm in all three dimensions. Tips were formed from Standard Tubing obtained from the Glass Company of America in precut 4-in. lengths. These short pieces of glass represent random samples from a great length of small tubing that has been redrawn from a much larger tubing. Only one tip was used from each pair formed, so each tip represents the results of a separate pull.

For this work gold coatings were applied by an ISI-5400 sputter coater. As described in Section III.2d of Chapter 6, thickness of the gold coating was measured by applying an initial gold coating to a group of tips and measuring them, followed by application of another coating and a second measurement of the tips. The increase of average tip size resulting from the second coating gives an accurate measurement of the thickness of the coating. Settings of the coating instrument were changed until the thickness of the gold coating, when measured in this manner, was 100 Å. This coating was then used for all tips and subtracted to obtain measurements of tip size.

For each group of tips, Table 6 gives the number of tips measured, the mean tip size in nm, and the standard deviation of tip size in nm. In this work we used the standard deviation as a measure of variability, because it is less influenced by single extreme values than is the range. Certain sources of variable tip size, such as variations in tip temperature, should cause the standard deviation to increase as tip size increases. Thus we also expressed the standard deviation as a decimal fraction of the mean (S.D./Mean), and these values are given in the final column of Table 6.

Tip groups A–G in Table 6 are arranged in the order of increasing tip size, and in Figure 82 the values of S.D./Mean are plotted as a function of tip size. If

Table 6. Variability of tip size (S.D./mean) as a function of tip size (OD$_t$). All tips formed from randomly selected 4-in. pieces of Standard Tubing, using our Model P-80C micropipette puller with a rectangular trough filament measuring 3 mm in all three dimensions

Group of tips	Number of tips measured	Mean tip size (OD$_t$) (nm)	Standard deviation of tip size (nm)	$\dfrac{\text{S.D.}}{\text{Mean}}$
A	15	48.3	24.0	0.497
B	13	58.4	11.3	0.193
C	14	105.4	10.9	0.103
D	15	130.0	10.8	0.083
E	15	159.0	12.2	0.077
F	14	215.0	20.0	0.093
G	15	442.0	39.6	0.090

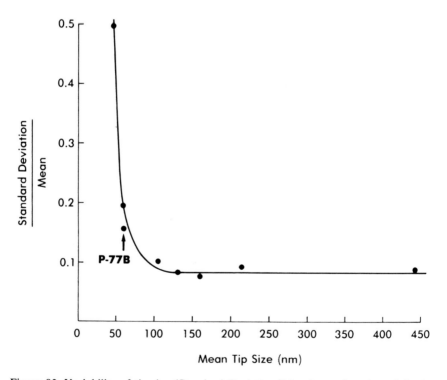

Figure 82. Variability of tip size (Standard Deviation/Mean) as a function of tip size, plotted from the data of Table 6. A smooth curve is fitted by eye through the data obtained when our Model P-80C micropipette puller was used to form tips from 4-inch pieces of glass that were randomly picked from a large amount of borosilicate tubing. For comparison, a single point is taken from Table 7 to show the result when tips were formed from similar material by our Model P-77B puller.

nonhomogeneities of the glass were equally important sources of variability of tip size throughout the range of tip sizes represented, then S.D./Mean should remain approximately constant as a function of tip size. Instead, it dropped markedly as tip size increased from 48.3 to 58.4 nm and then dropped further when tip size increased to 105.4 nm. Thereafter, there was no clear change in the value of S.D./Mean as tip size increased to 442.0 nm. These results closely confirm the predicted effects of nonhomogeneities of the glass, which should become ineffective above some critical tip size, and which should rapidly become more effective within the range below this critical tip size. These results also indicate that the critical tip size is in the vicinity of 100 nm (0.1 μm), which we have designated on other grounds as the border between ultrafine and fine tips.

IV.2c The reduced variability of tip size upon restricting the length of redrawn tubing used to form tips

If nonhomogeneities within glass contribute to the variability of tip size, it occurred to us that this variability might also be reduced by restricting the length of redrawn tubing from which pieces of glass to form tips are taken. As just mentioned, a great length of redrawn tubing is usually cut into 4-in. pieces, which become so intermixed that upon delivery they represent relatively random sites within the redrawn tubing. Alternatively, at least in the case of the Glass Company of America, 3-ft sections of tubing may be obtained. We thus compared the variability of tip size when the pieces of glass used to form tips were either

Table 7. The effect upon variability of tip size (S.D./mean) when all pieces of glass were taken from a single 3-ft length of tubing, compared with random selection from a much greater length of tubing. Results are shown at various tip sizes and with tips formed on both our Model P-80C and Model P-77B micropipette pullers. For details, see text

Group of tips	Glass used	Puller used	Number of tips measured	Mean tip size (OD_t) (nm)	Standard deviation of tip size (nm)	$\dfrac{S.D.}{Mean}$
Ia	Random	P-80C	15	48.3	24.0	0.497
Ib	3-ft length	P-80C	12	40.0	13.0	0.325
IIa	Random	P-80C	13	58.4	11.3	0.193
IIb	3-ft length	P-80C	11	59.5	5.6	0.094
IIIa	Random	P-77B	14	61.2	9.7	0.158
IIIb	3-ft length	P-77B	13	68.9	7.0	0.102
IVa	Random	P-80C	14	105.4	10.9	0.103
IVb	3-ft length	P-80C	12	108.0	11.5	0.106
Va	Random	P-80C	14	215.0	20.0	0.093
Vb	3-ft length	P-80C	13	220.8	22.2	0.101

from random sites within a great length of tubing or from a single 3-ft piece of tubing. For a given tip size, the tips formed from random glass and from a 3-ft piece of tubing were all pulled in a single session. The comparison was made at five different tip sizes, and our results are given in Table 7 in the order of increasing tip size.

The three groups of smallest tips were all in the ultrafine range, and they all exhibited similar marked reductions in the value of S.D./Mean when tips were taken from a single 3-ft section of tubing. In one case (Group II) the value of S.D./Mean dropped 51%, while Groups I and III both gave reductions of 35%. Thus Table 7 shows that the variability of tip size in the ultrafine range was consistently and markedly reduced by forming all tips from a 3-ft section of tubing. This could only occur if (1) there were significant differences in the glass itself over the length of a batch of redrawn tubing, and (2) these differences influenced the size of ultrafine tips. Hence these findings further indicate that nonhomogeneities within the glass are important factors influencing tip size.

Group I with the smallest tips (averaging slightly below 50 nm) yielded an S.D./Mean with random glass that was 0.497, by far the largest variability we have seen to date. Upon forming tips of this size from only 3-ft of tubing, the value fell to 0.325, which was still quite high. Thus, for tips of this size there are still nonhomogeneities within a 3-ft length of tubing that strongly influence tip size, and all groups of larger tips formed from only 3-ft of tubing gave values of S.D./Mean that were very close to 0.100. This suggests that only the Group I tips were small enough to be influenced by point-to-point variations of molecular structure within the glass. On the other hand, it is likely that changes of chemical composition occur over the great length of tubing formed by heating and redrawing, and nonhomogeneities of this type would be expected to influence somewhat larger tips. So it is hardly surprising that for the somewhat larger tips of Groups II and III, the greater nonhomogeneity represented by random glass remained a significant source of variability in tip size. In short, reduction of chemical nonhomogeneities probably accounts for the reduced variability of tip size which occurred for all three groups of ultrafine tips when they were formed from only a 3-ft section of tubing. When tip size was increased to just above the ultrafine range in Group IV, and then about doubled in Group V, the advantage of forming tips from only a 3-ft section of tubing disappeared. Hence tips in the fine range appear to be little if any influenced by either of the *main* factors that cause variability of tip size in the ultrafine range.

IV.3   The Minimum Variability of Tip Size

A remaining question is why the minimum value of S.D./Mean is consistently about 0.100 or slightly less. By the definition of standard deviation, assuming that tip sizes are normally distributed, this indicates that about 68% of all tips are within ±10% of the mean tip size. We are not aware of any applications of micropipettes in which this small variability is a significant problem. But the source of this remaining variability is of some interest.

One possibility is unidentified nonhomogeneities of glass that are equally significant within a 3-ft section of tubing as within an entire batch of tubing, and that influence even tips in the fine size range. When split tips are formed on dual-channel tubing made by fusing two pieces of Standard Tubing, the two tips often differ in size even when they are well above the ultrafine size range. In fact, the size differences under these conditions are sufficient to account for an S.D./Mean of about 0.100.

The other possibility is that the minimum variability of tip size results at least partly from slight differences between the pulling conditions when micropipettes are formed in succession by our puller. This is difficult to isolate, but the most likely source of such variability would be in the heating current. Most of the data in Table 7 were obtained with our P-80C puller, in which the heating current is much more stable than in our P-77B. For comparison, therefore, the Group III tips were formed with our Model P-77B. In Table 7 the results of this group fall closely in line with those obtained from the Model P-80C. This comparison may be seen best in Figure 82, where values of S.D./Mean as a function of tip size are plotted for tips formed from random glass with the P-80C puller. The point obtained from Table 7, using random glass with the P-77B puller, falls almost upon the smooth curve fitted by eye to the P-80C data. This indicates that even our P-77B puller contributes no significant variation of tip size resulting from inconsistency of the heating current, since the variability of tip size was not decreased when the stability of the heating current was greatly improved in our Model P-80C. (See Section III.1 of Chapter 18).

In short, these results strongly suggest that the minimum S.D./Mean of about 0.100 also results almost entirely from nonhomogeneities within borosilicate glass.

IV.4   Summary

Taken together, three different kinds of results provide compelling evidence that nonhomogeneities of borosilicate glass contribute to the variability of tip size among ultrafine tips. Further, this evidence indicates that when tips are formed by our puller, virtually all the variability of tip size results from nonhomogeneities within this complex glass. The variability of ultrafine tips may be decreased markedly by forming all tips from a single 3-ft section of tubing, instead of using pieces of glass randomly selected from a large batch of tubing. This strategy for reducing variability becomes ineffective, however, above the ultrafine range of tip size. When tips are formed from randomly selected pieces of glass, the variability of tip size also falls rapidly as tip size increases within the ultrafine range. It then becomes constant above a tip size of about 0.1 μm, the upper limit of the ultrafine range. Within the fine range of tip size (0.1–0.5 μm), the variability is so low that about 68% of all tips fall within ±10% of the mean tip size. Virtually all of this remaining variability also appears due to nonhomogeneities within borosilicate glass. Though theoretically our puller should contribute to this minimum variability of tip size, any contribution of this type has thus far proved too small to isolate.

These results indicate that if any further reduction in the variability of tip size is desired, particularly in the case of the smallest ultrafine tips, it will be necessary to use less complex glasses than borosilicate tubing. Our results to date have not shown any reduced variability of tip size when using aluminosilicate glass (see Section VII.2 of Chapter 18). Of course nonhomogeneities should be eliminated most effectively by quartz, since it consists of pure SiO_2 and has a highly regular molecular structure. Though quartz cannot be handled by available micropipette pullers, no critical need for it is apparent at this time. If such a need should develop, however, methods of handling quartz would merit careful investigation.

CHAPTER 16

Dual-Channel Micropipettes

PART I   APPLICATIONS AND REQUIREMENTS

Many types of research require dual-channel micropipettes. For example, in extracellular work a dual-channel micropipette may be placed close to a synapse, and a putative synaptic transmitter may be ejected from one channel by a brief current pulse, while the post-synaptic response is recorded through the other channel. For intracellular work, two channels may be needed for various purposes such as voltage clamping or ion-specific electrodes. If a cell is relatively large and can be visualized directly, the requirement of two intracellular channels may be met by penetrating it with two separate micropipettes. But if the cells studied are relatively small, or must be penetrated blindly by probing within tissue, dual-channel micropipettes are usually required.

In the case of small cells, which are typical of the retina and the vertebrate central nervous system, dual-channel micropipettes present some rather difficult and conflicting requirements. Ideally the outer tip diameter should be within the ultrafine range, to penetrate the small cells with minimal damage. Yet this ultrafine tip must contain two separate channels. The electrical independence of the two channels tends to be compromised by their close proximity, yet electrical independence is an essential requirement in most applications of dual-channel micropipettes. In addition, the channels are so small that the electrical resistance of each channel tends to be very high, but this must be held within reasonable limits.

A solution to these conflicting requirements has been found, thus extending the types of intracellular work that may be performed with ultrafine dual-channel micropipettes. Most of our work toward this goal has been reported previously (Brown and Flaming, 1977a), and it will be described here in greater detail.

PART II   TWO FUSED CAPILLARY TUBES

Dual-channel micropipettes are most commonly made by fusing together two similar capillary tubes. Some investigators have done this by heating and twisting the two tubes together prior to pulling the tips (Werblin, 1975), or by twisting the tubes together as the tips are formed. The twisting motion promotes fusion by holding the heated tubes firmly together. Of course the back ends of the capillary shafts must also be held together by some type of adhesive, both during and after pulling the tips, because fusion of the tips is quite fragile. Alternatively, pre-fused capillary tubes may be obtained from a glass supplier, and we have used this type of tubing from the Glass Company of America. It eliminates the need to bond the shafts together or to twist the tips during pulling. In addition, the orientation of the tubes in the shaft is well maintained at the tip, so the tip may be oriented accurately for beveling.

In experimenting with dual-channel micropipettes, we first formed tips on dual-channel tubing that consisted of two pre-fused lengths of Standard Tubing. Single-channel tips were also formed from Standard Tubing at the same puller settings. When compared in toad rods, using the methods described in Chapters 12–14, the single-channel tips were very satisfactory but the dual-channel tips were not. Cell penetrations were less frequent, while light-evoked responses after penetration were generally smaller and then deteriorated more rapidly. Thus the dual-channel tips encountered more resistance to penetration and caused more damage to the cell membrane. These effects probably resulted mainly from one dimension of the dual-channel tip being twice as great as the outer diameter of a single channel. Thus the dual-channel tip is larger, and asymmetric stretching of the cell membrane at the site of penetration may also be damaging. In addition, on either side of the line of fusion between the two channels, there are potential sites of leakage between the inside and outside of the cell.

In short, though dual-channel micropipettes of this type have been used successfully in many types of work, they have distinct shortcomings when used for intracellular work in small cells such as toad rods.

PART III   THIN-SEPTUM THETA TUBING

Based upon our experience with a pair of fused tubes, it appeared likely that a dual-channel tip with a smoothly rounded outer form would be more suitable for work in small cells. We thus turned to 'theta' tubing, so-called because its cross section resembles the Greek letter theta. This tubing is made by fusing a flat septum into a circular tube, using techniques described by Kump and Dehn (1975). A large piece of theta tubing (about one inch in diameter) is first assembled and then drawn out to make a great length of smaller tubing. In making the large assembly it proved unsatisfactory to use borosilicate plate glass as the septum in borosilicate tubing, because different batches of glass differ slightly in composition. As a result, a borosilicate plate glass septum consistently developed fine cracks when the assembly was drawn out to make small tubing. This problem was solved by also using borosilicate tubing for the septum. This was done by sawing longitudinally through a piece of tubing and then flattening the two hemi-tubes, which were then cut to size. Because of this requirement, the making of theta tubing has remained a hand process, and all of our theta tubing has been obtained from W.R. Dehn (R & D Scientific Glass Co., 15931 Batson Road, Spencerville, MD 20868, USA).

When we first tried theta tubing, in about 1976, the only type supplied contained a septum about two-thirds as thick as the outer wall, which we refer to as thin-septum theta tubing. Ultrafine tips were formed on this tubing and then tested by injecting only one channel, followed immediately by microscopic observation of the tip. Within a few minutes the injected channel was filled, but the other channel could also be seen filling from the tip backward. So fluid was crossing between the two channels at the tip. Under these conditions, of course, the two channels were not independent either electrically or in ionic composition. We speculated that the thin septum was attenuating and disappearing while the thicker outer rim extended somewhat farther, thus leaving a connection between the two channels at the tip (Brown and Flaming, 1977). This has now been confirmed (see Figure 85A).

PART IV   THICK-SEPTUM THETA TUBING

IV.1   Expected Advantages

If the septum were made thicker than the outer wall, major advantages could be expected. This should eliminate the connecting channel between the two tips. In addition, it seemed likely that the septum would then extend slightly beyond the outer rim. This should improve isolation of the ion pools utilized by the two tips, thus improving the electrical separation of the two channels.

Such an extension of the septum might also form enough of a spear to aid cell penetration.

IV.2   Design and Fabrication of Thick-septum Theta Tubing

Thick-septum theta tubing proved more difficult to fabricate, because of problems in fusing a thick septum with a flat edge into a round tube. But these problems were overcome by W. R. Dehn. After some experimentation, we settled upon thick-septum tubing with the type of cross section illustrated by the high contrast photograph of Figure 83. The thickness of the septum is about twice that of the outer wall. Since this tubing is made by hand, the outside diameter varied from about 1.3–1.9 mm, but most of a given batch varied only from 1.5–1.7 mm, and the average value was 1.6 mm. With these outer dimensions the channels were sufficiently large to be filled by injection with a 31-gauge stainless steel tubing. The cross section of each channel is shaped roughly like a half moon, and the acute angles at the tips of the half moon provide the necessary capillary action to fill the tip without requiring an Omega Dot.

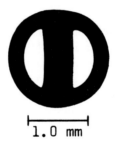

1.0 mm

Figure 83. Cross section of thick-septum theta tubing suitable for ultrafine dual-channel micropipettes. (From Brown and Flaming (1977a), reproduced by permission of Pergamon Press, Oxford, England)

IV.3   Electrical Isolation of Contacts with Dual-channel Tubing

Figure 84 shows our method of separating the back ends of the two channels of theta tubing, so that independent electrical contacts can be made with the fluids in the two channels. A high-speed Dremel tool is firmly mounted and used to rotate a wheel with diamond dust embedded in its rim and outer surface. Such wheels may be obtained from suppliers of dental instruments. As shown schematically in Figure 84, the theta tubing is advanced along this wheel so that all the glass on one side of the septum is cut down about 12 mm. This procedure abrades the surface of the septum, and these abrasions can permit fluid to creep by capillary action between the back ends of the two channels.

This may be prevented by applying a ring of silicone rubber (Dow Corning No. 734 RTV) all the way around the projecting longer channel. This nonconductive coating is permanent and also hydrophobic, so it resists being compromised by condensation upon its surface.

The back ends of dual-channel micropipettes formed from two fused tubes are easily separated by using the diamond wheel to cut across one of the tubes, the back end of which is then broken away. In this case an additional precaution is necessary because the capillary channels on either side of the line of fusion can draw fluid from the preparation up to the back end of the shorter tube, thus short-circuiting the shorter channel. This may be prevented by applying silicone rubber not only around the projecting longer tube but also over the back ends of these capillary channels. We are informed that another investigator has found vacuum grease an effective substitute for silicone rubber in these applications.

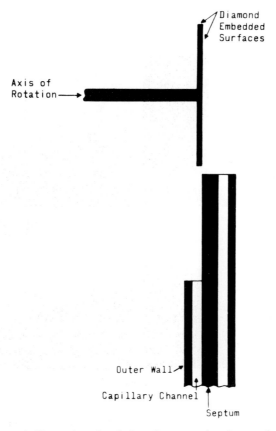

Figure 84. Schematic illustration of technique for separating the two channels at the back end of a micropipette formed from theta tubing. (From Brown and Flaming (1977a), reproduced by permission of Pergamon Press, Oxford, England)

IV.4   Characteristics of Micropipettes Formed from Thick-septum Theta Tubing

IV.4a   Tip form in end-on views

Though high quality end-on views are especially difficult to obtain, some sample tips formed upon theta tubing are shown in Figure 85. Relatively large tips are illustrated upon thin-septum tubing (B), tubing in which the septum and outer wall are of equal thickness (C), and thick-septum tubing (D). In all three cases the relative thickness of the tubing and outer wall remained constant out to the very tip. For example, in the case of thick-septum theta tubing the septum remained about twice as thick as the outer wall. But during tip formation the tips became more elliptical than the original tubing, as may be seen by comparing Figure 85(D) with Figure 83. This probably results from surface tension in the glass–air interface around the lumen of each channel. Surface tension at this site would cause the lumen of each channel to become more

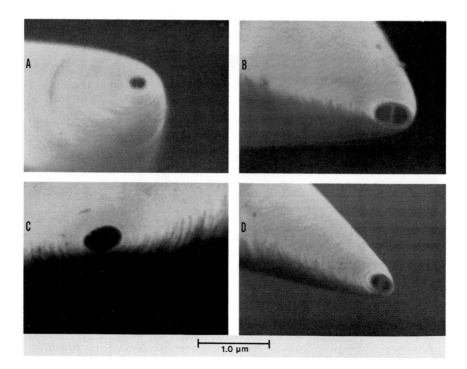

Figure 85. End-on SEM photographs of tips formed from theta tubing. (A) Relatively small tip formed from thin-septum theta tubing. Note that the septum fails to reach the tip. (B–D) Relatively large tips formed from theta tubing with a thin septum (B), a septum of the same thickness as the outer wall (C), and a thick septum (D).

rounded, thus altering the dual-channel tip toward an elliptical form. Of course surface tension around the outer margin of the tubing would oppose the change from a nearly round form to an elliptical one. But the lumen of each channel is much smaller than the outer boundary of the tubing, and surface tension becomes stronger as the diameter of an interface decreases (Sears, 1950). In addition, surface tensions around both channels act in concert, so they should dominate in determining the final form of the tip.

IV.4b   Septum failure in the smallest tips formed on thin-septum theta tubing

Figure 85(A) shows a tip formed upon thin-septum tubing to a size only slightly above the ultrafine range. Note that the central portion of the septum cannot be seen, a result that was obtained consistently under these conditions. This confirms our explanation of why fluid crosses between the two channels when ultrafine tips are formed upon thin-septum tubing. When the tip formed upon this tubing becomes as small as permitted by the thickness of the outer wall, the thinner septum attenuates and disappears before reaching the tip. The thin-septum tubing that we used gave this result up to tip sizes somewhat above the ultrafine range. When tip size exceeds some critical value, however, an adequate septum should be formed in thin-septum tubing, and this is confirmed by the larger tip of Figure 85(B). This explains why thin-septum theta tubing has long been used successfully for types of research permitting relatively large tips, though it fails within and slightly above the ultrafine range.

IV.4c   Ultrafine tips on thick-septum theta tubing

Our puller readily formed ultrafine tips on thick-septum theta tubing. Compared with Standard Tubing, it was only necessary to increase the heating current somewhat to soften the greater mass of glass. When short tips were desired, it was also necessary to increase airflow to cool the larger mass of glass with the requisite rapidity. After correcting for the gold coating, the outer diameters of these tips were usually about 0.07 μm, and the minimum tip size was about 0.055 μm. A side view of one of our smallest tips has been illustrated previously (Brown and Flaming, 1977a). We have thus far been unable to obtain high quality end-on views of dual-channel tips in the ultrafine range. But we have never observed an incomplete septum on a tip formed from thick-septum tubing. In addition, ultrafine tips formed on thick-septum tubing do not exhibit any cross-over of fluid at the tip when a single channel is filled, though this occurs consistently with thin-septum tubing (see Part III of this chapter). Hence a thick septum extends the use of theta tubing into the ultrafine range.

Just as a thin septum leads to an incomplete septum in ultrafine tips, it is ultrafine tips in which a thick septum would most likely protrude slightly and provide a kind of spear. Though the theoretical expectation of such a spear seems sound, we have been unable to demonstrate it by SEM, possibly because of the great difficulty in resolving the details of ultrafine tips.

IV.4d   Quality of cell penetration

When tested in toad rods, the thick-septum ultrafine tips penetrated even more readily than single-channel tips. Also, unlike dual-channel tips formed by fusing two tubes, the membrane potential and light responses were well maintained after penetration. Though the reason for penetrations being obtained so readily is not certain, it probably results from spear formation. Since the tip form is elliptical, penetration should also be much improved by beveling the long axis of the ellipse, and beveling should especially improve cell penetration for tips larger than the ultrafine range. We have not, however, studied the effects of beveling tips formed from thick-septum tubing.

IV.4e   Electrical isolation of the two channels in ultrafine micropipettes

As discussed in Section V.1 of Chapter 9, electrical interaction between the two channels of a dual-channel micropipette is conventionally measured by the coupling resistance, defined as $R_c = E_2/I_1$, where I_1 is the current passed through one channel and E_2 is the voltage measured across the other channel. Thus defined, coupling resistance decreases as electrical interaction between the two channels is decreased. For test purposes we filled both channels of ultrafine tips with 5 M K-acetate and then measured coupling resistance. Control tips formed from thin-septum theta tubing yielded high values ranging from 5–35 MΩ. When tips of similar size were formed from thick-septum theta tubing, coupling resistances were only 100–200 kΩ. These low values are similar to coupling resistances obtained by Werblin (1975) when dual-channel tips were formed from fused tubes and beveling was then used to separate the tips by 0.5–1.5 μm (see Section V.1 of Chapter 9). It is indeed surprising that thick-septum theta tubing can provide similarly low coupling resistances of ultrafine tips without beveling. This suggests that the ion pools at the two tips are effectively separated by a protruding spear, as well as by the thickness of the septum itself.

IV.4f   Single-channel electrical resistance in ultrafine dual-channel
micropipettes

Since an ultrafine tip formed from thick-septum tubing contains two channels and a thick septum, each channel must be much smaller than the lumen of a single-channel tip of similar outer diameter. This greatly increases the electrical resistance of each channel, and it is especially important to counter this effect for some applications. This is most readily done by minimizing tip length, and the airjet system of our puller permitted the length of these tips to be reduced to about 6 mm. The electrical resistance of a single channel filled with 5 M

K-acetate then averaged about 150 MΩ, which is satisfactory for most applications. By comparison, an average resistance of about 44 MΩ was obtained with single-channel tips of similar length and outer tip diameter.

IV.4g   Summary

In summary, the use of thick-septum theta tubing in our puller seems to solve all three of the main problems associated with ultrafine dual-channel micropipettes suitable for intracellular work in small cells. First, small cells such as toad rods may be readily penetrated with little or no damage. Second, electrical interaction between the two channels may be kept quite low. Third, by using our airjet system to minimize tip length, the electrical resistance of each channel may be kept low enough for the requirements of most work.

PART V   ION-SPECIFIC ELECTRODES

One of the main applications of dual-channel micropipettes is for measuring the concentrations of specific ions at highly localized sites. In this case one channel contains a ligand that generates a voltage signal, the amplitude of which is related to the concentration of a specific ion at the electrode tip, while the other channel serves as reference electrode. For intracellular work of this type it is important that the reference electrode also be intracellular to avoid unwanted signals resulting from resting membrane potentials or stimulus-evoked responses of the cell membrane. Ion-specific electrodes involve some specialized technical problems, two of which are especially important. One is the choice of a ligand offering maximum sensitivity to the ion species measured, while responding minimally to other ions that may be present. The other concerns how to silanize the ligand channel so that a small column of ligand may be drawn in by capillary action, while sparing the other channel from being silanized, since aqueous solutions would then fail to fill the tip of the reference channel. These problems have been treated in various publications and hence will not be dealt with here. Books in this field include those by Eisenmann (1967), Thomas (1978), Covington (1979), Lübbers *et al.* (1981), Morf (1981), Zeuthen (1981) and Koryta and Stulik (1983).

One point, however, is of special interest concerning the fabrication of dual-channel micropipettes for this type of work. Dr. Hiroshi Yamaguchi (Department of Physiology, University of Massachusetts Medical School, Worcester, MA 01605, USA) has found (personal communication) that aluminosilicate glass can provide improved results with ion-specific electrodes. He points out that Ca^{2+}-selective electrodes lose sensitivity at tip diameters smaller than about 1.0 μm, and this is believed due to properties of the glass itself. For example, when borosilicate glass becomes severely thinned in fine or ultrafine tips, electrical resistance across the column of Ca^{2+} ligand may approach the resistivity of the glass wall. Under these conditions a significant amount of the signal may be lost through the glass. In his work he thus fabricated the tips from aluminosilicate glass (Corning No. 1720 or 1724), which have volume re-sistivities that are respectively 2 and 6 orders of magnitude greater than that of borosilicate glass. Though his tubing was quite thin-walled (OD of 1.0 mm and ID of 0.72–0.86 mm), he was able to fabricate Ca^{2+}-selective electrodes with tip diameters of about 0.1 μm. In this work he used triple-channel tubing consisting of three tubes fused side-by-side. The outer tubes were used for the ligand channel and the reference channel, respectively, while the central channel was used as a spacer to improve the electrical separation between the outer channels. Under these conditions, he found that improved results could be obtained with Ca^{2+}-selective electrodes in small cells such as those of smooth muscle. Thus aluminosilicate glass offers distinct advantages for ion-specific electrodes, especially when small tips are required for intracellular work in small cells.

CHAPTER 17

The Burgeoning Field of Patch Clamping

PART I   THE BACKGROUND AND CAPABILITIES OF PATCH CLAMPING

I.1   Development of Basic Technique

A technique for studying membrane properties in small areas of a cell membrane was first developed by Strickholm (1961). A micropipette tip with an inner diameter of several μm was pulled, fire-polished, and pressed against the membrane of a skeletal muscle cell. Though the seal between glass and membrane was incomplete, it provided sufficient electrical isolation of a small patch of membrane from the remainder of the cell to measure membrane current, impedance, and capacitance in the membrane area enclosed by the micropipette.

A few subsequent studies employed this technique, but it was little applied until Neher and Sakmann (1976) made the necessary improvements permitting its use for studying single channels in cell membranes. Detection of the conductance change associated with opening or closing a single acetylcholine (ACh) channel in a skeletal muscle cell required that the seal resistance (between pipette interior and bath) be increased by a factor of at least four. This was done mainly by using collagenase and protease to enzymatically digest connective tissue and the basement membrane, which permitted closer contact between the pipette and membrane. The techniques and results of this work were described in further detail by Neher *et al.* (1978). Micropipettes were pulled and fire-polished to an inner diameter of 1–3 μm. Membrane current and conductance changes associated with discrete activations of ACh channels were then studied under voltage clamp conditions, which were provided by a pair of conventional micropipettes inserted through the cell membrane near the recording pipette.

The next step was a more dramatic increase of the seal resistance, which was first used by Sigworth and Neher (1980) to study single Na^+ channels in cultured muscle cells. Procedures for obtaining the higher seal resistances, and their main consequences, were then described by Hamill *et al.* (1981). When prescribed precautions were taken to assure cleanliness of the micropipette tip, and gentle suction was applied, a high resistance seal often developed within a few seconds. This technique increased the attainable seal resistance from about 50 MΩ, to 10–100 GΩ, thus carrying it upward by about three orders of magnitude, from the megohm to the gigaohm range. Such high resistance seals were called 'giga-seals'. They markedly decreased background noise from the cell membrane surrounding the micropipette tip, and signal loss through the seal was also reduced, thus improving the resolution of current recordings by an order of magnitude. The giga-seals also permitted voltage clamping a patch of membrane without separate intracellular microelectrodes, thus extending the application of voltage clamping to membrane patches in small cells.

I.2   Patch Clamp and Related Preparations

I.2a   Cell-attached patch

A giga-seal is not only electrically tight but mechanically strong. Once established, it permits the pipette to be pulled back from the cell without losing the seal. As shown in Figure 86, the combination of this manipulation with other simple procedures can provide several important extensions of patch clamping.

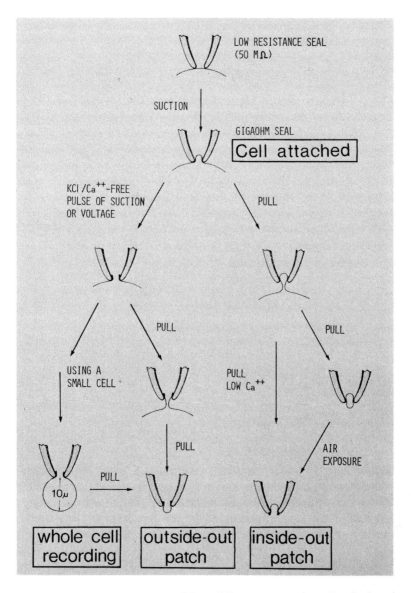

Figure 86. Schematic representation of four different preparations. Patch clamping is shown under 'cell attached' conditions and under 'cell-free' conditions with the patch either 'inside-out' or 'outside-out'. 'Whole cell recording' is also shown. Manipulations include drawing the pipette back from the cell ('pull'), short exposure of the pipette tip to air, and a brief pulse of either suction or voltage applied to the pipette interior during the 'cell attached' condition. For details, see text. (From Hamill *et al.* (1981), reproduced by permission of Springer-Verlag, New York, N.Y.)

At the top of Figure 86, a micropipette has been brought into contact with a cell membrane to establish a low resistance seal of about 50 MΩ. After applying gentle suction a gigaseal develops. This preparation is referred to as 'cell-attached' because the entire cell is still attached to the patch of membrane enclosed by the micropipette.

I.2b   Cell-free inside-out patch

As shown on the right of Figure 86, pulling back the micropipette first attenuates the connection of the membrane patch with the remainder of the cell; then the attenuated connection seals and pinches off, leaving a vesicle of cell membrane within the micropipette tip. If this vesicle is briefly exposed to air and then reinserted into the bath, the outer part of the vesicle may be disrupted. This leaves a cell-free 'inside-out patch', in which the cytoplasmic surface is directly exposed to the bathing solution. The outer part of the vesicle may also be made leaky by exposure to a low Ca^{2+} solution, but this procedure proved less satisfactory and less permanent.

I.2c   Cell-free outside-out patch

As shown on the left of Figure 86, a cell-free 'outside-out patch' may also be formed. In this case the membrane patch contained by the micropipette must first be disrupted by low Ca^{2+} or by a pulse of voltage or suction, among which the suction pulse seems preferred. Pulling then forms an attenuated connection with the cell, which seals and pinches off to form the outside-out patch. A great advantage of cell-free patches is that the bathing solution may be used to determine the effects upon single channel currents of presenting drugs or altered ion concentrations to either the cytoplasmic or extracellular surface of the cell membrane.

I.2d   Tight-seal whole-cell recording

Finally, Figure 86 shows that if the 'cell-attached' patch of membrane is disrupted without any further procedure, this preparation may be used for 'whole cell recording'. Membrane properties of almost the entire cell may thus be studied under voltage clamp conditions. According to Hamill *et al.* (1981), this procedure is restricted to cells less than about 30 μm in diameter. But it has the advantage that virtually the entire membrane of a small cell may be voltage clamped without the use of separate penetrating micropipettes. The original term for this preparation was rather unfortunate, since 'whole cell recording' may also be conducted by intracellular micropipettes. Thus Marty and Neher (1983) adopted the term 'tight-seal whole-cell recording'. Though awkward, this term seems more appropriate. When this preparation is used with voltage clamping, we suggest that 'whole cell clamp' might be even more appropriate. In addition to being brief, it would emphasize the relationship of this preparation to patch clamping.

I.2e   The loose patch clamp

In some cases it is desirable to record from patches that contain many channels but are still small enough to provide local recordings. For example, recordings of this type may be used to examine the distribution of channels over a cell surface, such as that of a muscle cell. A technique for this type of work, as described by Stühmer *et al.* (1983), has been called the 'loose patch clamp'. It employs pipette tips having inner diameters of 5–20 μm, which are pressed lightly against the cell membrane. Enzymatic cleaning of the cell membrane is avoided, and though suction improves the seal it is generally not required. Thus recordings may be made under more normal physiological conditions than those required for single-channel recordings. In fact, the basic recording conditions appear quite similar to those used in the early work of Strickholm (1961).

Of course the main limitation of a loose patch clamp is the relatively low seal resistance. This may be handled to some extent by careful compensation of the seal resistance in the recording circuitry (Stühmer *et al.*, 1983). More recently, Roberts and Almers (1984) described an improved solution employing concentric micropipettes. The inner barrel surrounds the patch of membrane within which membrane current is recorded. This inner patch of membrane, and the annular area of membrane between it and the outer pipette, are both held at the same potential. The inner patch is thus electrically isolated from the remainder of the cell membrane without requiring an exceptionally high seal resistance. Under these conditions the membrane current across the inner patch is neither lost by leakage through the seal resistance nor contaminated by activity of membrane areas outside the inner patch. Compared with compensation of the seal resistance by electronic circuitry, this method is more effective. It does not require measurement of the seal resistance, and the measurement of membrane current is not influenced by fluctuations or non-linearities of the seal resistance. On the other hand, fabrication of the requisite concentric patch clamp pipettes is notably difficult and time consuming.

I.2f   Suction recording of normal cell activity

Shortly after the work of Neher and Sakmann (1976), another variation of patch clamping was applied that was closely related to both the early work of Strickholm (1961) and to the loose patch clamp employed later. In this variation Yau *et al.* (1977) used a fire-polished suction electrode to record the membrane current of rod outer segments in the toad retina. This was done by sucking varying amounts of a rod outer segment into the electrode, so that membrane current could be recorded from the enclosed area of membrane. Voltage clamping was not applied, and normal light-evoked fluctuations of membrane current were recorded from a single rod outer segment. As later extended by Baylor and his co-workers, this method of recording from outer segments of vertebrate photoreceptors has proved very useful. For example, it has permitted the study of single photon absorptions in outer segments of toad rods (Baylor *et al.*, 1979) and it has provided a method of recording from the quite small outer segments of both rods and cones in a Macaque monkey (Nunn and Baylor, 1982; Nunn *et al.*, 1984).

I.3 The Growth of Patch Clamping and Related Techniques

Following demonstration of the main possibilities of patch clamping and closely related techniques, applications of these techniques have proliferated at an accelerated pace, and this promises to continue for some time. Like intracellular recording with micropipettes, patch clamping techniques permit critical results to be obtained upon a broad range of fundamental problems, and they have thus led to a second major flowering of research in the neural sciences. Patch clamping techniques are also similar to intracellular micropipettes in having broad applications to work on non-excitable cells. Perhaps the best single indication of the rapid growth of this field was the publication, only 7 years after the paper by Neher and Sakmann (1976), of a book edited by Sakmann and Neher (1983a) in which 25 chapters described the techniques and various applications of patch clamping. Since this book provides a definitive and detailed view of the field at that relatively recent time, our own treatment of most aspects of this subject has been kept brief.

I.4 The Relation of Patch Clamping Techniques to Intracellular Work with Penetrating Micropipettes

Though patch clamping and related techniques have many applications, there is one major limitation. These techniques require accessibility of the cell membrane to a micropipette with an outer tip diameter of about 1.0 μm or larger. Hence these techniques may be used on cultured or isolated cells, or cells that may be exposed by operative techniques, where they function most distinctively in research upon the properties of single channels in cell membranes. For *in situ* recording from cells that are buried in masses of tissue, such as the brain or spinal cord, penetrating intracellular micropipettes are still required to study membrane potentials at rest or in response to stimulation. Thus intracellular micropipettes and patch clamping pipettes are mainly complementary in the types of research that may be performed. For work on whole cells that are readily accessible, however, a choice may be made between these two general techniques.

PART II   PATCH CLAMPING TECHNIQUES

II.1   Glass–Membrane Seals

II.1a   During patch clamping

In all types of patch clamping and related techniques, a critical element is the quality of the seal between the tip of the glass pipette and a cell membrane. This seal appears to result from surface interactions between glass and membrane, and Corey and Stevens (1983) have identified four separate types of interaction that may be expected to contribute to this glass–membrane seal. A consistent observation is the capricious variation of seal formation from day to day, which Corey and Stevens attribute to extracellular matrix proteins. Suction is helpful in establishing a giga-seal, which usually develops within several seconds (Hamill *et al.*, 1981). Thereafter, it appears that suction is no longer critical, since the contained patch of membrane may be disrupted by a pulse of suction and the giga-seal may still be well maintained during 'whole cell recording' (see Figure 86).

II.1b   *During intracellular recording with penetrating micropipettes*

Though glass–membrane seals have been emphasized in patch clamping, where they are obviously critical, they play a less obvious but perhaps equally important role during intracellular work with penetrating micropipettes. For example, after penetrating toad rods we frequently note that over a short period the resting membrane potential increases and then stabilizes, and this phenomenon also occurs in the case of light-evoked responses. Similar experiences have been reported by many investigators in a variety of cell types. It thus appears that over a brief period the membrane sometimes seals around the micropipette tip. In cases where the initial resting membrane potential is quite low, probably owing to rather severe damage during penetration, such a seal does not develop. At the other extreme, the membrane potential is sometimes initially quite high and does not become higher, presumably because the penetration has caused so little damage that the seal requires no improvement. In short, our experience suggests that development of the seal is most apparent when minor damage has occurred. In such a case the glass tip must be in close enough contact with the membrane for the seal to develop quite well over a brief period, just as it does in patch clamping.

After obtaining a high membrane potential in a toad rod, we have noted that the micropipette can often be advanced or retracted many microns without disturbing the recording. An even more surprising observation was made while attempting to mark intracellular recordings in both inner and outer segments of toad rods by means of Procion yellow. Stains were readily recovered in inner segments. Procion yellow was also injected into outer segments on many occasions, following intracellular penetrations that were so close to the receptor surface that they could not have been in the inner segments. Yet no stained outer segment was ever recorded during careful histological searches. We were thus forced to conclude that attempted withdrawal of the micropipette from an outer segment was consistently breaking the outer segment away from the inner segment and removing it from the retina. In view of the extremely small area of contact between the membrane and a penetrating ultrafine micropipette, these observations imply that once the glass–membrane seal is established it is astonishingly strong. Hence this seal must be a major factor in maintaining stable intracellular recordings. It is probably especially helpful when there are unavoidable movements of the tissue such as muscle contractions, or during pulse and respiratory movements that are often encountered in the brain and spinal cord.

II.2   The Three-Step Fabrication of Patch Clamp Pipettes

A suction-type pipette is used for all types of research in this field, though in some cases suction is not actually applied. For work on single ion channels the inner diameter of the tip may be as small as about 0.5 μm, while for loose patch clamping it may be as large as 20 μm. Thus the tips are generally much larger than those of intracellular micropipettes and the range of tip size for various applications is also quite large. As described by Corey and Stevens (1983), these suction micropipettes are typically fabricated in three steps. After the tip is formed by a micropipette puller, it is coated with a nonconductor. This is often necessary to reduce capacitance to ground, because such capacitance introduces background noise in current recordings and it causes a brief current to enter the recording after each voltage step, which tends to obscure transient membrane currents. Sylgard $^{®}$ has become the favorite coating material, and with appropriate procedures it may be applied to within 10–50 μm of the tip. This greatly reduces capacitance to ground by thickening the non-conductive layer for all positions along the shank of the micropipette except for a short section just behind the tip itself. In the third step the tip is fire-polished. This smooths the tip and probably produces a cleaner surface by burning off contaminants such as a thin film of Sylgard $^{®}$. Though fire-polishing is not necessary to obtain giga-seals, it seems to provide giga-seals of greater stability.

II.3   Early Technique for Pulling Patch Clamp Pipettes

Methods of coating and fire-polishing tips have been fully described by Corey and Stevens (1983). We shall now treat in some detail how pipettes have been fabricated during early work in this field, partly as a background for the improved methods described in Chapter 18.

In forming patch clamp pipettes the tip must be relatively large (inner diameter about 0.5 μm or greater). Also, the cone angle in most cases should be quite large. Though many micropipette pullers can satisfy these requirements when appropriately modified and operated, a puller frequently used during the early years of patch clamping was the Kopf Model 700C. This is a two-stage vertical puller with basic capabilities similar to those of the Industrial Science Associates puller discussed in Sections III.3 and III.4 of Chapter 2. Following Corey and Stevens (1983), we shall describe the pulling of patch clamp pipettes with the Kopf instrument, which illustrates both the requirements of this work and the limitations of early pulling methods in this application.

In forming a patch clamp pipette with any puller, it has thus far been necessary to use at least two completely separate stages of pulling. During the first stage the glass is minimally heated and a relatively weak pull is exerted for a fixed distance to produce a very rapid taper. With the weak and slow pull required to do this, the glass becomes too cool to form an appropriate tip, so the glass must be reheated and pulled again. Unlike the more customary two-stage pull, in which the two stages involve sequential weak and strong pulls, the two stages in forming a patch clamp pipette are separated by a pause, and the pull strength is typically unchanged.

The Kopf puller has a fixed upper clamp and a moving lower clamp. For patch clamp pipettes, Corey and Stevens disconnect the moving element from the solenoid to reduce the strength of the gravity-powered pull. A stop must be introduced to control the length of the first pull, and a pushbutton switch should be added to turn off the heating current after the first pull, which attenuates the glass capillary to a diameter of 200–400 μm. Since there is only one moving element in the Kopf Puller, this attenuated part of the glass capillary will be below the heating filament. The capillary tubing must then be unclamped, moved upward to re-center the attenuated portion within the heating filament, and then re-clamped. The heating current is typically reduced for the second pull, and the final tip size is critically dependent upon the heating current used for this second pull. Thus Corey and Stevens recommend the design and use of a separate well regulated power supply for the heating current of this Kopf puller.

II.4 Patch Clamp Pipettes Formed by Early Pulling Techniques

Thus far, pipettes for patch clamping and related applications have been formed almost entirely from either soft or borosilicate glass. Pipettes formed as just described, using both types of glass, have been illustrated and discussed by Sakmann and Neher (1983b). The soft glass employed was Cee Bee ® capillaries with an OD of 1.6 mm and an ID of 1.0 mm (obtained from C. Bardram, Braunstien 4, 3460-Birkorod, Denmark). Compared with Standard Tubing, this glass has an OD/ID of only 1.6 and is thus thin-walled. A patch pipette formed from this tubing is shown in Figure 87. Its tip opening has a diameter of 1.1 μm, the wall thickness at the tip is 0.2 μm, and the cone angle at the tip is about 24°. A soft glass pipette of these dimensions is described as 'typical' of those used in cell-attached recordings. When filled with 150 m M KCl, its resistance was 2–2.5 MΩ, and Sakmann and Neher calculated the tip opening alone to have a resistance of about 1.2 MΩ. Thus the shank contributes significantly to the total pipette resistance, even when the cone angle is as large as 24°.

Sakmann and Neher found that thickening the wall at the tip offered three advantages. In addition to increasing the shunt resistance through the glass, the thicker-walled tips provided a higher success rate in obtaining giga-seals, and the stability of these giga-seals was improved.

They also investigated the use of hard glasses because of their higher electrical resistivity. The borosilicate tubing they used was obtained from Jencons Scientific (Leighton Buzzard, England). Having an OD of 1.8 mm and an ID of 0.8 mm, its OD/ID was 2.25 and it was thus slightly thick-walled. A tip formed

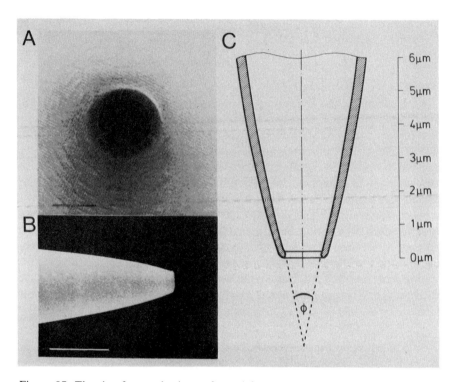

Figure 87. The tip of a patch pipette formed from thin-walled soft glass as described by Hamill *et al.* (1981). (A) End-on view by SEM. (B) Side view of the same pipette by SEM. Scale bars represent 1.0 μm in (A) and 4.0 μm in (B). (C) Reconstruction of longitudinal section of this pipette, which had a cone angle (ϕ) of 24°. (From Sakmann and Neher (1983b), reproduced by permission of Plenum Publishing Corporation, New York, N.Y.)

from this tubing is shown in Figure 88. The tip opening has a diameter of 0.98 μm, comparable to the tip opening of the soft glass pipette in Figure 87, but the thickness of the rim is about doubled, from 0.2 to 0.4 μm, while the cone angle is more than halved, from 24° to about 10°. As a result of the smaller cone angle, pipettes of the dimensions in Figure 88 (filled with 150 m M KCl) have typical electrical resistances of 8–11 MΩ. This is about 4 times the resistance of soft glass pipettes with similar tip openings. Hence this thick-walled borosilicate tubing increased the shunt resistance, and improved the thickness of the pipette rim, at the cost of a considerably higher electrical resistance of the pipette.

The importance of a low pipette resistance is probably greatest in the case of whole cell recording, when considerable current must be passed to voltage clamp the whole cell. Hence for whole cell recording, Sakmann and Neher used thick-walled borosilicate pipettes with relatively large tip openings (2–3 μm), which lowered the pipette resistance to 3–4 MΩ. As discussed in Section IV.2 of Chapter 18, the disadvantage of a reduced cone angle when using borosilicate

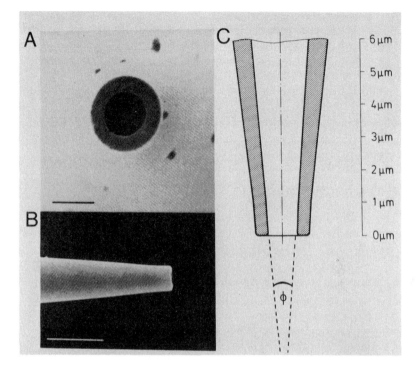

Figure 88. The tip of a patch pipette formed from thick-walled borosilicate glass as described by Hamill *et al.* (1981). (A) End-on view by SEM. (B) Side view of the same pipette by SEM. Scale bars represent 1.0 μm in (A) and 4.0 μm in (B). (C) Reconstruction of longitudinal section of this pipette. (From Sakmann and Neher (1983b), reproduced by permission of Plenum Publishing Corporation, New York, N.Y.)

tubing has now been alleviated by improved methods of forming patch clamp pipettes.

Sakmann and Neher also tried aluminosilicate tubing for patch clamping pipettes and found that tip dimensions could be obtained similar to those formed from soft glass and illustrated in Figure 87. Their aluminosilicate tubing was obtained from A-M Systems (Everett, WA 98024, USA), and they state that suitable results were obtained only when the tubing was thin-walled. By comparison with Standard Tubing, all aluminosilicate tubing available to date is thin-walled. But their best results were apparently obtained with a particularly thin-walled tubing. This result was not explained, and it does not follow the principle that pertained when patch clamp pipettes were formed from other types of glass. Hence it probably reflects the difficulty of handling the narrow working range of aluminosilicate glass (see Section II.4 of Chapter 15), which would be especially great when forming patch clamp pipettes from relatively thick-walled tubing. The problem of conveniently handling this type of glass has now been overcome in recent revisions of our micropipette puller (see Part V of Chapter 18).

II.5 Filling Patch Clamp Pipettes

Because of the relatively large tips, special methods such as an Omega Dot are not required to fill patch clamp pipettes. If the tips are immersed in the filling solution, they will usually fill by capillarity within about a minute. Suction is helpful if the filling solution is particularly viscous or if more rapid filling is desired. The remainder of the pipette is then backfilled by inserting a stainless steel needle as far as possible into the shaft and injecting filling solution. Further details of this procedure, and some precautions in special cases, have been discussed by Corey and Stevens (1983).

II.6 Suction Pipette Adapters

The suction pipette must be sealed into an adapter that makes electrical contact with the solution in the pipette and provides a connection for applying suction. A device for this purpose has been illustrated by Hamill *et al.* (1981). Adapters of similar design are now available from E. W. Wright (760 Dunham Rd., Guilford, CN 06437, USA) to fit any desired outer diameter of the pipette.

II.7 Patch Clamp Circuitry

The circuitry for this type of work must be designed carefully, and this subject has been treated extensively by Sigworth (1983). Among patch clamp amplifiers that have become available commercially, many investigators have used the List Model EPC-7 supplied by List-electronic (Pfungstaedter Strasse 18–20, D-6100 Darmstadt/Eberstadt, FRG). Recently a patch clamp amplifier with similar performance specifications and some convenient new features (the 'Axopatch') has become available from Axon Instruments, Inc. (1437 Rollins Road, Burlingame, CA 91010, USA).

CHAPTER 18

Extension of the Brown–Flaming Micropipette Puller to Patch Clamping and Conveniently Handling Aluminosilicate Glass

PART I   GOALS

In developing our puller the original goal of forming improved micropipettes for intracellular work in small cells had been attained, and further advantages had been realized. The new field of patch clamping, however, presented new requirements (see Sections II.3 and II.4 of Chapter 17). Since these requirements were not fully satisfied by available pullers, we next undertook to extend the capabilities of our instrument to better meet the needs of patch clamping.

For this purpose three limitations had to be overcome. First, the largest tips formed by our puller had remained about 1.0 μm, but patch clamping often requires considerably larger tips. Second, methods were required to form pipettes with the rapid tapers often desirable for patch clamping. This was particularly important for borosilicate glass, which offers advantages over soft glass for patch clamping, but which had yielded only relatively small cone angles by previous pulling methods (see Section II.4 of Chapter 17). Third, methods were required for conveniently handling aluminosilicate glass. It offers potential advantages for patch clamping because of its high electrical resistivity, but is more difficult to handle because of its narrow working range (see Section II.4 of Chapter 17).

PART II   REQUIREMENTS TO ATTAIN GOALS

The formation of larger tips, using a specific type of glass and a given OD/ID, requires reduction of the tip temperature (see Section IV.2 of Chapter 6). Increasing the rapidity of taper, however, requires a different approach. Forces of surface tension around both the outer boundary and lumen of the capillary tube will cause it to attenuate as it is heated and pulled (see Section I.3 of Chapter 6). While being drawn out over any given distance, a slower pull provides more time for surface tension to act, so the rapidity of taper increases. Increasing the cone angle will thus require a lowered *tip velocity*, defined as the pulling velocity during tip formation. For patch clamp pipettes, therefore, it is desirable to decrease both tip temperature and tip velocity, by comparison with values used for ultrafine and fine micropipettes. These requirements have been approached in previous work by lowering both the heating current and pull strength, procedures that have proved helpful but inadequate to provide ideal results.

If a patch clamp pipette is formed by only a single cycle of heating and attenuation, the pipette initially tapers rapidly, but as it attenuates the pull velocity increases rapidly and becomes greatest at the tip, resulting in a small cone angle. Thus patch clamp pipettes have typically been pulled in two separate cycles. By stopping the first pull at an appropriate point, and restarting the second cycle from zero velocity, the tip velocity is decreased and the cone angle correspondingly increased.

A second pull can also increase the attainable tip size if it is initiated by heating the glass only just enough to be further attenuated by the weak pulling force. By thus holding the glass temperature to a minimum at a point relatively close to the tip, the tip temperature may be decreased to increase tip size. If heating current is the same for both cycles, however, the full advantage of this procedure cannot be realized. Instead, at the onset of the second pull, the smaller mass of glass will heat rapidly and overshoot the desired tip temperature before the tip can be formed. For this reason, the heating current has typically been reduced for the second cycle (Corey and Stevens, 1983).

Since two pulling cycles are better than one, additional cycles should further increase the cone angles and tip sizes attainable. Three cycles have occasionally been used in previous work (Corey and Stevens, 1983), but the number of cycles available would ideally be unlimited.

In providing two or more pulling cycles, conventional single-sided pullers are awkward because the glass capillary must be recentered in the heating filament after each cycle. It is also necessary that each cycle be terminated while the tip is still tapering rapidly. If the first cycle is stopped after a fixed distance, the stopping point must be reset for each subsequent cycle except the final one. Since these procedures are inconvenient and time consuming, improved techniques were long needed for patch clamping. These problems were first avoided in the Sachs–Flaming puller, which is available from the Sutter Instrument Co. This instrument was designed mainly to form tips in the requisite size range for patch clamping. Though the pull is single-sided, the heating filament moves at half the speed of the pulling element, thus keeping the heating element centered upon the region of the forming tips. Multiple pulling cycles are then provided by programming the cycles to begin after a predetermined set of pulling distances.

The requirements of patch clamping reveal an additional advantage of a symmetrical two-sided pull, which assures that the forming tips are always centered within the heating filament. In addition, it became evident that a given pulling cycle would ideally be terminated when the pull velocity increases just enough to reduce the rapidity of taper. Since the velocity at which this occurs should change little between pulling cycles, it should not require resetting between pulling cycles. A preset pulling velocity, used to stop a pulling cycle or to control later events in tip formation, will henceforth be referred to as a *criterion velocity*.

A criterion velocity should likewise be better than a criterion distance for triggering the later events when forming ultrafine or fine micropipettes with a two-stage puller. In the traditional method a criterion distance controls the length of time during which heat is delivered after the onset of pulling, thus determining the temperature and viscosity of glass when the fast pull is activated. At any given moment, however, the pulling velocity is directly and strongly influenced by viscosity of the glass. Hence a criterion velocity offers distinct advantages.

For example, different types of glass heat at different rates during the weak pull, so a given criterion distance will yield different results whenever the type of glass is changed. If a criterion distance is established for a given result with borosilicate tubing, it will have to be altered for aluminosilicate glass, and the narrow working range of aluminosilicate glass can make the requisite value difficult to find. By contrast, if these two types of tubing were used with similar values of OD/ID, a given criterion velocity should assure similar viscosities at onset of the fast pull. The fast pull would thus be initiated at temperatures within the working ranges of both types of glass. Put another way, a criterion velocity should automatically adjust the length of the weak pull to provide the requisite viscosities and temperatures of different types of glass at the onset of the fast pull. This should permit interchanging types of glass without altering the criterion velocity, regardless of whether it is used to trigger the fast pull in forming ultrafine micropipettes, or to stop each pulling cycle when forming patch clamp pipettes.

When forming ultrafine or fine micropipettes, a criterion velocity should also provide automatic compensation for certain factors that can vary with a given type of tubing. For example, lowered heating current will heat the glass more slowly and require a greater length of slow pull to provide a given viscosity of the glass. A criterion velocity should thus permit a lowered heating current to lengthen the rapidly tapering segment, thereby reducing total tip length. This effect should supplement the airjet in further shortening tips, as desired in a variety of applications.

In summary, it appeared necessary to continuously monitor the pull velocity and to provide for triggering either the fast pull or the cessation of pulling at any desired pull velocity. These became the key requirements in extending our puller to form patch clamp pipettes and to conveniently handle aluminosilicate glass, while significantly improving the available capabilities for forming both patch clamp pipettes and intracellular micropipettes.

PART III OUR MODEL P-80B AND P-80C MICROPIPETTE PULLERS

III.1 Revisions of the Puller

Our first model of the new series (the P-80B) was altered in two major respects from the P-77B. An LVT (linear velocity transducer) was mounted upon the solenoid plunger (see Figure 11) to monitor the velocity of its fall during the weak pull. A microprocessor was also introduced to 'read' the output voltage of the LVT (which is linear with velocity), and to control the pulling cycle after a preset criterion voltage was attained. Though a microprocessor was not required for this purpose, it simplified the circuitry and increased the ease with which the pulling cycle could be altered. The microprocessor was not made accessible to external controls, but the pulling cycle could be changed readily by internal settings. Since these revisions permitted the weak pull to be terminated at a criterion velocity, previous controls for terminating it after a criterion distance were eliminated. As shown in Figure 89, the front panel was also changed. Separate controls and digital readouts were provided for the heating current ('heat index'), strength of fast pull ('pull index'), and criterion velocity ('velocity index'). Indicator lights were also provided to show the part of the pulling cycle in effect at any given time, and a 'reset' button was added to permit changing the puller settings between cycles.

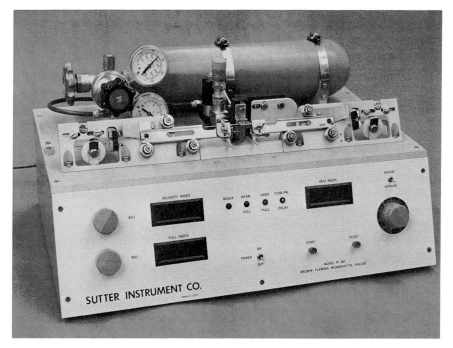

Figure 89. External appearance of the P-80B and P-80C models of the Brown–
Flaming micropipette puller.

Our Model P-80C remained the same except for the circuit controlling heating current. Though our control of heating current had been adequate for fine and ultrafine micropipettes, the heating current for patch clamp pipettes is sometimes much lower. A given current step will then represent a larger percentage change of heating current. In addition, the allowable percentage change of heating current becomes more critical when forming the large tips needed for certain applications of patch clamping. As a result, the sensitivity of setting the heating current proved marginal when some types of patch pipettes were formed by our Model P-80B. The potentiometer covering the full range of heating current was thus changed from a single turn to 10 turns, which provided more than enough sensitivity for patch clamp pipettes. Though stability of the heating current was already satisfactory, this was further improved by redesigning the circuit. This new circuit reduced the variation of heating current, during a 20 min period of monitoring, by at least a factor of 10.

III.2   The Pulling Cycle

III.2a   The traditional pulling cycle for micropipettes

When forming ultrafine or fine micropipettes, the basic pulling cycle remained the same as in our P-77 series of models, aside from the method of triggering the fast pull. The cycle was still started by pressing a button to turn on the heating current. When the criterion velocity was reached during the weak pull, the microprocessor immediately turned off the heating current and initiated the air pulse, then activated the strong pull after a delay of 40 msec. Duration of the air pulse remained at 300 msec, and the strong pull was turned off after 1.0 sec.

III.2b   The formation of patch clamp pipettes

The same pulling cycle may be readily adapted to meet the requirements of patch clamping. The strength of the fast pull is simply set at zero to prevent it from being activated. Thus, when the criterion velocity is reached during the weak pull, the heating current is turned off and only the air pulse is initiated. The function of the air pulse in this case is to stop the pulling cycle by cooling and hardening the glass. The slight delay in stopping the pull by this method may be taken into account by setting the criterion velocity low enough to stop the pulling cycle before the rapidity of taper decreases significantly.

A flag on the solenoid plunger, in conjunction with an optical switch, informs the microprocessor when the plunger has reached the lower limit of its travel. If this has been prevented by stopping pulling after the first cycle, the microprocessor delays 2.0 sec after the pulse activating the fast pull has been turned off; then the heating current is turned on to start a second pulling cycle. Additional pulling cycles are thus provided automatically until tips are formed on the final cycle. The solenoid plunger is then allowed to fall to its lower limit of travel, as sensed by the optical switch, and no further pulling cycle is initiated.

Many useful types of patch clamp pipettes may be obtained without changing puller settings between cycles, as illustrated in the following section of this chapter. For given settings of heating current, airflow, and criterion velocity, the puller will automatically provide the number of cycles required to form a tip under those conditions. Possibilities are increased, however, if puller settings can be changed between cycles. When the 'cooling-delay' indicator light shows that the 2.0 sec delay has been initiated, one has that long to press the 'reset' button. This resets the microprocessor and prevents it from starting a new cycle. Puller settings may then be changed at leisure and the next pulling cycle may be initiated with the 'start' button.

PART IV   PATCH CLAMP PIPETTES FORMED FROM BOROSILICATE GLASS

Since the higher electrical resistivity of borosilicate glass has important advantages for patch clamp pipettes, we have not experimented with soft glass but have explored some of the new possibilities with borosilicate glass. In this work we have used Standard Tubing, and the criterion velocity has been held constant for all pulling cycles used to form any given pipette.

IV.1   Range of Tip Size

In patch clamping the inner diameter of the tip is more critical than the outer diameter. Hence the inner diameter is usually given when stating the tip size of patch pipettes, and we shall follow this convention. The approximate range of tip sizes that we have now obtained with borosilicate tubing is shown in Figure 90. The smaller tip has an inner diameter of 0.50 μm, about the smallest size used in studying the properties of single ionic channels in cell membranes, while the larger tip has an inner diameter of 19 μm. This is about the largest tip size we have obtained to date, and it would be adequate for many applications requiring unusually large tips for patch clamping. Using previous methods, tips as large as about 10 μm have been obtained directly during pulling, but only with considerable difficulty. Tips with inner diameters up to 10 μm can now be formed easily and reliably, and considerably larger tips can be formed with lower reliability. For example, our 19 μm tips were obtained in about 1 out of 3 pulls. Since these large tips are readily measured under the light microscope, the reduced reliability in forming them is of little consequence. The upper limit of tip size that may be obtained directly during pulling is thus greatly increased. In many types of work requiring large tips, this should be a considerable convenience by eliminating the time-consuming and uncertain task of breaking tips to the desired size.

In obtaining tip sizes up to a few microns, it has proved unnecessary to reduce heating current significantly below the range of values used for ultrafine and fine tips. This undoubtedly results from the use of a velocity criterion and the capability of forming patch clamp pipettes by multiple pulling cycles. Heating current had to be lowered markedly, however, and air flow had to be increased, to obtain low enough tip temperatures to form the largest tips.

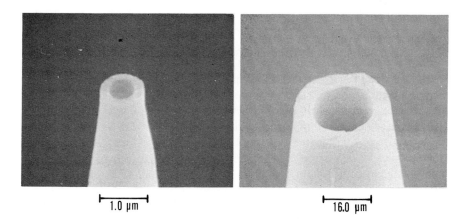

Figure 90. SEM photographs of the smallest and largest tips of patch clamp pipettes formed from borosilicate Standard Tubing by our Model P-80C micropipette puller. The respective inner tip diameters are 0.50 and 19.0 μm.

IV.2   Control of Tip Taper

Figure 91 shows a pair of pipettes formed respectively by 2 and 6 pulling cycles. The heating current and airflow settings were held constant, but the 6-cycle tip was obtained by lowering the criterion velocity to stop each cycle after a shorter distance and thus form a tip from more pulling cycles. The pipettes in Figure 91 are shown in both end-on and side views. The tip formed by 2 pulling cycles has a size of 3.5 μm. Though two cycles are better than one, the side view shows that this tip tapers rapidly at first and then much more slowly. In the tip formed by 6 pulling cycles the size was somewhat smaller, 2.4 μm. But this tip tapered rapidly and constantly, at an angle of 17.5°, over almost its entire length.

Of course the number of pulling cycles required to obtain a virtually constant taper will vary with a number of factors, but the 6 cycles required in the illustrated case is fairly typical. When conditions are used that provide such a constant taper, altered puller settings requiring even more cycles have little or no further advantage. In our experience to date, therefore, 6 is near the upper limit of the number of pulling cycles required to meet various needs.

The number of pulling cycles is controlled mainly by heating current, airflow, and criterion velocity. A decreased heating current decreases the delay in stopping a given pull, thus shortening each pull and requiring more cycles, and increased airflow has the same effect. The most critical factor, however, is criterion velocity, which upon lowering requires more cycles, as shown in Figure 91. It should also be noted that although a greater number of pulling cycles can be very helpful, it is not an end in itself. Instead, the convenient availability of an unlimited number of pulling cycles permits the use of pulling conditions that could not otherwise be used, including lower heating current, higher airflows and lower criterion velocities. Significant restrictions upon tip design are thereby removed.

In Figure 91 the magnification is too low to measure cone angles at the tips themselves. Thus Figure 92 shows tips formed with pulling variables constant, except for criterion velocity, which was progressively lowered to form tips from 3–6 pulling cycles. In the top row of pictures, these tips are shown at a high enough magnification to reveal tip sizes and cone angles. Note that the outer tip diameter approximately doubled between 3 and 4 pulling cycles and thereafter remained constant at about 3.3 μm. The cone angles measured 11° for the 3-cycle tip, 13.5° in the case of 4 cycles, and 12.5° for both the 5- and 6-cycle tips. The cone angles were thus quite similar to the 12° reported for borosilicate patch clamp pipettes by Sakmann and Neher (1983b). In addition, the cone angles changed little with the number of pulling cycles, though Figure 91 shows a greatly increased overall rapidity of taper when changing from 2 to 6 pulling cycles. This is because the 2-cycle tip in Figure 91, which tapers quite gradually over most of its length, shows an increased rapidity of taper at the tip itself, while 6-cycle tips exhibit the opposite effect. This is illustrated in Figure 92 by pictures of the 3- and 6-cycle tips at intermediate magnifications. While

Pulling Cycles

2 6

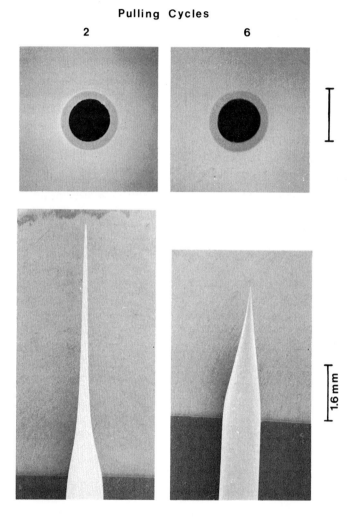

1.6 mm

Figure 91. SEM photographs showing end-on and side views of patch clamp pipettes formed from borosilicate Standard Tubing by our Model P-80C micropipette puller. Both tips formed at the same puller settings, except for criterion velocity, which was decreased to obtain the tip formed by 6 pulling cycles. The calibration mark for end-on views indicates 4.4 and 3.1 μm, respectively, when tips were formed by 2 and 6 pulling cycles. Note the marked shortening and increased rapidity of taper in the tip formed by the greater number of pulling cycles.

the outer boundaries of the 3-cycle tip are convex, those of the 6-cycle tip are concave.

In summary, our techniques for pulling patch clamp pipettes have thus far not significantly increased the obtainable cone angles of the tips when using borosilicate glass. On the other hand, much of the resistance of any micropipette is contributed by regions behind the tip itself. In Figure 91 our 6-cycle tip tapers rapidly, at an angle of $17.5°$, over its entire length except for the tip itself. To our knowledge this type of result has not been attained previously, but it is conveniently provided by our new puller design. This form of tip should be advantageous by significantly reducing the electrical resistance of patch clamp pipettes.

Pulling Cycles

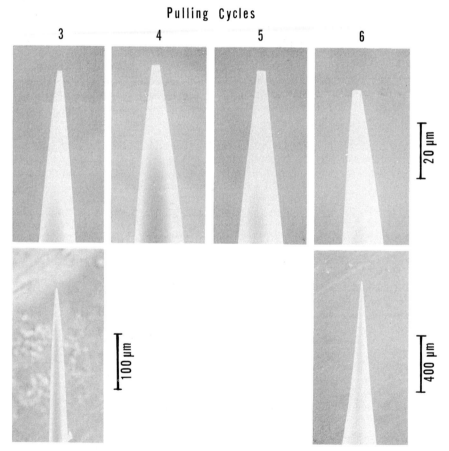

Figure 92. SEM photographs of patch clamp pipettes formed from borosilicate Standard Tubing by our Model P-80C micropipette puller. All tips pulled at the same settings, except for criterion velocity, which was decreased by steps to form tips by 3–6 pulling cycles (see text). In the top row, tips are shown at high enough magnification to illustrate their cone angles. Below, the tips formed by 3 and 6 pulling cycles are shown at lower magnification, to illustrate tip shape over a longer distance.

IV.3 Discussion

Though the Standard Tubing used in this work contained an Omega Dot, none can be seen at the tips in Figures 90 and 91, and this result proved typical. Thus the connection between the Omega Dot and wall must be broken as these tips are formed. This probably occurs because patch clamp tips are all relatively large, by comparison with ultrafine and fine tips, and they are formed at lower tip temperatures. The relatively large tip would not provide the strong fusion of the Omega Dot to the wall that occurs with fine tips (see Sections I.3 and II.1 of Chapter 7). In addition, the lower tip temperature would cause the connection that does exist to be more fragile at the moment of tip formation. Though this result is interesting, it has no significant consequence, since the Omega Dot is not needed to fill tips in the size range of patch clamp pipettes.

We have also noted that the decrease of outer/inner diameter as the tip is formed varies considerably with patch clamp pipettes. Using Standard Tubing with an OD/ID of about 2.0, the patch clamp tips in Figure 90 have values of OD_t/ID_t in the range of 1.7–1.8, while the tips in Figure 91 exhibit a value of about 1.4. By comparison, when fine micropipettes were formed from Standard Tubing with an OD/ID of 1.90, the average OD_t/ID_t was 1.51 (see Section III.3 of Chapter 6). Though our data are not extensive, we have the impression that the variability is greater with patch clamp pipettes, probably because of the large range of tip temperatures required to cover the range of tip sizes used in patch clamping. As shown in Figure 91, thinning of the walls is sometimes quite significant. This probably results from the relatively low temperatures at which patch clamp tips are often formed. Though only a weak pull is used, the low temperature and high viscosity of the glass would tend to produce a greater strain upon the glass and hence more thinning of the tubing wall.

In view of the new capabilities for using borosilicate glass to form patch clamp pipettes with high reliability and versatility, this type of glass would now seem preferable to soft glass for general purpose work in patch clamping. An exception may occur, however, when it is critical to lower the electrical resistance of a patch clamp pipette as far as possible. As reported by Sakmann and Neher (1983b), soft glass can provide cone angles up to 24°, and our method of obtaining rapid taper over the remainder of the tip should also apply to soft glass. Thus soft glass may still prove advantageous for minimizing the electrical resistance of patch clamp pipettes, but an accurate comparison remains to be made.

PART V PATCH CLAMP PIPETTES FORMED FROM ALUMINOSILICATE GLASS

Until recently, available aluminosilicate tubing was all much thinner-walled than borosilicate Standard Tubing. This appears to have resulted from the narrow working range of aluminosilicate glass. In such a case, thickening the wall can make it much more difficult to keep all of the glass within the narrow range of working temperatures while the tubing is pulled (see Section II.4 of Chapter 15). This is especially important when a large piece of tubing with a relatively high OD/ID ratio must be drawn out by a glass supplier to make a great length of smaller tubing. It is also important, though probably to a lesser extent, when tips are then formed by a micropipette puller.

Fortunately, an aluminosilicate tubing with an OD/ID of 1.67 has now become available from Clark Electromedical Instruments (P.O. Box 8, Pangbourne, Reading, RG8 7HU, England), and in the United States it is distributed by the Sutter Instrument Company. This tubing is significantly thicker-walled than previously available aluminosilicate tubings, so it seemed promising for patch clamping, since a thick-walled tip can improve the seal resistance. As shown in Sections III.1 and III.2 of Chapter 6, the higher OD/ID should also be helpful in forming exceptionally small tips. According to the supplier, this glass is composed of 51.9% SiO_2, 22.0% Al_2O_3, 7.8% P_2O_5, 7.7% MgO, 6.9% CaO, 2.1% B_2O_3, 1.4% BaO, and 0.2% As_2O_3.

When given puller settings were used to form patch clamp pipettes from borosilicate tubing, it was found unnecessary to change the settings to obtain patch clamp micropipettes from aluminosilicate tubing, a consequence of changing to a velocity criterion in our P-80 series of models. With constant puller settings, however, pipette dimensions and taper are different with the two types of glass.

Figure 93 shows typical patch clamp pipettes obtained from the described aluminosilicate tubing. Tip size can vary over a considerable range, but two features are striking. Compared with borosilicate glass, the tip tapers are usually much more rapid, and the cone angle can be somewhat greater than 24° (see Figure 93C). Also, the wall is always severely thinned at the tip (see Figure 93, A and B). A minor third point is that the Omega Dot continues to the tip, where it may always be seen.

It seems likely that all of these results stem from the stronger bonds in aluminosilicate glass (see Section II.4 of Chapter 15). With a constant weak pull, these stronger bonds probably slow the pulling velocity and thus increase the rapidity of taper. But this leaves unexplained the fact that especially high cone angles may also be obtained with soft glass, so this subject requires further analysis. With the weak pull constant, and the stronger aluminosilicate glass offering more resistance to being pulled, stress upon the glass will increase. During slower pulling this stress will also be applied for a longer time. These factors probably account in part for the much greater thinning of the walls at the tip. In any event, the stronger glass will not permit the two tips to separate at a given size unless the walls are more thinned than in the case of borosilicate glass. We have thus found the wall to be greatly thinned in all tip sizes obtained from aluminosilicate glass, and no means of preventing this has been found to date.

In summary, the described aluminosilicate tubing can be conveniently handled in forming patch clamp pipettes with tip sizes appropriate to many applications. In this type of work, aluminosilicate glass would offer higher resistivity.

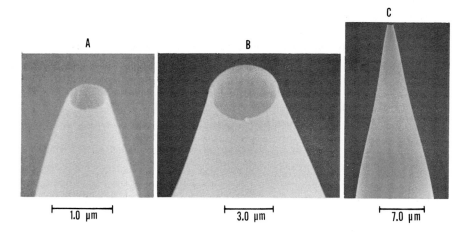

Figure 93. Sample SEM views of tips of patch clamp pipettes formed from aluminosilicate tubing by our Model P-80C micropipette puller. (A and B) Tips with respective inner diameters of 0.56 and 4.0 μm. (C) Side view of a tip tapering at an angle that remains virtually constant at somewhat greater than 24°.

Though wall thickness is decreased, electrical resistivity is increased by at least two orders of magnitude, when comparing Corning's aluminosilicate and borosilicate glasses. Thus the net effect may reduce signal loss and interference from membrane areas outside the tip. The more rapid tip taper would be an additional advantage by lowering the pipette's electrical resistance. The very thin-walled tips, however, may negate these advantages by compromising the quality of the glass-membrane seal required for all types of patch clamping. Perhaps an adequate seal resistance may be obtained with this type of glass, even when the wall is quite thin at the tip. It is also conceivable that a method may be found to prevent such severe thinning of the wall during tip formation. The most promising possibility, however, is thickening the wall by fire-polishing the tip. If one or more of these possibilities can be realized, as we would expect in the case of fire-polishing, then the potential advantages of aluminosilicate glass for making patch clamp pipettes should become useful in practice.

PART VI   MICROPIPETTES FORMED FROM BOROSILICATE GLASS

We have experimented extensively with ultrafine and fine micropipettes formed from borosilicate glass by our Model P-80C micropipette puller, using the conventional method of a weak pull suddenly shifting to a fast pull. This work is reported in part in Sections IV.2b and IV.2c of Chapter 15. Capabilities for forming micropipettes under these conditions have proved unchanged from those provided by our earlier Model P-77B. This was expected because the basic conditions of forming such micropipettes were not altered. Though a velocity index was substituted for the earlier distance index, results obtained by any given setting of the distance index should be duplicated by a velocity criterion selected to trigger later events of the pulling cycle after the same distance of weak pull. All capabilities of our Model P-77B puller were thus retained in the new design.

PART VII   ULTRAFINE MICROPIPETTES FORMED FROM ALUMINOSILICATE GLASS

We have also investigated using an aluminosilicate tubing, as described in Part V of this chapter, to make ultrafine micropipettes by the traditional method of a weak pull immediately followed by a fast pull. Unlike the case when using a distance criterion in our Model P-77B, the use of a velocity criterion in the Model P-80C yielded ultrafine tips on aluminosilicate glass while using the same settings that produced ultrafine tips on borosilicate tubing. More important, with appropriate adjustment of puller settings, even smaller and shorter tips were obtained than those formed from borosilicate tubings especially designed to minimize tip size.

VII.1   Minimum Tip Sizes (OD_t) of About 100 Å

Tip size and reliability were determined by adjusting puller settings for the smallest tips and measuring a group of 15 tips, each formed by a separate pull. The average tip size was 0.032 μm, and several of these tips measured only about 0.010 μm. By comparison, during extensive earlier work with borosilicate tubing, the smallest tips were provided by especially thick-walled glass, which gave an average tip size of 0.039 μm and an occasional tip as small as 0.029 μm (see Section I.2 of Chapter 8). Aluminosilicate glass thus reduced the average tip size from 0.039 to 0.032 μm. Furthermore, one of the aluminosilicate tips was much larger than any of the others, and the average of the remaining 14 tips was only 0.029 μm, the size of the smallest tip yet obtained from borosilicate glass. When comparing the occasional smallest tips obtained from the two types of glass, the results were even more striking. With aluminosilicate glass this was reduced by a factor of about 3, the smallest tips only measuring about 0.010 μm (10 nm or 100 Å). This tip size is only about 1.5 times the typical thickness of a cell membrane. Also, while the smallest tips formed from borosilicate glass were obtained quite rarely, the smallest aluminosilicate tips were obtained much more often. The described group of 15 micropipettes included at least three tips in the 100 Å size range, as shown in Figure 94.

With such small tips, of course thickness of the gold coating becomes exceptionally important in measuring tip size. As described in Section IV.2b of Chapter 15, our coating instrument had been adjusted to give 100 Å gold coatings, as determined by direct measurements. During this work with exceptionally

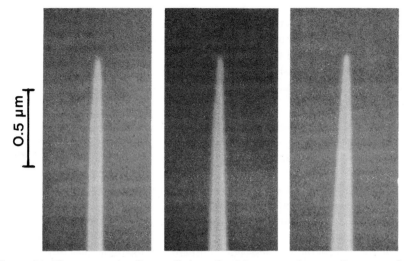

Figure 94. Three exceptionally small tips, all with measured outer diameters of only about 100 Å (0.01 μm), obtained from a group of 15 ultrafine tips formed from aluminosilicate tubing by our Model P-80C micropipette puller.

small tips, the coater settings were rechecked. A nominal 100 Å coating was applied to a group of 10 tips, which were measured, followed by a second nominal 100 Å coating and remeasurement of the tips. In this test the measured thickness of the gold coating was 98 Å. Since the smallest coated tips formed from aluminosilicate tubing measured about 300 Å, and since the coating was measured within a small margin of error, the value of 100 Å for the tips themselves is believed to be satisfactorily accurate.

In summary, aluminosilicate tubing can provide a significant reduction of both the average and minimum tip sizes obtainable with glass micropipettes, and tips with outer diameters of only about 100 Å may be obtained sufficiently often to be of practical value in experimental work.

VII.2   Reliability of Tip Size in the Ultrafine Range

Concerning reliability, the 15 aluminosilicate tips with an average tip size of 32 nm yielded an S.D./Mean of 0.637. As shown in Figure 82 of Chapter 15, the S.D./Mean of borosilicate glass rises rapidly for tip sizes under about 100 nm, and the smallest average tip size of about 48 nm gave an S.D./Mean of 0.497. Since the S.D./Mean is then rising very rapidly indeed, it is hardly surprising that when aluminosilicate glass reduced the average tip size to 32 nm, the associated S.D./Mean rose to 0.637. In fact, if this result for aluminosilicate glass were plotted in Figure 82, it would fit well to the results for borosilicate glass. Figure 82 also shows for borosilicate glass that the S.D./Mean remains constant, at a minimum value of about 0.100, for tip sizes exceeding about 100 nm. So we determined the reliability of aluminosilicate tubing, using 13 tips with an average tip size of 98 nm, which revealed an S.D./Mean of 0.104.

It thus appears that for tips of given size, the reliability of tip size is very nearly the same for the borosilicate and aluminosilicate glasses used in this work. Though such close similarity is probably coincidental, it is not surprising, because the chemical compositions of both types of glass are relatively complex.

VII.3   Shortening of Tips Compared with Borosilicate Glass

It was also observed that tips formed from aluminosilicate tubing were generally shorter than those obtained from borosilicate glass. For example, 10 tips each were formed from borosilicate Standard Tubing and from Clark Biomedical Instrument's aluminosilicate tubing, using identical settings on our Model P-80C puller. While tip length averaged 8.5 mm in the case of borosilicate glass, it was only 5.5 mm when tips were formed from the aluminosilicate tubing. When the shortest tips obtainable from these two types of tubing were compared, a similar advantage was noted for the aluminosilicate glass.

VII.4   The Physical Basis of Smaller and Shorter Tips

It is likely that the stronger molecular bonds in aluminosilicate glass, which are thus far a mixed blessing for patch clamp pipettes, are also the basis for the great advantages of aluminosilicate glass when forming ultrafine micropipettes. Compared with borosilicate glass, the stronger internal bonds require more thinning of the walls before a tip is formed, and this permits the formation of appreciably smaller tips. Likewise, these stronger bonds probably slow the pulling velocity (especially during the weak pull), thus producing a more rapid taper and a shorter tip.

VII.5   Advantages of Aluminosilicate Glass for Ultrafine Micropipettes

Of course the marked reduction of minimum tip size should improve the ease of penetrating small cells with minimum damage. Hence the efficiency of intracellular work in small cells should be further improved. In addition, work should become possible in some especially small structures, such as fine nerve fibers and intracellular organelles, which has not previously been possible. Though stiffness of the tip also influences the ease of cell penetration, this factor becomes less critical as tip size decreases. The stiffness of aluminosilicate glass will be decreased by the thinner wall, but increased by the stronger type of glass, and the net effect is difficult to predict.

For the intracellular recording of electrical activity, aluminosilicate glass should reduce electrical resistance of the micropipette by forming shorter tips. The effectiveness of shorter tips for lowering micropipette resistance has been demonstrated for borosilicate glass (see Table 1 of Chapter 5), so aluminosilicate glass should be a further advantage in this respect. Of course the capacitance of aluminosilicate tips will be increased by both the thinner walls and higher resistivity of the glass. The resulting effects upon the recording time constant will be mitigated, however, by the lowered micropipette resistance. Furthermore, with the negative capacitance provided by preamplifiers for biological recording, the time constant of a micropipette is seldom critical. But the higher capacitance of aluminosilicate tips may be significant in special cases, such as voltage clamping with a single electrode, or analyzing the time course of especially rapid signals.

Aluminosilicate glass is also especially promising for injecting material through ultrafine micropipettes. In the case of patch clamp pipettes, this glass thins severely as the tip is formed. Though we have not examined this with ultrafine tips, the same principle must hold, though perhaps to a lesser extent. Hence the inner tip diameter (ID_t) must represent a relatively large fraction of the outer tip diameter (OD_t). Just as this advantage may be obtained by using borosilicate tubing with a low OD/ID (see Section I.3 of Chapter 6 and Section II.2 of Chapter 14), it appears that an even greater advantage of this type can probably be obtained with aluminosilicate tubing. In addition, for any given tip size the aluminosilicate tubing can provide shorter tips. Since both of these factors should improve the ease of injecting material through a micropipette, aluminosilicate glass would appear ideal for this purpose.

In summary, when our redesigned P-80 series of pullers is used to form micropipettes from the described aluminosilicate tubing, major advantages may be expected for intracellular work. The significantly smaller tips that can be formed should increase the efficiency and extend the possibilities of penetrating especially small cells without significant damage. In addition, the combination of lowered OD_t/ID_t and shorter tips should decrease electrical resistance, and increase the ease of injecting materials into cells, when using tips of given outer diameter. Hence it would seem advisable to explore the possibilities of aluminosilicate glass in any investigation where these expected advantages would be helpful to the research goals.

VII.6   Limitations of Aluminosilicate Glass

Though ultrafine tips are readily formed, we have thus far not obtained micropipettes with fine tips in the range 0.1–0.5 μm. Since aluminosilicate glass can form both ultrafine tips and patch clamp pipettes, it seems unlikely that this is a fundamental restriction, but the requisite conditions for obtaining tips in the fine size range remain to be established.

When alumina is used as the abrasive, aluminosilicate glass bevels somewhat more slowly than borosilicate glass. Since alumina is the only abrasive of relatively high hardness that is available in particle sizes under 0.25 μm, beveling may not be feasible with ultrafine aluminosilicate tips. Beveling of such small tips is usually done to reduce electrical resistance or facilitate injections into cells. Since aluminosilicate glass offers strong advantages for such purposes, including a lowered OD_t/ID_t and shortened tips, ultrafine aluminosilica tips are probably superior to borosilicate glass for these purposes, even if they cannot be well beveled. Though untested to date, aluminosilicate glass should be beveled rapidly by diamond dust. Hence aluminosilicate tips larger than the ultrafine size range should be well beveled by using the various grades of diamond dust available (see Section IV.5 of Chapter 9).

PART VIII   THE FORMATION OF MICROPIPETTES BY MULTIPLE PULLING CYCLES

The introduction of new techniques for patch clamp pipettes also makes new possibilities available in the case of micropipettes. For example, one may use initial puller settings that produce a rapid taper, and allow them to operate over one or more pulling cycles, to produce a rapid taper over the desired distance. The reset button may then be used to stop pulling, and new settings may be introduced to form an ultrafine tip on the final pulling cycle. Though ultrafine tips have not yet been produced in this manner from borosilicate tubing, our experience with this procedure is quite limited. In the case of ultrafine tips, this procedure should further reduce electrical resistance and facilitate the injection of material into cells. A variety of other possibilities, using multiple pulling cycles, likewise remain to be explored in forming micropipettes for various applications. For instance, multiple pulling cycles may provide the key to the requisite conditions for obtaining fine tip sizes when using aluminosilicate glass.

PART IX   OUR MODEL P-80/PC PROGRAMMABLE MICROPIPETTE PULLER

IX.1   An Earlier Programmable Micropipette Puller

The use of a microprocessor to program and retain instructions for making micropipettes was first described by Bertrand *et al.* (1983). This feature was incorporated into an airjet puller using mechanical springs for the control of pull strength. Following a weak pull, triggering of later events in the pull cycle occurred after a preset distance, and two separate pulling cycles were used to form patch clamp pipettes. It was reported that 'fine' tips were also obtained with either high or low resistances, but the minimum tip size was not indicated, and only 77% of these tips 'were considered suitable for intracellular recordings'. As described by the authors, the main feature of this design was the microprocessor control, which permitted instructions to be stored for making micropipettes of different types; each type could then be obtained by activating the appropriate program. A micropipette puller based upon this description is marketed by W-P Instruments, Inc. (P.O. Box 3110, New Haven, CT 06515, USA).

IX.2   The Programmable Version of Our Micropipette Puller

After concentrating upon design features providing optimal performance and versatility, we introduced programmability as the final step. Our Model P-80/PC is thus a programmable version of the Model P-80C. The same types of results should be obtainable with these two pullers, but certain results are provided more conveniently by the programmable version. First, in forming tips from two or more pulling cycles, with puller settings varying between cycles, it is no longer necessary to stop and introduce new puller settings between cycles. Second, programs can be stored for forming various types of tips, and any one of these can be activated within a few moments. One may thus quickly and conveniently change between extremely different types of tips, from the smallest tips obtainable with aluminosilicate glass (minimum outer diameter about 100 Å) to patch clamp pipettes with inner tip diameters up to at least 19 μm.

In our Model P-80/PC a single pulling cycle contains settings for heating current, pull strength, and the criterion velocity to initiate later events in the cycle. A program to form a given type of tip can contain up to 16 pulling cycles, each with its own puller settings. Once established, an entire program is stored in memory, which can hold as many as 10 programs, each of which may be activated at will.

Though our basic design is not changed in the programmable model, the front panel is greatly altered, as shown in Figure 95. This version features an

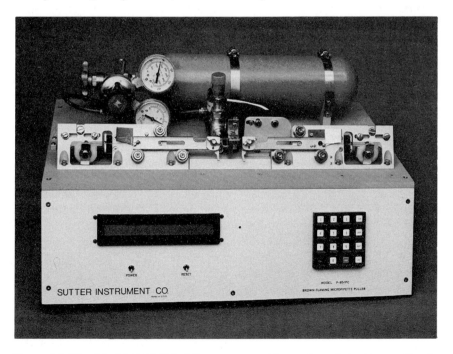

Figure 95. The Model P-80/PC fully programmable version of the Brown–Flaming micropipette puller.

expanded visual display and a keyboard, which may be used in combination for programming, storing, and activating various tip designs.

PART X   SUMMARY

The recent revisions of our micropipette puller appear to provide major advantages in forming micropipettes of all types. Patch clamp pipettes can now be formed with a high degree of reliability, even when using borosilicate or aluminosilicate tubing. By employing a velocity criterion to stop each pulling cycle, these patch clamp pipettes may readily be formed by an unlimited number of pulling cycles. This feature can provide a rapid and virtually constant taper over almost the entire length of the tip, which should markedly reduce the pipette's electrical resistance. In addition, the inner diameter of borosilicate patch clamp pipettes can vary from about 0.5 μm up to at least 19 μm, a considerably higher upper limit than provided by other pullers.

When forming ultrafine or fine micropipettes from borosilicate glass, all advantages of earlier versions of our puller are retained. In addition, the use of a velocity criterion permits these micropipettes to be formed by multiple stages of pulling. This provides increased possibilities for varying the profile of the tip to obtain improved performance in various applications.

The velocity criterion also provides a method of conveniently handling the narrow working range of aluminosilicate glass, which offers advantages of greater strength and higher electrical resistivity. Patch clamp pipettes have been formed from this glass which cover a considerable range of tip size and which taper at an angle of more than 24° for almost the entire length of the tip. When using this type of glass, however, the wall becomes severely thinned under the conditions required to form patch clamp pipettes. Though this may markedly reduce the seal resistance, it seems likely that this problem can be solved by thickening the wall of the tip during fire-polishing.

For ultrafine tips, aluminosilicate glass has now provided tips as small as about 100 Å. Compared with the smallest tips obtained from borosilicate tubings designed to minimize tip size, these tips are still smaller by a factor of about three. In addition, these tips are considerably shorter than those formed from borosilicate glass. Hence aluminosilicate glass is very promising for penetrating especially small cells without significant damage, thus expediting electrical recordings and the injection of experimental materials into these cells.

These capabilities are all available now in either a basic version of our puller, or in a fully programmable version that permits up to 10 tip designs to be programmed, stored, and activated at will.

PART XI   NOTES ADDED IN PROOF

XI.1   Fire-Polishing Tips with our P-80/PC Micropipette Puller

Since the manuscript of this book was completed, there have been further developments. First, the programmable version of our puller has proved capable of fire-polishing patch clamp pipettes, thus making it unnecessary to have a separate setup for this purpose.

After pulling a pair of pipettes, the tips must be moved forward to a predetermined location close to the heating filament. The criterion velocity must then be set to zero, so that the heating filament will be turned off after a given *time*, rather than after the pipette carriers attain a given velocity. The time divisions should be set at 10 msec/division, and the time of filament activation should be adjusted at 100 or more divisions, as determined by experience. The value for filament current must also be set by experience. Then the 'pull' button should be pressed for a single cycle of operation.

Once the conditions have been established for fire-polishing tips of given size that are formed from a given type of glass, the results have proved satisfactorily reliable. Tips in the typical size range for patch clamping applications have been fire-polished in the case of soft glass, and also in the cases of borosilicate and aluminosilicate glasses. Even larger tips suitable for holding cells by suction have also been fire-polished.

Though it might be thought that horizontally oriented tips would sag during fire-polishing, this has not proved to be a problem. In addition to the tip itself being closest to the heating filament, the thickness of the glass wall increases progressively behind the tip. Thus the glass at the tip itself will soften first, and if the time of filament activation is set appropriately, the tip will become fire-polished without any significant sagging. Of course, this requires controls to turn on the filament for an accurate preset time, as provided by our programmable puller.

XI.2 Patch Clamping with Aluminosilicate Glass

Our P-80 series of pullers has only recently become available, so little information has been received on patch clamping applications, but the initial personal communications are encouraging. Most notably, Luk Hondreghem (Cardiovascular Research Laboratories, CC-2209-MCN, Vanderbilt University School of Medicine, Nashville, TN 37232, USA) obtained our first Model P-80/PC. Using hematocrit tubing (a soft glass), pipettes have been formed and fire-polished that have functioned satisfactorily in patch clamp preparations. He notes especially that these pipettes are formed with high reliability by comparison with previous methods.

Unfortunately, we have not yet received reports of the relatively thick-walled aluminosilicate tubing (described in Part V of this chapter) being formed into patch clamp pipettes and then tested in preparations. As noted in Part V of this chapter, our only reservation about this glass for patch clamping is the marked thinning of the wall at the tip itself. But if this results mainly from the especially strong internal bonds in aluminosilicate glass, as we believe, then this problem should be common to various formulations of aluminosilicate glass. It would thus seem significant that other types of aluminosilicate glass have now been formed into pipettes, which after fire-polishing have been found to function well in patch clamping experiments. This has been done in two different research projects at our own institution. In addition, James L. Rae (Department of Physiology, Rush Medical College, 1750 W. Harrison, Chicago, IL 60612, USA) has reported similar results in a personal communication. Having tested various formulations of glass for patch clamping, he found Corning No. 1723 to be especially satisfactory. When this aluminosilicate tubing was formed into pipettes by a modified version of the Kopf puller (see Section II.3 of Chapter 17), and then fire-polished, high seal resistances were obtained that ranged up to 300 giga-ohms. Since fire-polishing was probably critical in solving the problem of wall thinning at the tip in this type of aluminosilicate glass, thus providing an adequately high seal resistance, it should be similarly helpful with the relatively thick-walled type of tubing described in Part V of this chapter.

XI.3   The Use of Aluminosilicate Glass for Intracellular Recording in Small Cells

Though aluminosilicate glass has thus far been little used for intracellular work, we have learned by personal communication of a recent notable application in the laboratory of W. Geoffrey Owen (Department of Biophysics & Medical Physics, University of California, Berkeley, CA 94720, USA). In the retina of the tiger salamander, intracellular recordings had long been attempted in bipolar cells, which are roughly spherical and 8–12 μm in diameter. In these attempts our puller (Model P-77B) had been used to form tips on borosilicate glass (Standard Tubing). But the requirements of this application proved so critical that only about 5% of the micropipettes penetrated cells, and the recordings were typically brief. Hence the rate of data acquisition was so low that the project was on the point of being abandoned. Upon switching to the aluminosilicate tubing described in Part V of this chapter, the situation improved dramatically. About 60% of the micropipettes then penetrated cells, and the recordings became much more stable, with some cells being held for 3–4 hours. The rate of acquiring useful data was thus improved by a factor of more than 10, and the project became quite feasible.

This result confirms our expectation, based upon the factors discussed in Section VII.5 of this chapter, that the described type of aluminosilicate tubing should have outstanding advantages for intracellular work in small cells. Since this tubing is also promising for patch clamping, it now seems possible that it will eventually be adopted as a new standard for a general purpose tubing that better meets many of the varied requirements of research in neurophysiology.

Acknowledgements

In conducting the work of this book, we incurred many debts. Virginia W. Brown derived the equations for tip size factors and made helpful comments on the manuscript. E. Kirk Roberts, of Stanford University, was consulted upon questions in physical chemistry. Victor G. Plumbo, of the Glass Company of America, provided the experimental tubings that were required especially for Chapters 6 and 7; these tubings were supplied without charge and were all within close tolerances of the dimensions requested. Experimental theta tubings were supplied without charge by William R. Dehn of the R & D Scientific Glass Company. The Sutter Instrument Company provided some of the components for recent experimental modifications of our micropipette puller, and their SEM facility was used for the scanning electron microscopy reported in Chapters 15 and 18. In constructing new instruments we have had the excellent services of James R. Wall for mechanical work. Seymour Winston assisted greatly with the electronics in our early instruments, and John Hudson gave helpful advice on electronics in recent revisions of our micropipette puller.

All work reported in this book, which has been conducted by the authors, has been supported by Research Grant No. EY OO468 from the National Eye Institute.

References

Alexander, J.T., and Nastuk, W.L. (1953). An instrument for the production of microelectrodes used in electrophysiological studies, *Rev. Scient. Instrum.*, **24**, 528–531.

Amthor, F. R. (1984). A modified slurry beveler for HRP-filled intracellular micropipettes, *J. Electrophysiol. Tech.*, **11**, 79–86.

Anderson, J.M., Kleinhaus, A., Manuelidis, L., and Prichard, J.W. (1974). Bevelled dual-channel microelectrodes, *IEEE Trans. Biomed. Engineering*, **21**, 482–485.

Baldwin, D.J. (1980a). Dry beveling of micropipette electrodes, *J. Neuroscience Methods*, **2**, 153–161.

Baldwin, D.J. (1980b). Non-destructive electron microscopic examination with rotation of beveled micropipette electrode tips, *J. Neuroscience Methods*, **2**, 163–167.

Barrett, J.N. (1973). Determination of neuronal membrane properties using intracellular staining techniques, in *Intracellular Staining in Neurobiology* (Eds. S.B. Kater and C. Nicholson), Springer-Verlag, New York.

Barrett, J.N., and Graubard, K. (1970). Fluorescent staining of cat motoneurons *in vivo* with beveled micropipettes, *Brain Res.*, **18**, 565–568.

Barrett, J., and Whitlock, D.G. (1973). Technique for beveling glass microelectrodes, in *Intracellular Staining in Neurobiology* (Eds. S.B. Kater and C. Nicholson), Springer-Verlag, New York.

Baylor, D.A., and Fuortes, M.G.F. (1970). Electrical responses of single cones in the retina of the turtle, *J. Physiol., Lond.*, **207**, 77–92.

Baylor, D.A., Fuortes, M.G.F., and O'Bryan, P.M. (1971). Receptive fields of cones in the retina of the turtle, *J. Physiol., Lond.*, **214**, 265–294.

Baylor, D.A., Lamb, T.D., and Yau, K-W. (1979). Responses of retinal rods to single photons, *J. Physiol., Lond.*, **288**, 613–634.

Berger, A.J., Averill, D.B., and Cameron, W.E. (1984). Morphology of inspiratory neurons located in the ventrolateral nucleus of the tractus solitarius of the cat, *J. Comp. Neurol.*, **224**, 60–70.

Bertrand, D., Cand, P., Henauer, R., and Bader, C.R. (1983). Fabrication of glass microelectrodes with microprocessor control, *J. Neuroscience Methods*, **7**, 171–183.

Bortoff, A. (1964). Localization of slow potential responses in the *Necturus* retina, *Vision Res.*, **4**, 627–636.

Bretag, A. (1983). Who did invent the intracellular microelectrode? *Trends in Neurosciences*, **6**, 365.

Brock, L.G., Coombs, J.S., and Eccles, J.C. (1952). The recording of potentials from motoneurons with an intracellular electrode, *J. Physiol., Lond.*, **117**, 431–460.

Brown, A.M., Wilson, D.L., and Tsuda, Y. (1984). Perfusion of small excitable cells using glass pipettes, in *Intracellular Perfusion of Excitable Cells* (Eds. P.G. Kostyuk and O.A. Krishtal) John Wiley & Sons, Chichester, England.

Brown, K.T. (1964). Optical stimulator, microelectrode advancer, and associated equipment for intraretinal neurophysiology in closed mammalian eyes, *J. Opt. Soc. Amer.*, **54**, 101–109.

Brown, K.T. (1968). The electroretinogram: Its components and their origins, *Vision Res.*, **8**, 633–677.

Brown, K.T. (1980). Physiology of the retina, in *Medical Physiology*, (Ed. V.B. Mountcastle), C. V. Mosby Co., St. Louis.

Brown, K.T., and Flaming, D.G. (1974). Beveling of fine micropipette electrodes by a rapid precision method, *Science*, **185**, 693–695.

Brown, K.T., and Flaming, D.G. (1975). Instrumentation and technique for beveling fine micropipette electrodes, *Brain Res.*, **86**,172–180.

Brown, K.T., and Flaming, D.G. (1977a). New microelectrode techniques for intracellular work in small cells, *Neuroscience*, **2**, 813–827.

Brown, K.T., and Flaming, D.G. (1977b). Intracellular recording in outer segments of red and green rods of the toad retina, *Soc. for Neuroscience Abstracts*, **3**, 554.

Brown, K.T., and Flaming, D.G. (1978). Opposing effects of calcium and barium in vertebrate rod photoreceptors, *Proc. Natl. Acad. Sci., USA*, **75**, 1587–1590.

Brown, K.T., and Flaming, D.G. (1979a). Technique for precision beveling of relatively large micropipettes, *J. Neuroscience Methods*, **1**, 25–34.

Brown, K.T., and Flaming, D.G. (1979b). Effects of Ba^{2+} upon the dark-adapted intensity-response curve of toad rods, *Vision Res.*, **19**, 395–398.

Brown, K.T., Watanabe, K., and Murakami, M. (1965). The early and late receptor potentials of monkey cones and rods, *Cold Spr. Harb. Symp. Quant. Biol.*, **30**, 457–482.

Brown, K.T., and Wiesel, T.N. (1958). Intraretinal recording in the unopened cat eye, *Amer. J. Ophthal.*, **46**, No. 3, Part II, 91–98.

Brown, K.T., and Wiesel, T.N. (1959). Intraretinal recording with micropipette electrodes in the intact cat eye, *J. Physiol., Lond.*, **149**, 537–562.

Brown, K.T., and Wiesel, T.N. (1961a). Analysis of the intraretinal electroretinogram in the intact cat eye, *J. Physiol., Lond.*, **158**, 229–256.

Brown, K.T., and Wiesel, T.N. (1961b). Localization of origins of electroretinogram components by intraretinal recording in the intact cat eye, *J. Physiol., Lond.*, **158**, 257–280.

Burke, R.E., and ten Bruggencate, G. (1971). Electronic characteristics of alpha motoneurons of varying size. *J. Physiol., Lond.*, **212**, 1–20.

Byzov, A.L., and Chernyshov, V.I. (1961). Automatic device for manufacturing microelectrodes, *Biofizika*, **6**, 485–489.

Charlton J.S., and Leeper, H.F. (1985). The arterially perfused eyecup of the tree squirrel, *Sciurus carolinensis*: a preparation for intracellular recording from mammalian retinal neurons, *J. Neuroscience Methods*, **13**, 153–162.

Chemical Engineer's Handbook (1973). (Eds. R.H. Perry and C.H. Chilton), McGraw-Hill, New York.

Chen, V.K.-H. (1978). A simple piezoelectric drive for glass microelectrodes, *J. Phys. E: Sci. Instrum.*, **11**, 1092–1093.

Chowdhury, T.K. (1969). Fabrication of extremely fine glass micropipette electrodes, *J. Scient. Instrum.*, Series 2, **2**, 1087–1090.

Clementz, B., and Grampp, W. (1976). A method for rapid bevelling of micropipette electrodes, *Acta Physiol. Scand.*, **96**, 286–288.

Copenhagen, D.R., and Owen, W.G. (1976). Functional characteristics of lateral interactions between rods in the retina of the snapping turtle, *J. Physiol., Lond.*, **259**, 251–282.

Corey, D.P., and Hudspeth, A.J. (1980). Mechanical stimulation and micromanipulation with peizoelectric bimorph elements, *J. Neuroscience Methods*, **3**, 183–202.

Corey, D.P., and Stevens, C.F. (1983). Science and technology of patch-recording electrodes, in *Single-Channel Recording* (Eds. B. Sakmann and E. Neher), Plenum Press, New York.

Covington, A.K. (1979). *Ion-Selective Electrode Methodology* (Vols. I and II), CRC Press, Boca Raton, Florida.

Del Castillo, J., and Katz, B. (1955). On the localization of acetylcholine receptors, *J. Physiol., Lond.*, **128**, 157–181.

Du Bois, D. (1931). A machine for pulling glass micropipettes and needles, *Science*, **73**, 344–345.

Eisenman, G., editor (1967). *Glass Electrodes for Hydrogen and Other Cations*, Marcel Dekker, Inc., New York.

Ellis, G.W. (1962). Piezoelectric micromanipulators, *Science*, **138**, 84–91.

Fish, R.M., Bryan, J.S., McReynolds, J.S., and Ries, J.J. (1971). A mechanical microelectrode pulsing device to facilitate the penetration of small cells, *IEEE Trans. Bio-Med. Engin.*, **18**, 240–241.

Flaming, D.G. (1982). A short review of current laboratory microcomputer systems and practice, *J. Neuroscience Methods*, **5**, 1–6.

Flaming, D.G., and Brown, K.T. (1979a). Effects of calcium on the intensity-response curve of toad rods, *Nature*, **278**, 852–853.

Flaming, D.G., and Brown, K.T. (1979b). Ca^{2+} and photoreceptor adaptation: Reply to Lipton, Ostroy and Dowling, *Nature*, **281**, 407–408.

Flaming, D.G., and Brown, K.T. (1982). Micropipette puller design: form of the heating filament and effects of filament width on tip length and diameter, *J. Neuroscience Methods*, **6**, 91–102.

Frank, K., and Becker, M.C. (1964). Microelectrodes for recording and stimulation, in *Physical Techniques in Biological Research*, Vol. V (Ed. W.L. Nastuk), pp. 22–87, Academic Press, New York.

Fromm, M., and Schultz, S.G. (1981). Some properties of KCl-filled microelectrodes: Correlation of potassium 'leakage' with tip resistance, *J. Membrane Biol.*, **62**, 239–244.

Fromm, M., Weskamp, P., and Hegel, U. (1980). Versatile piezoelectric driver for cell puncture, *Pflüg. Arch.*, **384**, 69–73.

Gardner, R.L. (1978). Production of chimeras by injecting cells or tissue into the blastocyst, in *Methods in Mammalian Reproduction* (Ed. J.C. Daniel, Jr.), Academic Press, New York.

Gordon, J., and Hood, D.C. (1976). Anatomy and physiology of the frog retina, in *The Amphibian Visual System* (Ed. K.V. Fite), Academic Press, New York.

Graham, J., and Gerard, R.W. (1946). Membrane potentials and excitation of impaled single muscle fibers, *J. Cell. Comp. Physiol.*, **28**, 99–117.

Hamill, O.P., Marty, A., Neher, E., Sakmann, B., and Sigworth F.J. (1981). Improved patch-clamp techniques for high-resolution current recording from cells and cell-free membrane patches, *Pflüg. Arch.*, **391**, 85–100.

Handbook of Chemistry and Physics (1972-1973), 53rd Edition, CRC Press, The Chemical Rubber Co., Cleveland.

Hengstenberg, R. (1981). A piezoelectric device to aid penetration of small nerve fibers with microelectrodes, *J. Neuroscience Methods*, **4**, 249–255.

Hodgkin, A.L., and Huxley, A.F. (1945). Resting and action potentials in single nerve fibers, *J. Physiol., Lond.*, **104**, 176–195.

Hoppe, P.C., and Illmensee, K. (1977). Microsurgically produced homozygous-diploid uniparental mice, *Proc. Natl. Acad. Sci., USA*, **74**, 5657–5661.

Howell, B.J., Baumgardner, F.W., Bondi, K., and Rahn, H. (1970). Acid–base balance in cold-blooded vertebrates as a function of body temperature, *Am. J. Physiol.*, **218**, 600–606.

Hudspeth, A.J., and Corey, D.P. (1978). Controlled bending of high-resistance glass microelectrodes, *Am. J. Physiol.*, **234** (1), C56–C57.

Isard, J.O. (1967). The dependence of glass-electrode properties on composition, in *Glass Electrodes for Hydrogen and Other Cations* (Ed. G. Eisenman), Marcel Dekker, Inc., New York.

Jacobson, S.L., and Mealing, G.A.R. (1980). A method for producing very low resistance micropipettes for intracellular measurements, *Electroenceph. Clin. Neurophysiol.*, **48**, 106–108.

Kelly, J.S. (1975). Microiontophoretic application of drugs onto single neurons, in *Handbook of Psychopharmacology*, Vol. 2 (Eds. L.L. Iversen, S.D. Iversen, and S.H. Snyder), Plenum Press, New York.

Koryta, J., and Stulik, K. (1983). *Ion-Selective Electrodes* (2nd Edition), Cambridge University Press, Cambridge, England.

Kripke, B.R., and Ogden, T.E. (1974). A technique for beveling fine micropipettes, *Electroenceph. Clin. Neurophysiol.*, **36**, 323–326.

Kump, W.R., and Dehn, W.R. (1975). Fabrication techniques for multichannel microelectrodes, *Fusion*, **22**, Book II, 9–11.

Lassen, U.V., and Sten-Knudsen, O. (1968). Direct measurements of membrane potential and membrane resistance of human red cells, *J. Physiol., Lond.*, **195**, 681–696.

Lederer, W.J., Spindler, A.J., and Eisner, D.A. (1979). Thick slurry bevelling, *Pflüg. Arch.*, **381**, 287–288.

Leeper, H.F., and Charlton, J.S. (1985). Response properties of horizontal cells and photoreceptor cells in the retina of the tree squirrel, *Sciurus carolinensis*, *J. Neurophysiol.*, **54**, 1157–1166.

Ling, G., and Gerard, R.W. (1949). The normal membrane potential of frog sartorius fibers, *J. Cell. Comp. Physiol.*, **34**, 383–396.

Lipton, S.A., Ostroy, S.E., and Dowling, J.E. (1977). Electrical and adaptive properties of rod photoreceptors in *Bufo marinus*—I. Effects of altered extracellular Ca^{2+} levels, *J. Gen. Physiol.*, **70**, 747–770.

Livingston, L.G., and Duggar, B.M. (1934). Experimental procedures in a study of the location and concentration within the host cell of the virus of tobacco mosaic, *Biol. Bull.*, **67**, 504–512.

Lübbers, D.W., Acker, H., Buck, R.P., Eisenman, G., Kessler, M., and Simon, W., editors (1981). *Progress in Enzyme and Ion-Selective Electrodes*, Springer-Verlag, Berlin.

Lutz, A., and Wagman, I.H. (1965). A rolling diaphragm hydraulic micromanipulator, *Electroenceph. Clin. Neurophysiol.*, **18**, 184–186.

Lux, D. (1960). Microelectrodes of higher stability, *Electroenceph. Clin. Neurophysiol.*, **12**, 928–929.

Marty, A., and Neher, E. (1983). Tight-seal whole-cell recording, in *Single-Channel Recording* (Eds. B. Sakmann and E. Neher), Plenum Press, New York.

McGrath, J., and Solter, D. (1985). Nuclear and cytoplasmic transfer in mammalian embryos, in *Manipulation of Mammalian Development* (Ed. R.B.L. Gwatkin), Plenum Press, New York.

McGraw-Hill Encyclopedia of Science & Technology (1982), 5th Edition, McGraw-Hill, New York.

Morey, G.W. (1954). *Properties of Glass*, Reinhold Publishing Corp. New York.

Morf, W.E. (1981). *The Principles of Ion-Selective Electrodes and of Membrane Transport*, Elsevier Scientific Publishing Co., Amsterdam.

Nastuk, W.L. (1951). Membrane potential changes at a single muscle end plate produced by acetylcholine. *Fed. Proc.*, **10**, 96.

Nastuk, W.L. (1953). Membrane potential changes at a single muscle end-plate produced by transitory application of acetylcholine with an electrically controlled microjet, *Fed. Proc.*, **12**, 102.

Nastuk, W.L., and Hodgkin, A.L. (1950). The electrical activity of single muscle fibers, *J. Cell Comp. Physiol.*, **35**, 39–73.

Neher, E., and Sakmann, B. (1976). Single-channel currents recorded from membrane of denervated frog muscle fibres, *Nature*, **260**, 799–802.

Neher, E., Sakmann, B., and Steinbach, J.H. (1978). The extracellular patch clamp: A method for resolving currents through individual open channels in biological membranes, *Pflüg. Arch.*, **375**, 219–228.

Nunn, B.J., and Baylor, D.A. (1982). Visual transduction in retinal rods of the monkey *Macaca fascicularis*, *Nature*, **299**, 726–728.

Nunn, B.J., Schnapf, J.L., and Baylor, D.A. (1984). Spectral sensitivity of single cones in the retina of *Macaca fascicularis*, *Nature*, **309**, 264–266.

Oakley, Burks H, Flaming, D.G., and Brown, K.T. (1979). Effects of the rod receptor potential upon retinal extracellular potassium concentration, *J. Gen. Physiol.*, **74**, 713–737.

Ogden, T.E., Citron, M.C., and Pierantoni, R. (1978). The jet stream microbeveler: An inexpensive way to bevel ultrafine glass micropipettes, *Science*, **201**, 469–470.

Pascoe, J.E. (1955). A technique for the introduction of intracellular electrodes, *J. Physiol., Lond.*, **128**, 26P–27P.

Peters, M., and Tetzel, H.D. (1980). Piezoelectric drive for step-by-step microelectrode advancement, *J. Exp. Biol.*, **86**, 333–336.

Plamondon, R., Gagne, S., and Poussert, D. (1976). Low resistance and tip potential of glass microelectrode: improvement through a new filling method, *Vision Res.*, **16**, 1355–1357.

Prazma, J. (1978). Penetration of cells membrane by the piezoelectric driver, *Experientia*, **34**, 1387–1388.

Purves, R.D. (1980). The mechanics of pulling a glass micropipette, *Biophys. J.*, **29**, 523–530.

Purves, R.D. (1981). *Microelectrode Methods for Intracellular Recording and Ionophoresis*, Academic Press, London.

Rikmenspoel, R., and Lindemann, C. (1971). Improved piezoelectric driver for glass microelectrodes, *Rev. Sci. Instr.*, **42**, 717–718.

Roberts, W.M., and Almers, W. (1984). An improved loose patch voltage clamp method using concentric pipettes, *Pflüg. Arch.*, **402**, 190–196.

Sakmann, B., and Neher, E., editors (1983a). *Single-Channel Recording*, Plenum Press, New York.

Sakmann, B., and Neher, E. (1983b). Geometric parameters of pipettes and membrane patches, in *Single-Channel Recording* (Eds. B. Sakmann and E. Neher), Plenum Press, New York.

Sears, F.W. (1950). *Mechanics, Heat and Sound*. Addison-Wesley Press, Cambridge, Massachusetts.

Shaw, M.L., and Lee, D.R. (1973). Micropipette sharpener with audio and hydraulic readouts, *J. Appl. Physiol.*, **34**, 523–524.

Sigworth, F.J. (1983). Electronic design of the patch clamp, in *Single-Channel Recording* (Eds. B. Sakmann and E. Neher), Plenum Press, New York.

Sigworth, F.J., and Neher, E. (1980). Single Na^+ channel currents observed in cultured rat muscle cells, *Nature*, **287**, 447–449.

Sonnhof, U., Förderer, R., Schneider, W., and Kettenmann, H. (1982). Cell puncturing with a step motor driven manipulator with simultaneous measurement of displacement, *Pflüg. Arch.*, **392**, 295–300.

Steinberg, R.H. (1973). Scanning electron microscopy of the bullfrog's retina and pigment epithelium, *Z. Zellforsch.*, **143**, 451–463.

Stoner, L.C., Natke, E. Jr., and Dixon, M.K. (1984). Direct measurement of potassium leak from single 3 M KCl microelectrodes, *Am. J. Physiol.*, **246**, F343–F348.

Strickholm, A. (1961). Impedance of a small electrically isolated area of the muscle cell surface, *J. Gen. Physiol.*, **44**, 1073–1088.

Stretton, A.O.W., and Kravitz, E.A. (1968). Neuronal geometry: Determination with a technique of intracellular dye injection, *Science*, **162**, 132–134.

Stühmer, W., Roberts, W.M., and Almers, W. (1983). The loose patch clamp, in *Single-Channel Recording* (Eds. B. Sakmann and E. Neher), Plenum Press, New York.

Tasaki, K., Tsukahara, Y., Ito, S., Wayner, M.J., and Yu, W.Y. (1968). A simple, direct and rapid method for filling microelectrodes, *Physiol. and Behavior*, **3**, 1009–1010.

Tauchi, M., and Kikuchi, R. (1977). A simple method for beveling micropipettes for intracellular recording and current injection, *Pflüg. Arch.*, **368**, 153–155.

Thomas, R.C. (1978). *Ion-Sensitive Intracellular Microelectrodes: How to Make and Use Them*, Academic Press, London.

Tomita, T. (1965). Electrophysiological study of the mechanisms subserving color coding in the fish retina, *Cold Spring Harb. Symp. Quant. Biol.*, **30**, 559–566.

Tupper, J.T., and Rikmenspoel, R. (1969). Piezoelectric driving device for glass capillary microelectrodes *Rev. Sci. Instr.*, **40**, 851–852.

Ujec, E., Vit, Z., Vyskocil, F., and Kralik, O. (1973). Analysis of geometrical and electrical parameters of the tips of glass microelectrodes, *Physiologia Bohemoslovaca*, **22**, 329–336.

Van der Pers, J.N.C. (1980). An electromagnetic microelectrode holder for pulsating penetration of brain tissue, *J. Neuroscience Methods,*, **2**, 319–321.

Van Essen, D., and Kelly, J. (1973). Morphological identification of simple, complex and hypercomplex cells in the visual cortex of the cat, in *Intracellular Staining in Neurobiology* (Eds. S.B. Kater and C. Nicholson), Springer-Verlag, New York.

Volf, M.B. (1961). *Technical Glasses*, Sir Isaac Pitman and Sons, Ltd., London.

Walls, G.L. (1963). *The Vertebrate Eye and its Adaptive Radiation*, Hafner Publishing Co., New York.

Warren, B.E. (1940). X-ray diffraction study of the structure of glass, *Chem. Reviews*, **26**, 237–255.

Warren, B.E., and Biscoe, J. (1938). Fourier analysis of x-ray patterns of soda-silica glass, *J. Amer. Ceramic Soc.*, **21**, 259–265.

Werblin, F.S. (1975). Regenerative hyperpolarization in rods, *J. Physiol. Lond.*, **244**, 53–81.

Whitten, D.N., and Brown, K.T. (1973). Photopic suppression of monkey's rod receptor potential, apparently by a cone-initiated lateral inhibition, *Vision Res.*, **13**, 1629–1658.

Winsbury, G.J. (1956). Machine for the production of microelectrodes, *Rev. Scient. Instrum.*, **27**, 514–516.

Yau, K.-W., Lamb, T.D., and Baylor, D.A. (1977). Light-induced fluctuations in membrane current of single toad rod outer segments, *Nature*, **269**, 78–80.

Yoshikami, S., and Hagins, W.A. (1971). Light, calcium, & the photocurrent of rods & cones, *Biophys. J.*, **11**, 47a.

Zachariasen, W.H. (1932). The atomic arrangement in glass, *J. Am. Chem. Soc.*, **54**, 3841–3851.

Zeuthen, T., editor (1981). *The Application of Ion-Selective Microelectrodes*, Elsevier/North Holland Biomedical Press, Amsterdam.

APPENDIX I

Personal Historical Notes (by K.T.B.)

It may interest some readers that three pioneers in microelectrode techniques, namely Ralph W. Gerard, Stephen W. Kuffler and L.G. Livingston, contributed to the work of this book by having a strong and direct influence upon my career.

At The University of Chicago, in the spring of 1949, I took Gerard's course in neurophysiology. I was then a graduate student in psychology, with a developing interest in vision, which psychologists of that time studied almost exclusively by psychophysical techniques. Gerard's introduction to neurophysiology was illuminating and indeed fascinating, owing largely to his enthusiasm for the field and his dramatic style of presentation. His course convinced me that although psychophysics can contribute much to studies of the special senses, neurophysiology is an even more powerful tool. In fact, psychophysical studies define problems that can only be studied by physiological methods such as those of neurophysiology. For example, the dark adaptation curve is a psychophysical determination of how sensitivity to light increases as a function of time in the dark. It thus answers an important question, but it poses further questions about the underlying mechanisms that can only be answered by direct physiological studies of the visual system. So I decided to pursue psychophysical studies of vision for a few years, as a useful background, and then undertake long term neurophysiological work in the visual system. Though my contact with Gerard was only as a student in his large class (which included all the first-year medical students), this decision was strongly influenced by his outstanding teaching.

By 1949, as is now well known, Gerard's laboratory had introduced micropuncture techniques and proved their usefulness for intracellular studies of excitable cells. But I have no memory of this technique having even been mentioned in his neurophysiology course. Perhaps it was described and I forgot it, along with most of the other details of the course. Other possibilities are that he considered this too advanced for an introductory course, or that he thought discussion of the subject would be immodest, or that he was still unsure how important the technique would become.

After completing graduate work and studying vision by psychophysical methods for several additional years, I was especially fortunate to work in Kuffler's laboratory from 1955–1958. By that time the importance of microelectrode work in neurophysiology had become well established, and Kuffler had contributed to that process through significant contributions to a variety of important problems. Torsten Wiesel arrived in Kuffler's laboratory at the same time, and we were provided a fine opportunity to learn microelectrode techniques while conducting studies of the cat retina (Brown and Wiesel, 1958; 1959; 1961a; 1961b).

During that period I became acquainted with the Livingston micropipette puller, and later visited Swarthmore College, where my undergraduate work had been completed after the interruption of World War II. While visiting a former biology teacher, I was startled to see a Livingston micropipette puller on his shelf. Only then did I realize that the designer of the first notably successful micropipette puller was the same Livingston whose introductory biology course had initiated my enduring fascination with that field.

APPENDIX II

Derivation of Equations for Tip Size Factors

The three equations presented in Section I.4 of Chapter 6 are derived below.

PART I DEFINITIONS OF TERMS

OD = outside diameter of capillary tubing
ID = inside diameter of capillary tubing
OD_t = outside diameter of tip
ID_t = inside diameter of tip
OD_{ts} = outside diameter of tip, Standard Tubing
ID_{ts} = inside diameter of tip, Standard Tubing
u = twice the wall thickness of tubing
u_t = the value of u at the tip, assumed constant as OD/ID varies
F_o = factor by which outside tip diameter is changed relative to that of Standard Tubing, i.e.,

$$F_o = \frac{OD_t}{OD_{ts}}$$

F_i = factor by which inside tip diameter is changed relative to that of Standard Tubing, i.e.,

$$F_i = \frac{ID_t}{ID_{ts}}$$

PART II ASSUMPTIONS

Assumption 1: That the ratio of outer/inner diameter remains constant throughout the length of a micropipette, i.e.,

$$\frac{OD}{ID} = \frac{OD_t}{ID_t}$$

288

Assumption 2: That the absolute thickness of the glass wall at the tip will be constant and independent of the OD/ID ratio, providing that the type of glass and the pulling conditions at the tip remain constant.

PART III   DERIVATION OF EQUATIONS

Let us first derive an equation for F_o as a function of OD and ID. It is obvious that in the general case $OD_t = ID_t + u_t$, and for Standard Tubing $OD_{ts} = 2u_t$. Since we have defined

$$F_o = \frac{OD_t}{OD_{ts}}$$

then $OD_t = F_o \cdot OD_{ts}$. Substituting $2u_t$ for OD_{ts}, we have $OD_t = 2F_o u_t$. Similarly, since $ID_t = OD_t - u_t$, we find by substitution that $ID_t = 2F_o u_t - u_t$. We may thus say that:

$$\frac{OD_t}{ID_t} = \frac{2F_o u_t}{(2F_o - 1)u_t}$$

Since

$$\frac{OD}{ID} = \frac{OD_t}{ID_t}$$

by assumption 1, we have

$$\frac{OD}{ID} = \frac{2F_o}{2F_o - 1}$$

Solving this equation for F_o, then

$$F_o = \frac{OD}{2(OD - ID)} \qquad \text{(EQUATION 1)}$$

Let us next derive an equation for F_i as a function of F_o. By definition,

$$F_i = \frac{ID_t}{ID_{ts}}$$

From assumption 1 and the definition of Standard Tubing, $ID_{ts} = u_t$. We also know that $OD_t = ID_t + u_t$ and $OD_t = 2F_o u_t$. Therefore, $ID_t + u_t = 2F_o u_t$. Solving for ID_t, we get $ID_t = (2F_o - 1)u_t$. By substitution we obtain

$$F_i = \frac{(2F_o - 1)u_t}{u_t}$$

which reduces to:

$$F_i = 2F_o - 1 \qquad \text{(EQUATION 2)}$$

Using Equation 1 to substitute for F_o in Equation 2, we also obtain:

$$F_i = \frac{ID}{OD - ID} \qquad \text{(EQUATION 3)}$$

Subject Index